FITNESS FOR COLLEGE

AND LIFE

CHARLES A. BUCHER, A.B., M.A., Ed.D.

Director, School of Health, Physical Education,
Recreation and Dance, The University of Nevada at Las Vegas,
Las Vegas, Nevada; Consultant, President's Council on Physical Fitness
and Sports; Consultant, National Fitness Foundation

WILLIAM E. PRENTICE, Ph.D. A.T.,C. L.P.T.

Assistant Professor, Department of Physical Education,
The University of North Carolina,
Chapel Hill, North Carolina

With 145 illustrations

TIMES MIRROR/MOSBY
COLLEGE PUBLISHING

ST. LOUIS • TORONTO • SANTA CLARA   1985

Editor: Nancy K. Roberson
Developmental Editor: Michelle Turenne
Project Editor: Susan K. Hume
Manuscript Editor: Mark Spann
Designer: Diane M. Beasley
Production: Margaret B. Bridenbaugh
Cover photo: Four by Five Inc.

Library of Congress Cataloging in Publication Data

Bucher, Charles Augustus, 1912-
Fitness for college and life.

Includes index.
1. Physical fitness.   I. Prentice, William E.
II. Title.
GV481.B83   1985   613.7′07′11   84-22672
ISBN 0-8016-0884-8

GW/VH/VH 9 8 7 6 5 4 3 2 1   01/A/082

FITNESS FOR COLLEGE AND LIFE

PREFACE

Physically Fit. During the past decade this term has taken on a new meaning. In many respects, physical fitness has become a way of American life. We eat, sleep, go to school or work, and exercise. The term *physical fitness* appears on television and radio and in magazines, books, and newspapers. The concept of the attractive, healthy, physically fit person is used to sell food and drug products, clothing, sports equipment, and memberships to health and fitness clubs. In essence, it is almost impossible to go through an entire day without being exposed to something that involves physical fitness.

This national preoccupation with fitness has affected every segment of our society. People of all ages and backgrounds have decided to take responsibility for their own physical and in some cases mental well-being by becoming physically active. Perhaps nowhere is this obsession with physical activity more evident than on college or university campuses, which on any given day are crowded with people jogging, walking, or bicycling. The gymnasiums and playing fields are likely even more crowded. In many cases these college students are establishing patterns of living that may well affect their long-term health and leisurely pursuits.

Because of the tremendous number of people who are involved in some type of physical activity, there are a host of self-proclaimed fitness "experts" who tend to disseminate a wealth of misinformation regarding strength training, improvement of cardiorespiratory endurance and flexibility, weight control, nutrition, and injury and stress management. Although it is true that there are many different approaches that will ultimately lead to physical fitness, there are certain principles and guidelines that tend to make the pursuit of physical fitness much safer and more effective.

This text is directed specifically at college students. It has been specially designed for use in classes that are aimed at acquainting the student with the nature and scope of fitness by providing information that will show the student the importance of and the scientific foundations for engaging in a sound physical fitness program. It describes the component parts and basic principles that should be known and followed if a student wishes to become physically fit for college and life. It also outlines exercises, activities, and resources that can be utilized in developing a well-rounded physical fitness program.

In writing this text, we have attempted to blend theory with practical application by providing a general discussion of the various fitness-related topics followed by worksheets and specific activities to which the theory can be applied.

There are a number of reasons why you should use this textbook:

Comprehensive and Systematic Coverage

This text covers the essential elements of fitness for the college student. First, it introduces the reader to the meaning of fitness and its value and popularity in today's world. It then sets forth basic principles that should be adhered to by students who aspire to be physically fit. It continues with a discussion of the basic components of fitness: cardiorespiratory endurance, strength, flexibility, body composition, and nutrition. Next, it provides basic guidelines for the safe participation in a fitness program and how to prevent and care for common injuries. Because the management of stress is an important aspect of any fitness program, this subject is also discussed with suggestions as to how one can successfully cope with stress. Finally, a series of lifetime fitness activities suitable for each person's program are described together with a discussion of resources that are available on college campuses to assist the student in his or her fitness program.

Based on Scientific Theory

To the extent possible, this text discusses various concepts, principles, and theories that are supported by scientific research, factual evidence, and sound logic. These have been drawn from disciplines such as exercise physiology, nutrition, athletic training, biomechanics, and physical therapy. It is important for anyone involved in a physical activity program to have at least a basic understanding of why it is more efficient to make use of a specific technique to maximize results. This text then deals not only with practical application but also with theory to support it.

Timely and Practical Material

As the first chapter of this book points out, a "fitness boom" exists in this country. People of all ages are realizing the values of being physically fit. Therefore they are interested in finding the right formulas, activities, and procedures for achieving health and fitness. College students are no exception. They are realizing that being physically fit can contribute to their success in college, getting a job, and the achievement of their educational and life goals. This text provides essential and contemporary information for achieving the goal of optimal physical fitness for college and life. It is timely and practical for today's young person attending college and desiring to make the most of his or her life.

The manuscript for the text was carefully reviewed by exercise physiologists and fitness experts. This, together with considerable market research, was done in order to make sure the subject matter content was accurate, practical, and relevant to today's college students.

The text is concerned with those key components and dimensions of physical fitness with which young people should be concerned, such as cardiorespiratory endurance, strength, flexibility, and body composition, as well as the activities and training programs essential to the optimal development of these components.

In light of the increasing importance being given to stress management, a chapter is also devoted to this subject. The nature and scope of stress management is presented, with particular attention being given to the impact stress has on the physiologic functioning of the human body. The role of physical activity and relaxation techniques are then discussed as means of alleviating stress.

Because nutrition plays an important role in achieving physical fitness, this subject is also included together with appendices that include the nutritive values of various types of foods.

Readable and Interesting

The subject of fitness is presented in a lively, readable style at the college student's level of understanding. Fitness is a fascinating subject, and we have tried to communicate our enthusiasm for the subject. Worksheets, techniques for assessing specific fitness components, and suggestions for specific training are provided in the text so that the student can easily apply what is being discussed.

Pedagogical Aids

The aids this text utilizes to facilitate its use by students and instructors include:

Objectives: Listed at the beginning of each chapter to introduce to students the points that will be highlighted. Accomplishing the objectives indicates fulfilling the chapter's intent.

Figures, Tables, Photos: Essential points in each chapter are illustrated with clear visual materials.

Self-Assessment Tools: These include worksheets and evaluation forms that students and instructors can use in developing and assessing an awareness of students' personal fitness habits and needs. Blank copies are duplicated at the end of the text for convenience of use.

Summary: Each chapter has a summary outlining the major points covered.

Glossary of Key Terms: Each chapter contains a glossary of terms for quick reference.

References and Suggested Readings: Lists of up-to-date references and suggested readings are provided at the end of each chapter for the student who wishes to read further on the subject being discussed.

Appendices: These include a table on the nutritive value of food, a supplementary table on the nutritive value of fast foods, resources to assist students with a fitness program, and duplications of the self-evaluation forms and worksheets to be completed by the students.

Supplements

An *Instructor's Manual* is also available. It provides suggestions on how to utilize the text to its fullest potential. The manual includes chapter overviews, key terms, learning objectives, a topical teaching outline, key teaching points, a test bank of true-false, multiple-choice, and discussion questions for each chapter. Also included is a list of additional reading and audiovisual resources.

Probably the most valuable information for the instructor will be two instructional plans outlining suggested activities that can be utilized in a 10-week (4 sessions a week) and a 14-week (3 sessions a week) college class pattern. Activities will include such things as lectures, physical activities, testing, and demonstrations. Instructors will be able to use the instructional plans as outlined to plan their classes, or they can adapt them in a way that will better fit into their own college pattern of instruction.

ACKNOWLEDGMENTS

If you have never been involved in the production of a textbook, it is difficult to understand the magnitude of such an undertaking. Dozens of persons have been involved with this project from its inception and all have contributed in their own way, but a few deserve special thanks.

The secretarial staffs of the Department of Physical Education at the University of North Carolina at Chapel Hill, particularly Kaye Buchanan and Linda Prather, and the School of Health, Physical Education, Recreation and Dance at the University of Nevada, Las Vegas, particularly Joan Burns and Lana de Mille, have been most patient and helpful in typing and retyping this manuscript.

Michelle Turenne, the developmental editor at Times Mirror/Mosby, was responsible for coordinating the efforts between the authors. She offered nothing but encouragement, constructive suggestions, and a significant amount of self-control toward the completion of this project.

We would also like to express our sincere appreciation to the publisher's reviewers—Kenneth Ackerman, M.A., Southern Illinois University at Carbondale; Joy Cavanaugh, Ph.D., San Jose State University; Sister Janice Iverson, O.S.B., M.S., South Dakota State University; G. E. Landwer, Ph.D., Texas Christian University; JoAnn Otte, M.S., Weber State College; John R. Webster, M.S., Central Connecticut State University; and Anthony Wilcox, Ph.D., Kansas State University—for their critical reading of earlier drafts of this text. Their suggestions for improvement greatly influenced the final draft. We also wish to express our gratitude to Bob Henchal, Jr., Exercise Physiologist and Director of Health and Physical Education for YMCA, Las Vegas, for his contribution to the development of this text.

Finally, we would like to thank our wives, Jackie and Tena, for being there.

CONTENTS

1

THE FITNESS BOOM

After completing this chapter, you will be able to:

- Describe the nature and scope of the fitness boom.
- Define the terms *fitness* and *physical fitness*.
- Describe some of the misconceptions about physical fitness.
- Explain the role of physical activity in achieving an optimal state of physical fitness.
- List the component parts of physical fitness.
- Describe the relation of the body systems to fitness.
- Explain why an optimal state of physical fitness is important to college students.

The fitness boom has consumed the thinking of the American public, and the human body has become an obsession for many Americans. Today, health spas and fitness centers abound in shopping centers, industrial complexes, hotels, and educational institutions. The *New York Times* best-seller list usually includes several books that relate to exercise, diet, and fitness—how to slim down, shape up, and achieve that svelte look.

Americans spend annually an estimated $1 billion on sport shoes, $50 million on exercise and diet books, $140 million on roller skates, and much more than $200 million on weight-training equipment.[1]

The President's Council on Physical Fitness and Sports indicates that the number of adults who exercise regularly has doubled in the last 20 years. The council also points out that 70 million Americans bicycle, 27 million adults swim, and millions of college students compete in collegiate sports.[2] Clearly times have changed, and the public's conception of the proper physical dimensions of the human body is not what it was years ago.

1

Take the test America!™

1 Three-Minute Step Test

A strong heart and healthy lungs are essential for a long and productive life, and help to decrease the risk of cardiovascular disease.

The step test measures the heart and lungs' response to endurance activities.

GOAL: By stepping up and down on a 12" bench in rhythm with a metronome, your heart rate is measured and compared against nationally recognized fitness standards.

3-MINUTE STEP FITNESS STANDARDS (Heart Rate)

AGE	18-29		30-39		40-49		50-59		60 & Over	
SEX	F	M	F	M	F	M	F	M	F	M
GOLD	<80	<75	<84	<78	<88	<80	<92	<85	<95	<90
SILVER	80-110	75-100	84-115	78-109	88-118	80-112	92-123	85-115	95-127	90-118
BRONZE	>110	>100	>115	>109	>118	>112	>123	>115	>127	>118

< = less than   > = more than

2 Sit & Reach

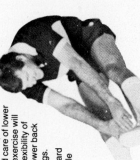

The sit and reach test is important for the prevention and care of lower back problems. This exercise will help to evaluate the flexibility of your muscles in the lower back and the back of the legs.

GOAL: To reach forward as far as possible while in a sitting position.

SIT & REACH FITNESS STANDARDS (Inches)

AGE	18-29		30-39		40-49		50-59		60 & Over	
SEX	F	M	F	M	F	M	F	M	F	M
GOLD	>22	>21	>22	>21	>21	>20	>20	>19	>20	>19
SILVER	17-22	13-21	17-22	13-21	15-21	13-20	14-20	12-19	14-20	12-19
BRONZE	<17	<13	<17	<13	<15	<13	<14	<12	<14	<12

< = less than   > = more than

3 Arm Hang

The arm hang is included in the National Fitness Test to evaluate muscular strength and endurance of the hands, arms and shoulders. A regular program of arm hangs helps to develop these areas as well as grip strength.

GOAL: To hang from the horizontal bar as long as possible.

ARM HANG FITNESS STANDARDS (Minutes)

AGE	18-29		30-39		40-49		50-59		60 & Over	
SEX	F	M	F	M	F	M	F	M	F	M
GOLD	>1:30	>2:00	>1:20	>1:50	>1:10	>1:35	>1:00	>1:20	>:50	>1:10
SILVER	:46	1:30	1:00	1:20	:30	1:10	:30	1:00	:21	1:10
		:46		:40		:45		:35		:30
BRONZE	<:46	<1:00	<:40	<:50	<:30	<:45	<:30	<:30	<:21	<:30

< = less than   > = more than

Curl-Ups

Curl-ups provide support for your lower back and help to improve posture while trimming and toning stomach muscles.

This test is effective in determining the muscular strength and endurance of your abdominal area.

GOAL: To do as many correct curl-ups as possible in one minute.

CURL-UPS FITNESS STANDARDS (Number Completed)

AGE	18-29		30-39		40-49		50-59		60 & Over	
SEX	F	M	F	M	F	M	F	M	F	M
GOLD	>45	>50	>40	>45	>35	>40	>30	>35	>25	>30
SILVER	25-45	30-50	20-40	22-45	16-35	21-40	12-30	18-35	11-25	15-30
BRONZE	<25	<30	<20	<22	<16	<21	<12	<18	<11	<15

< = less than   > = more than

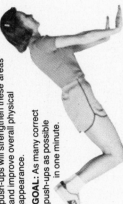

(For Women)

This portion of the National Fitness Test will help us to evaluate muscular strength and endurance in your arms, shoulders and chest.

These muscle groups are used every day to lift, carry, push and press. A continued program of push-ups will strengthen these areas and improve overall physical appearance.

GOAL: As many correct push-ups as possible in one minute.

PUSH-UPS FITNESS STANDARDS FOR WOMEN (Number Completed)

AGE	18-29	30-39	40-49	50-59	60 & Over
GOLD	>45	>40	>35	>30	>25
SILVER	17-45	12-40	8-35	6-30	5-25
BRONZE	<17	<12	<8	<6	<5

< = less than   > = more than

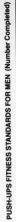

(For Men)

These muscle groups are used every day to lift, carry, push and press. A continued program of push-ups will strengthen these areas and improve overall physical appearance.

GOAL: As many correct push-ups as possible in one minute.

PUSH-UPS FITNESS STANDARDS FOR MEN (Number Completed)

AGE	18-29	30-39	40-49	50-59	60 & Over
GOLD	>50	>45	>40	>35	>30
SILVER	25-50	22-45	19-40	15-35	10-30
BRONZE	<25	<22	<19	<15	<10

< = less than   > = more than

Optional Challenge Series

These tests are recommended to anyone who has maintained a regular fitness program for at least six weeks.

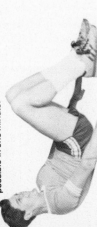

1-1/2 MILE RUN
GOAL: To run 1-1/2 mile

The Optional Challenge Series is a three-part test which will be administered by the honor system, since these tests are to be taken before the National Fitness Test.

Further information and score sheets are available at all test centers.

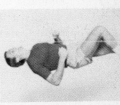

THREE-MILE WALK
GOAL: To walk three miles

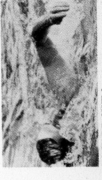

600-YARD SWIM
GOAL: To swim 600 yards as quickly as possible.

Source: National Fitness Foundation

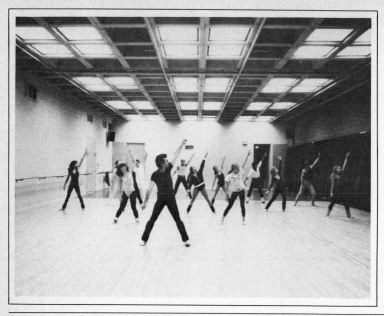

Aerobic dancing.

Yet with all the emphasis on physical fitness today, some questions can be raised regarding the health status of our young people, particularly college students. On one hand, we hear that students are taller and healthier than their parents were years ago. On the other hand, some surveys, such as that by Updyke,[3] indicate that the physical fitness of both high school and college students leaves much to be desired.

Updyke,[3] led a research team that compiled a study entitled "Fitness Profile of American Youth." Updyke and his team administered fitness tests to selected young persons from 1979 to 1981.* He indicates that although performance should continue to increase as young people grow older, the research indicates that fitness levels seem to peak at age 14 and then flatten out or decline from that age on. For example, he points out that the average 17-year-old boy takes 12.8 seconds to run 100 yards, whereas the average 14-year-old boy can cover the distance in 12.6 seconds. Also, the typical 17-year-old girl can do only 38 modified push-ups in 2 minutes, compared with 43 such push-ups by 12-year-old girls.[3]

Furthermore, some of the surveys and polls that indicate adults are physically fit are suspect. For example, a recent Harris survey showed that 59% of adults questioned indicated they exercised regularly. However, another item on the same survey that was not stressed was that only 15% of those persons surveyed said they were physically active enough to achieve physical fitness.[2]

A recent *Washington Post*-ABC public opinion poll showed that 53% of Amer-

*Another Updyke study (1983-1984) showed that 2 out of 3 young persons could not meet desirable physical fitness standards.

ican adults 18 years of age and older exercised *strongly* on a daily basis, that is, their heart and breathing rates increased rapidly and with greater intensity. However, when some of these same persons were questioned more closely, they indicated their work was a source of sufficient exercise. Moreover, further analysis showed that some of these same persons were working in undemanding jobs.[4]

One conclusion that can be drawn regarding the fitness of college-age men and women is that in most cases there is room for improvement. And as you will discover in the following section, there is some confusion among young people as to what is meant by the term *physical fitness*.

THE MEANING OF PHYSICAL FITNESS

What College Students Say

Talks and class discussions reveal how some college students define the term *physical fitness:* "being able to physically do what you want to do", "a body with toned muscles"; "a state in which your body has sufficient strength and endurance for all physical activities"; "being able to participate in any sport or exercise with ease"; or "the ability to use your body effectively."

Although these definitions cover some aspects of physical fitness, they do not tell the whole story. Unless students know and are able to accurately conceptualize what the term means, it may be difficult for them to achieve a state of fitness because their goals will not be clear. Consequently, the life-style they establish may not help them achieve the desired results. There are also other misconceptions about physical fitness.

The Athlete as a Model

Some students view outstanding athletes as examples of "physically fit" persons. They do not seem to realize that physical activity is not only for the superfit athlete but that everyone can benefit from activity and achieve levels of fitness conducive to her or her life-style.

Fitness and Individual Differences

It is now an established fact, contrary to past misconceptions, that women are capable of strenuous physical activity and may achieve superior levels of physical fitness and motor skill. Furthermore, handicapped persons, including visually impaired, physically impaired, or hearing impaired persons, can achieve a high degree of physical fitness and athletic skill.

Age and Fitness

Just as you are never too sedentary to begin a fitness program, you are never too old, either. It is wise to begin a fitness program early in life, but everyone can benefit from exercise no matter when they begin. Although everyone can

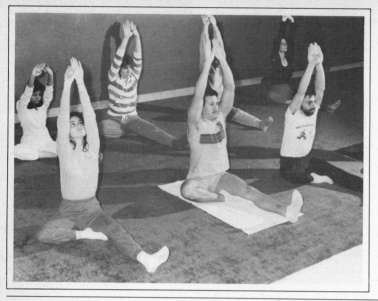

Flexibility is important to achieving physical fitness.

begin an exercise program, it is especially important to monitor the effects of any program. If you have not exercised for 5 years, you will not achieve fitness in 2 weeks. As will be pointed out later, the program should start with a medical examination, commence at your own tolerance level, and be administered progressively.

Physical Effort and Fitness

Any physical fitness program requires effort to produce results. Steam baths, sauna baths, fitness machines, and gimmicks such as body wraps or fad diets may be relaxing or demonstrate short-term effects, but it is necessary to exert effort to achieve the lasting benefits of physical fitness. The body must do the work. Too often, students look for the easy way to achieve their goal. Physical fitness can be attained, but only after a commitment to an ongoing exercise program and months of work. There is no shortcut to physical fitness. You can't sit and be fit.

The Commercialization of Physical Fitness

This is an age in which physical fitness is often packaged and sold. Because many people are reluctant to participate in fitness programs on their own, a multimillion-dollar business of "providing" fitness has been established. These fitness programs are provided by a multitude of spas, exercise clubs, steam

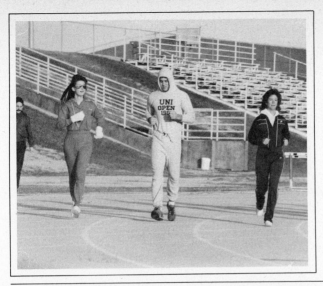

Jogging is an excellent way to develop physical fitness.

baths, health clubs, and numerous other establishments. Some are legitimate, but others are more interested in your money than your fitness. Some are fly-by-night organizations that are in and out of business within months and may reappear in a different part of the country after filing bankruptcy in one area. If you are considering becoming a member of one of these clubs, carefully check the legitimacy of the establishment and ask about the programs that are offered before you join.

The True Meaning of Physical Fitness

Fitness is a broad term denoting dynamic qualities that allow you to satisfy your needs regarding mental and emotional stability, social consciousness and adaptability, spiritual and moral fiber, and organic health consistent with your heredity. *Physical fitness* means that the organic systems of the body are healthy and function efficiently so as to enable the fit person to engage in vigorous tasks and leisure activities. Beyond organic development, muscular strength, and stamina, physical fitness implies efficient performance in exercise or work and a reasonable measure of motor skill in the performance of selected physical activities. This doesn't mean that you have to be a skilled performer athletically.

The same degree of physical fitness is not essential for everyone. It depends on factors such as the tasks you must perform and your potential for physical effort. Physical fitness is very individualized and will vary according to the demands and requirements of a specific task. The collegiate athlete must con-

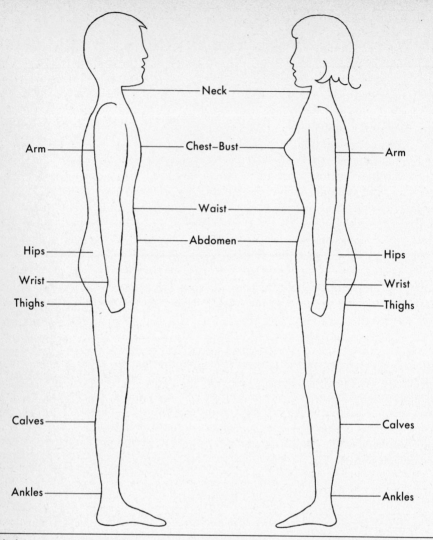

It is important to measure your body now and during your physical fitness program. Measure the parts of your body that are indicated while in a standing position. Measure your neck just below your chin; your chest or bust at the nipple line; your arms, hips, and calves where those features are largest in circumference; wrist at minimal circumference; waist ½ inch above your navel; your thigh just below the curve of your buttocks; and your ankle just above the ankle bone. Be sure that the tape is not pulled so tight that it depresses the skin and thus distorts the measurement.

In general, proper girth proportions suggest that chest or bust should have a similar measurement as hips, upper arm about twice the size of wrist, waist less than chest or bust and hips, hips same as chest or bust, thighs less than waist, calves less than thighs, and ankles less than calves.

stantly work to improve his or her strength, endurance, flexibility, speed, and cardiorespiratory efficiency, whereas the student who cycles to class will require less effort to maintain his or her level of physical fitness. The weekend golfer needs a different level of physical fitness than the mountain climber or wheelchair athlete, and a 40-year-old mother requires a different physical fitness level than her daughter. Physical fitness varies according to the circumstances of a person at different times in his or her life. Because no set standard of physical fitness applies to all people, an optimal level depends on your age, sex, body type, vocation, or physical limitations such as those associated with diabetes or asthma.

Physical fitness is not entirely dependent on exercise. Desirable health practices also play an important role. The road to physical fitness includes proper medical care, the right kind of food and in the right amounts, good oral hygiene, appropriate physical activity adapted to your individual needs, satisfying work and study, healthy play and recreation, and proper amounts of rest and relaxation.

Physical fitness among collegiate men and women, as among people in general, exists in varying degrees. Practically anyone can improve his or her fitness status, but physical activity is essential to achieving physical fitness. There are no shortcuts; physical fitness cannot be stored up. It requires daily attention. The sprinter who fails to run after the track season ends will backslide in respect to

Daily Fitness Schedule

It is important to regularly appraise your daily schedule to determine if you are devoting the proper amount of time to keeping fit. Keep a daily record for 1 week, four times a year. Compare and adjust schedule when necessary.

Physical Activity	Dates	S	M	T	W	T	F	S	Average
List the number of hours you participate in any form of physical activity in or out of school.									

Recreation									
List the number of hours you spend in nonphysically active leisure time activities such as television, knitting, or card playing.									

Health Requirements									
List the number of hours you spend eating, sleeping, and on personal grooming.									

his physical fitness level. The person who plays tennis all summer and then gives up all physical activity when school starts will not remain physically fit.

The Role of Physical Activity

Physical activity is as natural and essential to humans as is eating. Whether you are awake or asleep, muscular contractions permit your lungs to breathe, your heart to beat, your eyes to move, and your body to turn.

Movement of a body part or of the whole body is the primary function of the human muscular system, but because no system operates independently, movement also involves the skeletal, nervous, circulatory, and respiratory systems. These systems support muscular movement, and conversely physical activity contributes to their own effective functioning and well-being.

Although the significance of strength, stamina, and physical prowess for daily living might be questioned by some now that our "pioneer" days have given way to a more comfortable existence, biologists, physiologists, and physicians agree that our need for physical activity and body strength and stamina still exists. Biologically, we have the same basic need for movement to grow and live effectively that our ancestors had.

The means of attaining physical strength and stamina necessarily differ today. Study, work, and home maintenance demand less activity and by themselves do not fulfill activity needs. You must make some conscious effort to supply the necessary vigorous, large-muscle activity your body needs.

THE COMPONENT PARTS OF PHYSICAL FITNESS

Although complete consensus on the components of physical fitness does not exist, most authorities agree that the following are basic elements.

Muscular Strength

Muscular strength is the ability or capacity of a muscle or muscle group for exerting force against resistance. It refers to the muscle's ability to exert maximal force in a single effort. Strength is needed in all kinds of work and physical activity. Muscles that are strong result in better protection of body joints and fewer sprains, strains, and other muscular difficulties. Furthermore, muscle strength helps in maintaining proper posture and provides greater endurance, power, and resistance to fatigue. The strength of abdominal muscles, or lack thereof, is a primary cause of lower back problems. Weak abdominal muscles and inflexible posterior thigh muscles allow the pelvis to tip forward, thus causing an abnormal arch in the lower back that results in lower back pain. Strength is also an important element of athletic activity. The best athletes pay particular attention to developing strength in various muscle groups.

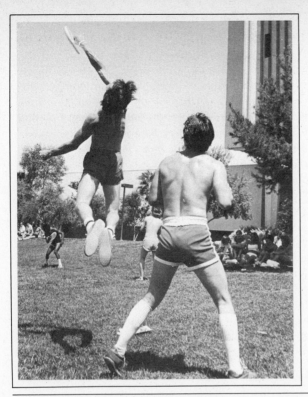

College students playing with a Frisbee.

Muscular Endurance

Muscular endurance is the ability of muscles to repeat or sustain a muscle contraction. Three variations of muscular endurance exercises are recognized: *isometric* exercise, in which a maximal static muscular contraction is held; *isotonic* exercise, in which the muscles continue to raise and lower a submaximal load (as in weight training or performing push-ups); and *isokinetic* exercise. In the isometric form, the muscles maintain a fixed length; in the isotonic form, they alternately shorten and lengthen. Isokinetic exercise is that type of activity in which the strength-training regimen involves using muscle contractions that are executed throughout a full range of movement against a constant resistance. It is a contraction at constant velocity, with the resistance changing to accomodate the force created by the muscles, which changes throughout the range of motion.

Muscular endurance must assume some muscular strength. However, there are distinctions between the two; muscle groups of the same strength may possess different degrees of endurance.

Cardiorespiratory Endurance

Cardiorespiratory endurance is the ability to persist in a physical activity that requires oxygen for physical exertion. The student who runs 2 miles or swims 2000 yards is displaying cardiorespiratory endurance. The functioning of the heart, lungs, and blood vessels is essential to distribute oxygen and nutrients and remove wastes from the body. To perform vigorous activities, efficient functioning of the heart and lungs is necessary. The more efficiently they function, the easier it will be to walk, run, study, and concentrate for longer periods of time. If success is measured by effort, the more efficient student will be able to maintain that effort for a longer time.

Cardiorespiratory endurance is characterized by moderate contractions of large muscle groups for a relatively long time, during which adjustments of the cardiorespiratory system to the activity are necessary, as in distance running or swimming. Exercise of this nature involves the heart, the vessels supplying blood to all parts of the body, and the oxygen-carrying capacity of the blood. Cardiorespiratory endurance can be assessed by various technical measurements, including blood pressure, heart rate, stroke volume of the heart, and oxygen consumption. These tests are often taken during a resting state and then again after exercise.

Flexibility

Flexibility is the quality that permits freedom of movement. It is a measure of the range of motion allowed by the body's joint or joints. Flexibility is important for performance in most active sports; it is also important for maintaining good posture. Furthermore, it is essential for carrying on many daily activities. It can help to prevent muscle strain and orthopedic problems such as backaches.

Body Composition

Body composition relates to the makeup of the body in terms of muscle, bone, fat, and other elements. In respect to physical fitness it particularly refers to percentages of fat in the body as they relate to the fat-free content. Approximately 50% of all adults can be considered to be overweight. An excess of fat in the body is unhealthy because it requires more energy for movement and may reflect a diet high in saturated fat. The demand on the cardiorespiratory system is greater when percent body fat is high. Furthermore, it is believed that obesity contributes to degenerative diseases such as high blood pressure and atherosclerosis. Obesity can also result in psychologic maladjustments and may shorten life. A balance between caloric intake and caloric expenditure is necessary to maintain proper body fat content. Exercise is effective in controlling body fat.

Relation to a Physical Fitness Program

When designing an individualized physical fitness program, you must first decide what it is you are trying to accomplish and then select those specific components of fitness that ultimately help you reach your goal. For example, the goals of fitness improvement for a 55-year-old person would likely differ considerably from a 20-year-old college student who is preparing to compete in varsity gymnastics. Our 55-year-old would be more concerned with such fitness components as cardiorespiratory endurance, flexibility, and body composition. Improvement in these three specific areas would enhance performance in daily tasks without undue fatigue, as stated in our definition of physical fitness.

On the other hand, the 20-year-old gymnast must not only be concerned with those components that have been mentioned but also with components such as strength, speed, power, balance, and agility. If he or she does not include activities in the training regimen that specifically address these various skill-

---

Some Activities to Help You Develop Components of Physical Fitness

Muscular Strength

Swimming	Gymnastics	Racquetball
Weight training	Karate	Backpacking
Judo	Cycling	Mountain climbing

Calisthenic exercises (such as push-ups, leg raises, bench step-ups, flutter kicks)

Muscular Endurance

Jogging	Cycling	Mountain climbing
Running	Cross-country skiing	Fencing
Swimming	Backpacking	Handball
Weight training	Dancing	Hiking
Rowing	Ice skating	Calisthenics

Cardiorespiratory Endurance

Aerobic dancing	Swimming	Handball
Skipping rope	Cross-country skiing	Hiking
Running	Cycling	Mountain climbing
Jogging	Backpacking	Rowing

Flexibility

Calisthenics	Karate
Gymnastics	Swimming
Judo	Modern dancing

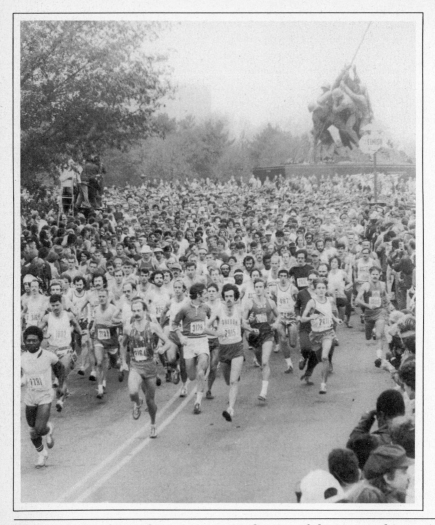

The popularity of marathon runs is one indication of the increased interest in physical fitness.
From Bucher, C. (1982). *Administration of physical education and athletic programs* (8th ed.). St. Louis: C.V. Mosby.

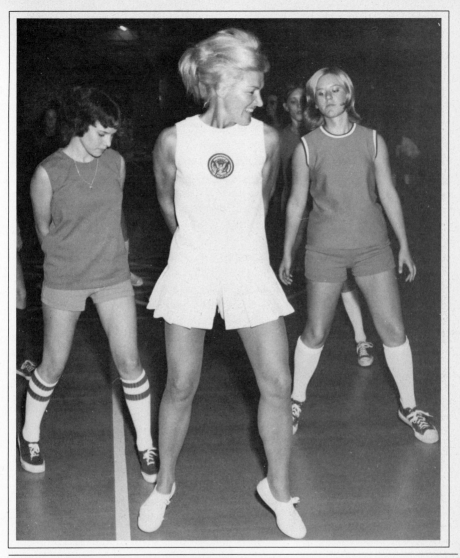

The President's Council on Physical Fitness and Sports conducts physical
fitness clinics throughout the United States.
From Bucher, C. (1982). *The administration of physical education and athletic programs* (8th ed.). St. Louis: C.V. Mosby.

related fitness components, chances are that he or she will be unsuccessful in a competitive situation.

BODY SYSTEMS AND PHYSICAL FITNESS

Muscular and Skeletal Systems

The body's muscular and skeletal systems are responsible for all human locomotion and movement. The condition of these systems depends in large measure on the demands advanced by regular activity; conversely, your muscular strength, stamina, and efficiency determine the effectiveness of your activity.

Muscles become more efficient as they perform the work of contraction, especially if the work is performed regularly and in gradually increasing loads. The demands of contraction inherent in exercise increase the size and strength of individual muscles and groups of muscles. Intensive activity involving body movement can increase joint range, improve general coordination, improve general postural tone, increase endurance, and develop specific performance skill.[5]

The size and strength of muscles increase as a result of exercise. They also gain endurance. This is a result of the *sarcolemma* (the connective tissue surrounding each fiber sheath) becoming thicker and stronger and also a thickening of the connective tissue within the muscle. There is a chemical change in the muscle as a result of exercise, with increases in phosphocreatine content, glycogen, nonnitrogenous substances, and hemoglobin, all of which help the muscles work more efficiently. The rate of lactic acid formation in physically fit persons is lower while exercising than in sedentary persons. The more lactic acid in the system, the more fatigued a person becomes.

Heart and Circulatory System

Exercise strengthens the heart muscle. Greater demands placed on the heart cause it to increase in size and get stronger through use. The volume of blood per beat of the heart increases, bringing better nourishment to all parts of the body. Continued and regular exercise develops the heart's network of small vessels that supply oxygen to the cells and remove waste products. The person who exercises regularly has a lower pulse rate, and this rate returns to normal more quickly after exercise than does the pulse rate of the sedentary person. The increase in blood pressure is less in the physically fit person. The number of red corpuscles (the oxygen-carrying part of the blood) is greater. Cholesterol formation in the walls of the arteries appears to be less in the person who exercises regularly.

Lungs and Respiratory System

Exercise improves the functioning of the lungs by deepening the respiration process. The rate of breathing is slower in the physically fit person, who may take as few as 6 to 8 breaths per minute, as compared to 18 or 20 in the sedentary person. There is deeper diaphragmatic breathing as a result of physical activity, and the blood is exposed to oxygen over a greater area. In the sedentary person, a greater portion of the lungs becomes closed off to air that is inhaled. Thus regular exercise will result in greater economy in respiration; the physically fit person takes in larger amounts of air and absorbs oxygen from the air in greater amounts than the person who is out of shape.

Digestive and Excretory Systems

Exercise helps to keep the digestive and excretory organs in good condition. The nerves and muscles of the stomach and intestines become well-toned and function more efficiently.

Nervous System

The muscles are controlled by nerves. Messages are relayed by the nerves to the muscles, which in turn react in the way the person wishes, whether by running, playing a musical instrument, or hitting a tennis ball. Consequently, muscular exercise enhances nerve-muscle coordination. Furthermore, nervous fatigue may be lessened by pleasant physical activity because the nervous fatigue that has accumulated through anxiety or mental work is offset through muscular activity.

IMPORTANCE OF PHYSICAL FITNESS

Before outlining some reasons why physical fitness is important to college students, it is helpful to sample the different reasons they have for wanting to be physically fit.

What College Students Say

College students, on being asked why physical fitness is important to them, have said: "I think physical fitness is important. I've been active in sports all my life and the main purpose of my taking a physical education class is to stay in shape. Physical fitness is needed for a variety of reasons, the most important being physically and mentally sound. I feel if you're healthy and physically fit, you have a better outlook on life. You also feel better about yourself as well as about other people." "It's important for survival." "Certain activities like gymnastics contribute needed skills to my major, which is theater." "College students should endeavor to be renaissance persons, and that means you need to be physically fit." "It makes you feel better." "Physical fitness is one of the best ways to relax and relieve tension physically and mentally." "It helps to get rid of frustrations and releases mental stress."

Importance of Physical Fitness to Students

I want to be physically fit to:

Lose weight	Yes	No
Feel better	Yes	No
Lessen the risk of heart attack	Yes	No
Have a better self-image	Yes	No
Be more successful in sports	Yes	No
Have more strength	Yes	No
Relieve stress	Yes	No
Increase efficiency for study, work, and other responsibilities I have as a college student	Yes	No
Help my sleep pattern	Yes	No
Reduce tension	Yes	No
Increase energy	Yes	No
Have a better-looking figure	Yes	No
Contribute to my health	Yes	No
Have greater resistance to illness and disease	Yes	No
Improve cardiorespiratory function	Yes	No
Increase flexibility	Yes	No
Improve my posture and appearance	Yes	No
Improve my outlook on life	Yes	No
Increase my social outlets	Yes	No

Physical Fitness and Success in College

To be successful in a higher educational experience, an optimal level of fitness is necessary. Physical ailments and emotional depression or a lack of stamina that detract from mental effort are drains on the student and can result in decreased functioning or failure in college.

As philosopher Will Durant advised, "Health is mostly within each person's will. In many cases sickness is a crime. We have done something physiologically foolish, and nature is being hard put to it to repair our mistakes. The pain we endure is the tuition we pay for our instruction in living." Good health and physical vitality, on the other hand, enhance intellectual vitality and thus ensure greater academic accomplishments. Optimally, a fit student will be more productive, more vigorous, and live a more rewarding life.

Fitness is the capacity for a task. The task you as a college student are concerned with at the moment is to be a success in college. A lifetime of ambition and hope lies ahead for you. The degree to which you achieve your goals will be enhanced by how fit you are to accomplish the tasks that college and life demand. Many freshmen do not complete 4 years of college and attain a degree. If a lack of fitness for the task is one of the reasons for these dropouts, students

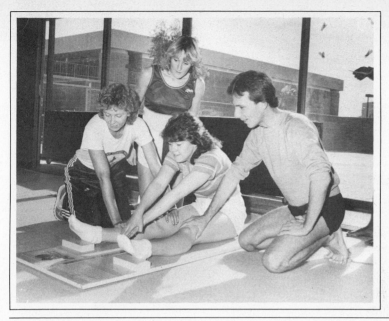

Flexibility is a component of physical fitness. College students being checked for flexibility.

can better ensure their success by preparing themselves physically as well as mentally for the demands of college.

Fitness is not developed in a day or in one easy lesson. It takes time and hard work. If you have overlooked this essential to success, a good start would be to determine the contribution that physical fitness can make to you as a college student.

Technologic Advances Encourage Inactivity

Many college students live a sedentary existence and gear their exercise to the demands of everyday life. Because the physiologic demands of today's society are relatively easy, little activity is experienced. Because of this lack of activity, body processes may deteriorate. Medical problems such as coronary heart disease, hypertension, obesity, lower back pain, and insufficient rest may be directly or indirectly linked with a lack of physical fitness activity.

The concept of physical fitness is not new. Primitive humans relied primarily on speed, agility, and strength in the fight for survival. Life was a constant struggle that could only be met through physical prowess. Without knowing the scientific benefits of fitness, primitive humans existed, adapted to a variety of environmental conditions, and lived vigorous lives. In contrast, we now rely

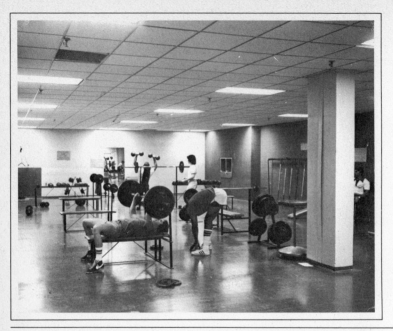

Weight training at Sinclair College, Dayton, Ohio, helps develop strength, a
component of physical fitness.
From Bucher, C. (1982). *Foundations of physical education and sport* (9th ed.). St.
Louis: C.V. Mosby.

largely on our intellect. Whereas cognitive activity is essential for many work-
related skills, little physical effort is required in much of our modern society.
In fact, the modern life-style fosters a lack of physical fitness. Technologic
advances such as the automobile, television, elevators, escalators, and moving
sidewalks eliminate the need for physical exertion and contribute to a sedentary
life-style. Too often our society is so concerned with developing superiority of
the intellect that there is a danger of neglecting the development of the whole
person. Physical fitness affects the total person: our intellect, emotional stability,
and physical conditioning.

In addition, our society is characterized by a fast-paced life-style, with ob-
ligations and stresses that affect our physical and emotional fitness. A common
misconception among college students is that daily living incorporates enough
exercise to maintain an adequate level of fitness. Walking back and forth to
class, participating in intramural activity, or working in a part-time job usually
provide a limited amount of physical exertion that in most cases is not adequate
to produce physical fitness or eliminate tension.

A physical fitness program should be initiated on a regular basis to overcome
inactivity and maintain an optimal level of fitness. Furthermore, an adequate

Suggestions For Making Physical Activity More Attractive

Some students find physical activity dull. Here are some ways to make it more inviting:

1. Exercise to music.
2. Exercise with classmates.
3. Keep your program simple.
4. Instill variety into activity: for example, dancing, hiking, tennis, and swimming.
5. Reward yourself when fitness goals are met.
6. Don't become upset when goals are not met and benefits are not immediate.
7. Keep a record of things such as your weight and distance you jog.
8. Take a break whenever you wish.
9. Plan the program to fit into your daily life.

amount of such things as rest, social and emotional outlets, and diet are also required for an appropriate level of fitness.

College Years Are Formative Years

The period between 18 and 30 years of age are the formative years for establishing physical fitness. At this time, the body reaches the peak of maturity and physiologic functioning. However, during this period students may be preoccupied in starting their life's work, socializing, or exerting minimal amounts of physical and mental effort. Instead of establishing and maintaining optimal levels of activity, students may become less active, marry, start a job, and normally forget about a physical fitness program until age 35 or 40, when they may be beset with obesity, cardiac disorders, or decreased vitality.

Activities such as swimming, mountain climbing, skiing, backpacking, or scuba diving may become prohibitive to the student because of the lack of physical fitness. Even if an unfit student is participating in these activities, the safety, proficiency of skill, or enjoyment may be increased immensely by a higher level of physical fitness. Nothing is more enjoyable than skiing on new snow, but if the skier fatigues after only a short time on the slopes, he or she misses hours of enjoyment.

The Social Rewards

With the loss of physical fitness necessary to participate in physical activity comes a decrease in social outlets. The feelings associated with vigorous activity and companionship inherent in such activities are missing because of the unwillingness to acquire or maintain a satisfactory level of physical fitness. Students who do maintain ongoing fitness programs may be more able to cope with the intellectual demands of college as well as enjoy the physical and social benefits of being physically fit. Students may have too often concentrated on developing only their minds and forget to develop their total selves. Physical fitness affects the entire person, and you will find that rich dividends accrue when you concentrate on the development of not only the mind but also the body.

Summary of Benefits

The following is a summary of some of the general benefits of vigorous activity and physical fitness for college students.

Biologically, human beings are designed to be active creatures. Although changes in civilization have resulted in a decrease in the amount of activity needed in accomplishing the basic tasks associated with living, the human body has not changed. Therefore it is important to be aware of the requirements for good health and recognize the importance of vigorous physical activity in your life. If you do not, your health, productivity, and effectiveness are likely to suffer.

Regular, vigorous activity increases muscle size, strength, and power and develops endurance for sustaining work. The increase in muscle tissue is not an increase in number of muscle cells, but rather a condition of *hypertrophy*—the result of an increase of cytoplasm within individual muscle cells. The greatest increase in muscle growth is brought about by those activities that make the muscle work to full capacity.

Exercise taxes the circulatory and respiratory systems. Muscular activity demands that an increased amount of oxygen be delivered to the working muscle cells. This increase is brought about by more rapid and deeper breathing, by increased heart rate, and by elevated blood pressure. These normal physiologic responses become quicker and more efficient when the demands are made with regularity. A severe, infrequent demand, such as that made on the circulatory system by a person who participates in athletic activity only occasionally, can be extremely fatiguing and place too much strain on the heart. Vigorous daily activity develops a cardiovascular fitness that produces the quality of physical reserve power and stamina called endurance.

Besides organic vigor and fitness, physical activity contributes to improvement in agility, speed, coordination, and skill. A primary objective of collegiate physical education programs is the acquisition of skills that lead to enjoyable recreational sporting performance not only during collegiate years but also throughout life.

Exercise helps you maintain a healthy body weight by using excess calories. Loss of body weight is best brought about by a reducing diet; but weight control involves more than merely reducing caloric intake to compensate for sedentary habits and overeating. Regular physical activity takes care of some of our dietary excesses and prevents the adding on of undesired adipose tissue. Excess body fat results in undue stress on normal body functions, particularly those of the heart. Being overweight shortens life. Among persons whose weight exceeds normal by only 15% to 25%, death rates increase by an estimated 30%.

What Makes Your Physical Activity Most Enjoyable?

		Yes	No
1.	Involves other students	✓	✓
2.	Can participate in alone		✓
3.	Is a sport or game		✓
4.	Involves competition		✓
5.	Provides a good physical workout	✓	
6.	Provides an opportunity to excel	✓	
7.	Helps relax	✓	
8.	Is fun	✓	
9.	Contributes to weight control	✓	
10.	Contributes to feeling better physically	✓	
11.	Can be done in a minimum of time	✓	
12.	Requires little space and equipment	✓	

Physical activity is not a panacea for all that ails us, but many people use regular exercise, especially of a recreational nature, as a means of mental relaxation. It is usually not difficult to find a sporting or recreational activity to fit into your daily regimen.

Physical exercise contributes to improved posture and appearance through the development of proper muscle tone, more flexible joints, and a feeling of well-being.

Physical activity results in more energy and thus contributes to greater individual productivity for both physical and mental tasks.

Physical activity helps to develop your kinesthetic intelligence. (*Kine* means movement and *esthetic* means beautiful. Kinesthetic intelligence results in more efficient, functional, and attractive movement.)

People who become physically active may pay more attention to such things as proper nutrition, rest, and relaxation and also drink less alcohol and stop smoking because they do not want to undo the benefits that accrue from physical activity. They are committed to engaging in health-promoting rather than health-harming behavior.

The period from 18 to 30 years of age has been referred to as the period when we possess the greatest amount of physical and mental vitality. In most cases, after age 30 qualities such as muscular endurance, coordination, and strength tend to decrease. Furthermore, as we age, recovery from vigorous exercise requires a longer time. Regular physical activity, however, tends to delay and in some cases prevent the appearance of some degenerative processes. For best results, control of the aging process should start early, before the aging process sets in, that is, before a person's physical development has been completed, which in most cases is between the ages of 14 and 22. Although physical

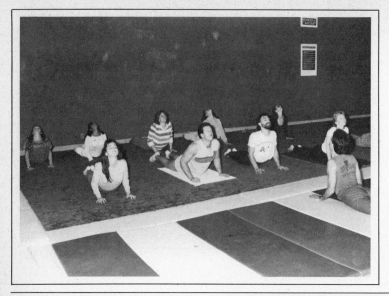

The period between 18 and 30 years of age are the formative years for establishing fitness. College students practicing yoga.

capacities decrease with age, these capacities can be maintained at acceptable levels if you continue to be active. If you stay physically fit throughout your life, you will retain more strength, flexibility, cardiorespiratory health, and a more desirable body composition than if you become sedentary.

The benefits of physical fitness for the college student are numerous. The student who is physically fit has greater amounts of strength, energy, and stamina; an improved sense of well-being; better protection from injury because strong, well-developed muscles safeguard bones, internal organs, and joints and keep moving parts limber; and improved cardiorespiratory function.

CONCLUSION

The collegiate years are important years during which to lay the foundations of physical fitness for a lifetime. During these years, problems such as extra weight often appear. Students become preoccupied with studies, dating, and preparing for careers. As a result, they often forget about fitness requirements. The collegiate years should be the time for incorporating regular physical activity as part of your life-style. It's also a time for establishing a personal daily regimen that will help to guarantee a productive, healthy, happy, and interesting life.

College students have many demands on their time. Classes, long hours of study, extracurricular activities, work, and other responsibilities take their physical and mental toll. Unless you are in good physical condition, academic studies may suffer, sickness can result, and college life may become a struggle. On the other hand, if you are in good physical condition, you have a better chance of achieving academically and having a more enjoyable college career than your physically unfit classmates.

For the tasks that college students face today and tomorrow there is no substitute for being in optimal physical condition. At every stage, from freshman year through postgraduate study, success depends on the way you use your personal resources and develop your physical and mental talents.

This text will provide the knowledge and understanding about various aspects of fitness that you will need to make a success of college. It is designed to show the importance of and essential ingredients for fitness. It will explain how students can assess, develop, and maintain their fitness. Further, it will describe various fitness activities and point out how tobacco, alcohol abuse, drugs, and self-medication are deterrents to fitness. Finally, it will show students how to plan and develop a personalized fitness program.

SUMMARY

- The emphasis on physical fitness is widespread throughout the United States.
- The public's concept of the physical dimension of the human body has changed over the years. In the past, people didn't understand the relationship between physical activity and physical fitness; today, the public in general is much more fitness conscious.
- The physical fitness of many college students leaves much to be desired.
- There is confusion among young people as to the true meaning of physical fitness, its component parts, and how it is assessed and developed.
- Anyone can benefit from physical exercise throughout his or her entire lifetime.
- There is no shortcut to fitness.
- The totally fit person is one who has developed all aspects of fitness, including fitness of all the body systems.
- Physical fitness is individualized and varies according to the demands of a specific task.
- Physical fitness depends on factors such as good nutrition, medical care, rest, relaxation, recreation and exercise.
- Component parts of physical fitness include muscular strength, muscular endurance, cardiorespiratory endurance, flexibility, and body composition.
- Biologically, human beings are designed to be active creatures.
- To be successful in higher education, an optimal level of fitness is necessary.
- Fitness is the capacity of a person for a task, and the task a student is concerned with is making a success of college.
- Modern life-styles, with the emphasis on technologic advances, luxury, and the "good life," provide deterrents to fitness.
- Medical problems such as coronary heart disease, hypertension, obesity, and lower

back pain are often either directly or indirectly linked with a lack of physical fitness activity.
- The period between 18 and 30 years of age has often been referred to as the formative years for establishing fitness.
- College students list many reasons why they consider physical fitness to be important, such as providing better outlook on life, providing an excellent way to relieve tensions, and contributing to a healthy mind.
- The organic systems of the body depend in large measure on regular physical activity.
- There are many general benefits of vigorous activity and physical fitness, including muscular strength, cardiovascular fitness, agility, skill, proper body weight, mental relaxation, improved posture, and greater energy.

GLOSSARY

body composition The percentage of total body weight composed of fat vs. the percentage of total body weight composed of lean tissue

cardiorespiratory endurance The ability to perform physical activities for extended periods of time as oxygen is supplied to the various tissues of the body

fitness A broad term denoting dynamic qualities that allow a person to satisfy his or her own needs, such as mental and emotional stability, social consciousness and adaptability, spiritual and moral fiber, and organic health consistent with a person's heredity

flexibility The range of movement that is possible about a given point or through a series of articulations

hypertrophy Increase in muscle bulk, as by thickening of muscle fibers; exaggerated growth

isokinetic exercise The changing of the length of the muscle as muscle contraction is performed at a constant velocity against resistance

isometric exercise Involves a muscle contraction in which the length of the muscle remains constant while tension develops toward a maximum creating force against an immovable resistance

isotonic exercise Involves a muscle contraction in which force is generated while the muscle is changing in length

muscular endurance The ability to perform repetitive muscle contractions against a resistance

muscular strength The maximal force that can be applied by a muscle during a single maximal contraction

organic systems Refers to various organic systems that make up the human body, such as circulatory and digestive systems

physical fitness An important component of total fitness, it is the ability to perform daily tasks with sufficient strength and vigor without experiencing undue fatigue, and to have enough strength, energy, and stamina left over to enjoy recreational pursuits and be able to meet unforeseen emergencies

sarcolemma Thin, transparent, homogeneous sheath enclosing striated muscle fibers.

REFERENCES

1. Conrad, C.C. (1982, October). *Direction of the National Program of Physical Fitness and Sports*. Annual Conference of Sports, Medicine and Physical Fitness, New Jersey.
2. President's Council on Physical Fitness and Sports. (1982, November). *Newsletter*. Washington, DC: U.S. Government Printing Office.
3. Updyke, W. (1982). *Profile of youth reveals fitness levels lower than desirable*. News release. Washington, DC: Nabisco Brands.
4. Lamb, D.R. (1984). *Physiology of exercise* (2nd ed.). New York: Macmillan.

SUGGESTED READINGS

deVries, H.A. (1980). *Physiology of exercise for physical education and athletics*. (2nd ed.). Dubuque, IA: Wm. C. Brown.

Falls, H.B., & others. (1980). *Essentials of fitness*. Philadelphia: Saunders College.

Fox, E.L., (1984). *Sports physiology*. Philadelphia: CBS College Publishing.

Griffiths, M. (1974). *Introduction to human physiology*. New York: Macmillan.

Johnson, W.R., & Buskirk, E.R., (1974). *Science and medicine of exercise and sport*. New York: Harper & Row.

Lamb, David R. (1984). *Physiology of exercise* (2nd ed.). New York: Macmillan.

Mathews, D.K., and Fox, E.L. (1981). *The physiological basis of physical education and athletics*. Philadelphia: W.B. Saunders.

McArdle, W.D. & others. (1981). *Exercise physiology*. Philadelphia: Lea & Febiger.

Morehouse, L.E. & Miller, A.T., Jr. (1976). *Physiology of exercise*. St. Louis: C.V. Mosby.

Strauss, R.H. (1979). *Sports medicine and physiology*. Philadelphia: W.B. Saunders.

2

BASIC PRINCIPLES FOR
A TRAINING PROGRAM

After completing this chapter, you will be able to:

- Explain the need to observe basic principles concerning the right kind of training program needed to be physically fit.
- Recognize initial considerations such as attitude, reasons for wanting to be physically fit, and present level of physical activity in planning a training program.
- Describe the role of exercise tolerance, goals, specificity, fun, overload, progression, consistency, individuality, and safety in planning a training program.
- Identify the importance and role of warm-up, workout, and cool-down in a training program.

Some college students think of health and fitness as the responsibility of physicians, hospitals, clinics, insurance companies, and the government. They believe that fitness is someone else's responsibility, not their's. If they become sick, they reason that a physician will prescribe the right medicine or send them to the hospital or to a specialist who will provide the proper remedy. Students should realize, however, that fitness cannot be purchased or the responsibility relegated to some other person or agency. As Dr. John Knowles,[1] former president of the Rockefeller Foundation, has pointed out, health is a moral obligation on the part of each person. It is erroneous to equate more health services with better health. Instead, people must take responsibility for their own health and fitness. Part of that responsibility is following a sound training program.

The decisions that you make now will affect your physical fitness in the future. You are the one who decides what to eat, when and if to exercise, drink, engage in drug abuse, smoke, see a physician, and engage in a sound training program. In some cases, if you are sick, you have only yourself to blame.

Years ago problems such as poor nutrition and sanitation, factors over which we have control, were causes of much sickness and poor physical fitness, with the result that entire populations were often affected. Today, modern science

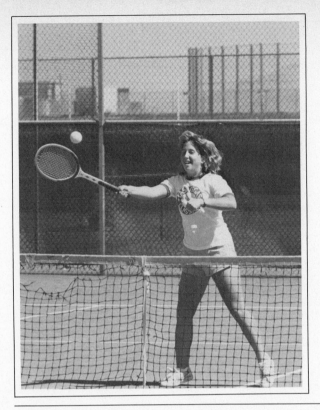

Tennis.

has eliminated many health scourges and provided humans with knowledge concerning basic principles that should be observed to maintain health and physical fitness. However, this knowledge must be applied to be effective. For example, seat belts are placed in automobiles because research shows that many deaths and injuries can be prevented if they are worn. Although this knowledge is readily available, some people still insist on ignoring this protective device. As a result, many people are needlessly injured or killed each year in automobile accidents.

Much information has been generated regarding principles that should be observed to design the right kind of training program needed to be physically fit. The realization that fitness is a personal responsibility has prompted many conscientious people to observe these principles, and in so doing achieve an optimal state of physical fitness. College students are discovering that the responsibility for physical fitness does not rest with physicians, hospitals, and health services; each person has a responsibility for his or her own fitness.

This chapter sets forth basic principles for a training program to help college students who want to be physically fit.

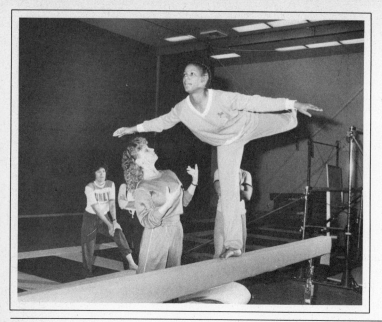

The balance beam.

INITIAL CONSIDERATIONS

Before starting your personal training program, it may be helpful to examine your attitude toward physical fitness, your reasons for wanting to be physically fit, and your present level of activity. Identifying your reasons for starting a physical fitness program and what you expect the program to achieve will help you determine the degree to which you are motivated and aspire to a desirable fitness level, which in part determines how successful you will be in developing and maintaining a satisfactory degree of fitness.

Determining Your Attitude

To determine your attitude toward physical fitness, ask yourself the following questions:

Do I enjoy exercising?
Do I feel that being fit makes me look better?
Do my parents and friends encourage me to exercise?
Do I avoid making excuses for not engaging regularly in physical activity?
Do I feel better after a vigorous physical workout?
Am I the right weight?

Do I want to be in good physical shape?

Do I enjoy engaging in active sports?

Do I find exercise to be invigorating and not boring?

Am I inclined to live an active and not a sedentary existence?

Do I have a guilty feeling if I do not exercise regularly?

Do I really want to be physically fit?

If you answered "yes" to these questions, you will probably benefit from a planned training program and, as a result, you will improve your self-concept, enjoy physical exercise, have a more attractive figure, and maintain control of your life. However, if you answered "no" to these questions, you may not be as successful as you could be in your quest to achieve a satisfactory state of fitness and the dividends that accrue from such a state of being.

Determining Your Reasons For Wanting to Be Physically Fit

All of us are concerned about physical fitness, but our concern develops as the result of different motivations. Some people want to be physically fit because of the effect that physical fitness can have on their appearance. Others want to be physically fit because of the benefits that it can offer toward healthful living. Still others desire physical fitness because of the implications it has for leisure time or recreational pursuits.

Whatever your motivation for starting an individualized training program, your first consideration should be to determine exactly what it is that you are trying to accomplish. For example, are you simply trying to improve your general health by becoming involved in some type of physical activity, or are you interested in training for some event or activity involving competition?

Your answer to this question will largely determine the training techniques that will most effectively help you achieve your goals of fitness improvement. For example, if one of your reasons is to improve cardiorespiratory function, then you will want to include activities in your program such as jogging, skipping rope, or swimming. If one of your reasons is weight control, you will want to engage in physical activity for a sufficient length of time and on a regular basis as well as watch your food intake so that you will burn up the necessary calories to achieve this goal. If you want to develop strength in your shoulder girdle, you may want to start a weight-training program.

Determining Your Present Level of Physical Activity

To plan your training program, it will also be helpful to look at your present activity level. This can be done by determining the accuracy of the following statements:

I exercise for 15 minutes each day.

I participate in some sport once a week.

I engage in 1 hour of physical activity in the college gymnasium twice a week.

Because of my demanding study schedule, I only exercise on weekends.

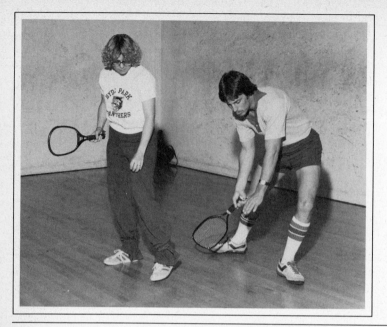

Racquetball.

I never exercise during the school year, only in the summer.

I know what my resting heart rate is.

I am enrolled in physical education classes that meet twice a week.

I am a spectator of college sports and not an active participant.

I jog every other day for 20 minutes at a time, getting my heart rate up to approximately 75% of 220 minus my age.*

I use my car to go from the dormitory to my classes.

I use the elevators rather than walking up the stairs.

Your answers to these questions will help to determine whether exercise on a regular basis and the degree to which you are participating in a desirable training program. It will also be helpful to match the goals you have previously established for wanting to engage in a fitness program with your present level of activity to determine what changes need to be made, if any, to achieve your objectives.

A representative sample of college students was surveyed at a western university† to determine their present level of activity. This survey found that 9% of them did not spend any time in physical activity such as jogging, running, engaging in sports, calisthenics, aerobics, and swimming; 37% spent 3 hours or less each week; 24% spent 6 hours or less each week; and 30% spent more than 6 hours per week. When asked the question "do you feel that you spend

*See discussion of target heart rate on pp. 56-57.

†Based on random sample of 250 students at the University of Nevada—Las Vegas in 1983.

Checklist For Training Program

1. Have you determined your exercise tolerance to physical activity?   Yes   No
2. Have you identified the physical fitness goals you wish to accomplish?   Yes   No
3. Are the activities you select enjoyable?   Yes   No
4. Do you gradually increase the intensity of some of your physical activities to achieve the benefits of overload?   Yes   No
5. Do you provide for progression in your training program, adding a little each time in terms of repetitions of an exercise, speed, and endurance required?   Yes   No
6. Do you set aside a definite time during the day and week to pursue your physical fitness program?   Yes   No
7. Is your training program suited to your individual needs?   Yes   No
8. Do you observe safety procedures in the implementation of your fitness program?   Yes   No
9. Do you engage in warm-up exercises before working out?   Yes   No
10. Does your workout help in developing and maintaining the qualities of muscular strength and endurance, cardiorespiratory endurance, and flexibility?   Yes   No
11. After working out, do you engage in a cool-down period?   Yes   No
12. Do you keep a record of your training and periodically check the progress you are making?   Yes   No

NOTE: If you have developed a sound training program, your answer to each question should be "Yes."

sufficient time each week engaging in physical fitness activities?", 36% of the students said "yes"; 62% said "no", and 2% said they didn't know. Some typical comments were: "I don't have enough time due to work and school studies," "I lack motivation or am lazy," "I need encouragement," "I should do more," "I'm slim but not in good shape," and "I don't work out enough in the winter."

These same students were asked to make a subjective assessment of their own physical fitness. The result: a majority of students believed that their state of physical fitness left much to be desired. They also believed that factors such as the following were deterrents to their physical fitness: lack of proper physical exercise, drug abuse, stress, smoking, diet, alcohol abuse, and lack of sleep. This survey may or may not be representative of college students in general.

PLANNING THE TRAINING PROGRAM

After assessing the initial considerations regarding their physical fitness, some students may feel they have achieved a satisfactory state of physical fitness, one that is compatible with their goals. In this case these students should follow a

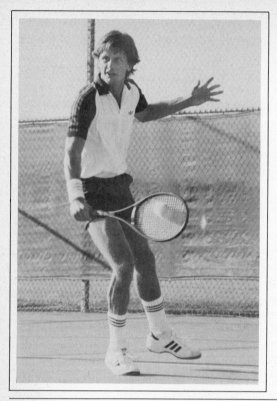

Tennis.

program of maintenance. However, we suspect that a majority of college students, after carefully evaluating their physical fitness, will not be satisfied with their condition and will want to improve their situation. For some of these students a medical examination by a physician is next in order. This is particularly true if a student has not exercised regularly for a number of years, is overweight, and is not in sound physical condition.

In some cases it may be wise to take a *stress exercise test*. Such an evaluation is conducted while the person is walking or running on a motor-driven treadmill. The test is intended to reveal how healthy the heart is and the range of desirable limits of exercise. Heart rate, blood pressure, and sometimes the amount of oxygen consumed are monitored. During the test, exercise is gradually made more strenuous every 1 to 3 minutes by increasing the speed of the treadmill to at least the level at which the person plans to do his or her exercise program. The test, however, usually goes beyond this level (for further information, see Chapter 3).

Determining Your Exercise Tolerance

Exercise tolerance means the manner in which the body responds to exercise. Physical activity should not produce prolonged fatigue and pain; instead, the body should respond favorably to exercise. Afterward, you should feel invigorated and relaxed. In other words, exercise should be adapted to your tolerance level. The response of the body to physical activity will indicate what the tolerance level is. All things being equal, if there is a positive reaction to the physical activity, then it represents a suitable part of your training program.

Matching Your Goals with Specific Activities

Your fitness goals should be taken into consideration when planning a training program. The exercise program you choose should be one that results in the development of the component(s) of fitness that you desire. This means that activities selected should be specific to goals. For example, your goal might be the development and strengthening of the abdominal muscles. You realize that the muscular system in the pelvic region is important because the abdominal muscles support the vital organs of the viscera, keeping them in proper and efficient relation to one another, and furthermore that chronic back pain frequently has its origin in this area. Therefore you want to engage in exercise that will strengthen the abdominal and back muscles. If your goal is to develop shoulder girdle strength, you may want to include high-resistance exercises such as lifting heavy weights. If your goal is increasing stamina or endurance, this may be achieved effectively by engaging in activities such as running, swimming, skating, or cycling, in which the circulatory system is brought into maximal use.

Having Fun

Enjoying yourself may be one of the most critical factors in a successful training program. The activity you select must be one that you enjoy.

A quick look at the streets on a sunny spring day will show how popular running is as a physical activity. There is no question that a running program will result in significant improvement in cardiorespiratory endurance over a period of time. But some people simply hate to run and would prefer to do anything else. If these people select running as their activity because it is "in" and not because they enjoy doing it, then chances are that they will not stick with that activity for very long. You should select the type of activity that will allow you to do two things: (1) achieve the ultimate goals of physical fitness improvement that you have established for yourself and (2) maintain your interest and motivation for a long time (weeks or months), so that physical improvement may be realized as a result of that activity.

Motivation can play an important role in your ability to stick with an exercise program, even though you may not totally enjoy the particular activity you are being forced to do. The varsity athlete is motivated to achieve a high level of

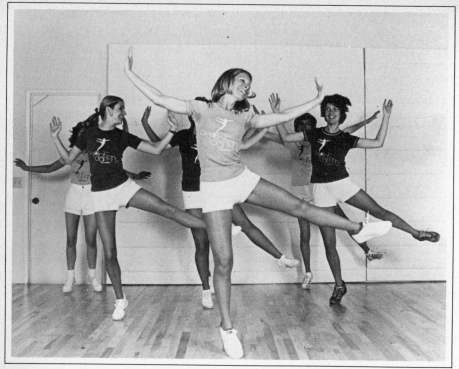

FIGURE 2-1

Aerobic dancing contributes to cardiovascular fitness, muscular fitness, and flexibility.
Courtesy President's Council on Physical Fitness and Sports. From Bucher, C. (1982). *Foundations of physical education and sport.* (9th ed.). St. Louis: C.V. Mosby.

fitness through training by coaches and peers as well as by the challenge of competition. Conversely, if you are a recreational athlete, you probably don't have the same type of competitive motivation; in this case it becomes even more critical that you derive some pleasure and enjoyment from the activity in which you participate.

Overload

To achieve the greatest benefits from the exercise program, you should recognize the principle of *overload*. Overload is a gradual increase in the intensity of the physical activity that is a part of the training program, for example, extending yourself by running for a longer time or distance or increasing the speed of the

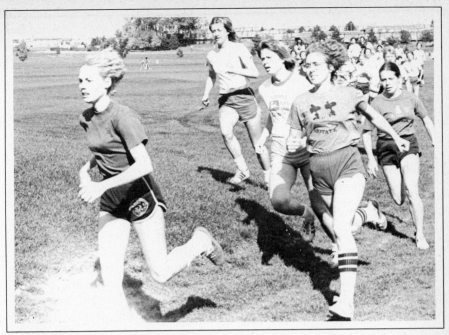

FIGURE 2-2

Cross-country is an excellent example of the training benefits of utilizing the principle of overload.
From Bucher, C. (1982). *Foundations of physical education and sport*. (9th ed.). St. Louis: C.V. Mosby.

exercise. In so doing the cardiorespiratory rate will be stepped up, thus causing an overload on these organic systems with resultant beneficial effects.

This is one of the most critical factors in any activities program. For a physiologic component of fitness to improve, the system must work harder than it is used to working. Stress must be presented to a given system so that over a period of time the system will improve to the point at which it can easily accommodate the additional stress. For example, if you are on a running program to improve cardiorespiratory endurance, and you go out and run 1 mile in 10 minutes, the cardiorespiratory system will be able to accommodate this distance and intensity very easily. However, if the long-range goal of your training program is to run the Boston Marathon, it is foolish to believe that you could finish a race of this distance and intensity by running only one 10-minute mile a day. By gradually overloading the system by running farther at a faster pace, you force the cardiorespiratory system to work more efficiently to keep up with increased physiologic demands. It is not unreasonable to expect that overloading the system over a long period of time is capable of producing significant improvement in the ability of that system to handle a stressful exercise bout. (See also Chapter 3 on cardiorespiratory endurance.)

Progression

Progression is closely related to overload. It is essential that you make progress in your exercise program. But more important, the rate of progression should be within your capabilities to adapt physiologically. Without overloading the system, progression does not occur. For example, in weight training, exercises are commonly referred to as progressive resistance exercise (PRE). In a PRE program, a particular muscle is exercised through a full range of motion against resistance. Improvement in strength occurs only when the muscle is overloaded; progression in weight should occur only when the muscle has adapted to the increased overload.

Progression is also important for motivation. Interest level in an activity remains high as long as you continue to see improvement in your physical ability. Even though weight increases may be minimal in strength training, a progression of even 1 pound is often enough to maintain interest and motivation.

A little today and a little more tomorrow is a good principle to follow in any training program. You should start gradually and add a little each day in terms of such factors as repetitions of an exercise, speed, or endurance required. In other words, the workout should gradually become a little longer or more intense until you reach the desired level of physical fitness.

Consistency

One of the biggest problems with beginning a training program is finding time during the day to fit in an hour or so of activity. For the competitive varsity athlete, *consistency* is not a problem because a specific hour is assigned for practice, and everyone is required to be there at that time. The recreational athlete frequently has a problem finding a specific time unless he or she is involved in a class that meets on a scheduled basis. It is important to select a specific period of time for exercising each day and stick to it.

The number of days per week you are involved with a specific activity will vary depending on a number of personal factors. However, it is recommended that you should try to work out at least 3 days per week to see minimal improvement. For the competitive athlete, three times per week is usually insufficient; he or she should attempt to work out five or six times per week.

Individuality

When you become involved in an activity program, it is important to remember that no two persons are exactly the same; therefore training regimens should meet the criterion of *individuality*. Not all persons involved in similar activities will progress at the same rates, nor will they be able to overload their systems to the same degree. It is extremely important to push competitive athletes to the limits of both their physical and mental capabilities. But there is a fine line between pushing athletes *to* limits at which improvement in performance continues and pushing athletes *beyond* their limits, after which physical activity becomes detrimental to their well-being. A successful coach has the ability to push an athlete to the individual limits of physical ability without going beyond them.

It is important to consider the degree of stress in your life. Some people tend to see physical activity as an outlet for stress that is built up during the day. However, for competitive athletes, the competition itself may provide a stressful situation that may in some cases be detrimental to their total well-being. This further emphasizes the point that before beginning a training program of any type it is necessary to decide what you are trying to accomplish.

People differ in terms of things such as fitness goals, makeup of their physical resources, motivations, body build, and state of physical fitness. Therefore a training program for one person will not necessarily satisfy the needs of another person. Exercise is good, but it must be adapted to individual needs and abilities. Just as a medical prescription must be relative to a person's health needs, so should a physical fitness prescription be relative to a person's exercise needs based on individual objectives, needs, functional capacity, and interests.

The time of day in which you engage in physical activity is not important. The important thing is to set aside a definite time for a fitness program and make it part of your daily routine. The least desirable times are probably after a meal, when activity may make you uncomfortable, and just before bedtime, when activity may make it difficult to sleep.

Safety

Another factor to consider when planning a training program is safety. The purpose of the activity program should be to improve selected components of fitness through physical exercise. Unfortunately, injuries often occur as the result of poorly planned activity programs. Too often people who have been sedentary for long periods of time overestimate their physical abilities and "overdo" it. This overdoing may result in musculoskeletal injuries or other health problems.

The rule of thumb to follow is to start out slowly and progress according to your own capabilities. If you are involved in a personal exercise program and are unsure of how to get started or perhaps how quickly to progress, seek professional advice from persons with some background in training and conditioning, such as certified athletic trainers, physical educators, or physicians (see Appendix C for other sources of help).

Three Basic Elements of Every Training Program

You should be aware of the three basic elements of any physical fitness program, namely, *warm-up, workout,* and *cool-down.*

The Warm-Up

Take from 10 to 20 minutes to warm up.

Engage in exercises that stretch muscles and put body joints through a full range of motion.

Exercise all body segments and muscle groups, including neck, shoulder girdle and joints, trunk, thigh joints, thighs, knees, and legs.

Engage in exercises that stimulate a gradual increase in heart and circulatory system action.

Warm-up. A period of warm-up exercises should take place before the workout. The warm-up increases body temperature, stretches ligaments and muscles, and increases flexibility. Related warm-ups, those similar to the activity engaged in, are preferable to unrelated ones because of the practice effect that results.

Warm-ups have been found to be important in preventing injury and muscle soreness. It appears that muscle injury can result when vigorous exercises are not preceded by a related warm-up. An effective, quick warm-up can also be an effective motivator. If you get satisfaction from a warm-up, you probably will have a stronger desire to participate in the activity. By contrast, a poor warm-up can lead to fatigue and boredom, limiting your attention and ultimately resulting in a poor program.

The function of the warm-up is to prepare the body physiologically for some upcoming physical work bout. Most professionals view the warm-up period as a precaution against unnecessary musculoskeletal injury and possible muscle soreness. The purpose is to very gradually stimulate the cardiorespiratory system to a moderate degree, thus producing an increased blood flow to working skeletal muscles and resulting in an increase in muscle temperature.

Moderate activity speeds up the metabolic processes that produce an increase in core body temperature (a 13% increase in metabolic rate causes a 1° C increase in body temperature). An increase in the temperature of skeletal muscle causes an increased speed of contraction and relaxation, probably because nerve impulse conduction velocity is increased. The elastic properties (the length of stretch) of the muscle are increased, whereas the viscous properties (the rate at which the muscle can change shape) are decreased.

The warm-up should be generalized total body activity as opposed to a localized warm-up. Again, the main function of the warm-up is to increase core temperature as well as the temperature in the muscles that are going to be active. A generalized warm-up will more effectively accomplish this objective.

The type of warm-up should be related to the activity. For example, a soccer player uses the upper extremity considerably less than a lower extremity, so his or her warm-up should be directed more toward the lower extremity, perhaps by adding some stretching exercises for the lower extremity. The warm-up should

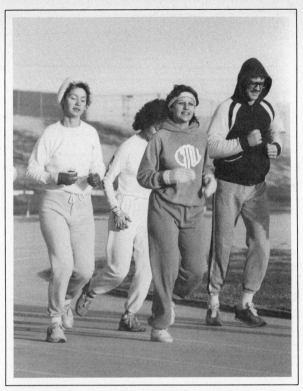

FIGURE 2-3

After a warm-up period there should be a vigorous workout.

also be sport-specific; for example, a basketball player should warm up by shooting lay-ups and jump shots and dribbling; a tennis player should hit forehand and backhand shots and serves.

The warm-up should last approximately 10 to 15 minutes. You shouldn't wait longer than 15 minutes to get started in the activity following the warm-up, although the effects will generally last up to about 45 minutes. Thus the third-string football player who warms up before the game and then does nothing more than stand around until he gets into the game during the fourth quarter is running a much higher risk of injury. This player should be encouraged to stay warmed up and ready to play throughout the course of a game. In general, sweating is a good indication that the body has been sufficiently warmed up and is ready for more strenuous activity.

The warm-up should begin with 2 or 3 minutes of light jogging to increase metabolic rate and core temperature. This should be followed by a period of flexibility exercises in which the muscles are stretched to take advantage of the increase in muscle elasticity. Finally, the intensity of the warm-up should be

The Workout

Take from 30 minutes to 1 hour to work out.
Engage in exercises and activities that will develop muscular strength and endurance, cardiorespiratory endurance, and flexibility.
Adapt to individual needs.
Alternate work and rest periods.
As a beginner, increase duration of exercise intervals and keep exercise intensity constant.
Monitor heart rate (see Chapter 3).

The Cool-Down

Take from 5 to 10 minutes to cool down after working out.
Engage in relaxing forms of exercise.
Activities can include slow jogging, walking, and stretching exercises.
Check heart rate, which should show recovery from acceleration during the workout.

increased gradually by performing body movements and skills associated with the specific activity in which you are going to participate.

Workout. You should dress appropriately for the workout in clothes that will enable you to move freely and safely.

Some exercise physiologists have suggested that a workout, or conditioning period, might consist of the following:

 10 minutes of warm-up
 10 minutes of strength exercises
 20 minutes of cardiorespiratory exercises
  5 minutes of cool-down

Specific exercises for the workout are discussed in Chapters 3, 4, 5, and 11.

Cool-down. After a vigorous workout, a cool-down period is essential. This part of the training program helps in returning the blood to the heart for reoxygenation, thus preventing a pooling of the blood in the muscles of the arms and the legs. After vigorous activity, enough blood may not circulate back to the brain, heart, and intestines, and symptoms such as dizziness or faintness may occur without a cool-down period. The cool-down period enables the body to cool and return to a resting state. Such a period should last about 5 to 10 minutes.

Although the value of warm-up and workout periods is well accepted, the importance of a cool-down period afterward is often ignored. Again, experience and observation seem to indicate that persons who stretch during the cool-down period tend to have fewer problems with muscle soreness after strenuous activity which can result from ischemia in the working tissues.

Testing Your Physical Fitness

Students should know whether or not they meet desirable physical fitness standards. This can be determined by an assessment that utilizes scientific tests of measurement and evaluation (see Chapter 3 for tests of cardiorespiratory endurance and Chapter 6 for calculation of percent body fat using skinfold measurements).

Test results serve you in several ways. They offer you an assessment of your physical fitness and identify your weaknesses and strengths. In those cases in which norms are provided, they show how you compare with your peers. Becoming aware of how you compare with criterion standards and with peers can provide motivation toward achieving your personal fitness goals. Such standards indicate where special attention should be directed within an individualized program and where fitness counseling and help are needed so that appropriate procedures can be followed for improvement. Most important, they provide information for the planning of a meaningful training program.

PRECAUTIONS

A general assessment of the training program you are following might be indicated by your reaction to exercise. Ten minutes after exercise, breathing and heart rate should have returned to normal and you should not be physically drained and experience extreme fatigue. Furthermore, you should not experience broken sleep as a result of the physical activity and you should not have excessive fatigue the next day. If any of these conditions prevail, the exercise probably was too severe or too prolonged in light of your present physical condition.

If you experience difficulty in breathing, lose coordination, become dizzy, have chest pains, or become nauseated or faint, you should stop or modify the exercise. If such symptoms persist, consult a physician.

If the weather is hot and humid, you should be careful not to become overheated and dehydrated. During such weather, workouts should be moderate and you should drink lots of water.

The training program should not be hurried. Start slowly and gradually increase the intensity and duration of the workout. It is natural to experience some muscle soreness at first. However, this will disappear as you gradually achieve a state of physical fitness.

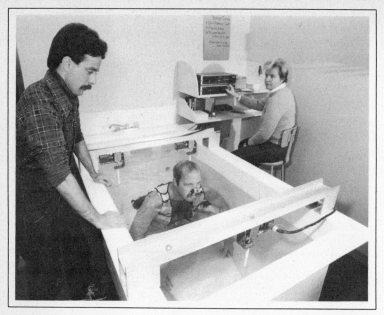

FIGURE 2-4

Students should know whether or not they meet desirable physical fitness standards. College student being tested for percentage of fat in relation to percentage of nonfat in his total body mass.

HOW QUICKLY CAN YOU EXPECT RESULTS?

There is no shortcut to fitness; it takes time. You should not expect results in a matter of hours or even days. After a month of appropriate activity on a regular basis, some improvement should be noted, depending on what your physical fitness condition was when you started. After an extended period of gradual improvement, you may reach a plateau at which you experience no improvement, but instead seem to stay at the same level of fitness. This is a natural phenomenon. In time, with regular workouts, improvement will occur; after several months, the desired results will be attained. Make a commitment to the training program and keep at it; you will feel better, and this will in turn motivate you to continue. Once you have attained a desirable physical fitness level, you will be strongly motivated to maintain this level through regular workouts.

HELP FOR THE SEDENTARY STUDENT

If you find you are not fit, you need help and guidance in planning a physical fitness program. Effort must be directed toward eliminating the cause or causes of your poor condition. And it should be remembered that the causes of poor fitness vary widely. They can involve problems such as being overweight or underweight, a poor diet, illness, emotional disturbances, or an unhealthy lifestyle. A fitness program should address such a cause or causes. If the cause involves infection and illness, then the help of a physician is necessary. If the cause is an emotional disorder or a psychologic maladjustment, the college guidance or health services can help. If the cause relates to an unhealthy lifestyle, health and physical education personnel may be of help. If the cause is lack of the right kind and amount of physical activity, your school's physical education staff can help. (See Appendix C for a discussion of college resources that can assist you in planning in a fitness program.)

SUMMARY

- Fitness is a personal responsibility.
- Much scientific knowledge has been generated regarding principles that should be observed when designing the right kind of training program needed to be physically fit.
- Before starting a personal training program, it is helpful to examine your attitude toward physical fitness, reasons for wanting to be physically fit, and present level of activity.
- Most college students, after careful analysis, are not satisfied with their physical condition.
- Some students should have a medical examination or take a stress test before engaging in a training program.
- Exercise tolerance refers to the manner in which the body responds to exercise.
- Your fitness goals should be considered when planning a training program.
- Physical activities should be enjoyable.
- To achieve the greatest benefits from the exercise program, you should recognize and employ the principle of overload.
- The training program should be progressive and within your capabilities to adapt physiologically.
- Consistency in exercising is important.
- Training programs should be individualized.
- Safety should be a consideration in the training program.
- Three basic elements of every training program are warm-up, workout, and cool-down.
- Students should know whether or not they meet desirable physical fitness standards as determined by scientific methods of measurement and evaluation.
- A general assessment of the training program you are following may be obtained by monitoring your reaction to exercise.
- There is no shortcut to fitness. It takes time; you should not expect results in a matter of hours or even days.
- The causes of poor fitness vary widely and can involve problems such as poor diet, illness, emotional disturbances, and obesity.

GLOSSARY

consistency To engage in a physical routine and activity on a frequent and regular basis

cool-down The period following a vigorous workout when the muscles function to aid the cardiovascular system in returning blood to the heart for reoxygenation, preventing a pooling of blood in the extremities and helping to reduce muscle soreness

exercise tolerance The manner in which the body responds to exercise

heart rate (HR) The number of heart beats in 1 minute

individuality The criterion that training regimens meet the individual needs of the students

metabolism The chemical processes of a cell, tissue, or organism by which food substances are transformed into chemical nutrients and energy

overload An increase in the intensity of the physical activity resulting in the cardiorespiratory rate being stepped up thus causing an overload on these organic systems with resultant beneficial effects

progression A sequence in which progress is made in the exercise program within the scope of the person's ability to adapt physiologically

stress exercise test A test in which heart rate, blood pressure, and sometimes the amount of oxygen consumed are monitored to determine how healthy the heart is and the range of desirable limits of exercise

warm-up Exercise before the work-out to increase body temperature, stretch ligaments and muscles, and increase flexibility

workout The vigorous exercise period that follows a warm-up and may involve exercises designed to develop elements such as strength and cardiorespiratory endurance

SUGGESTED READINGS

Allsen, P., & others. (1983). *Fitness for life—an individualized approach* (3rd ed.). Dubuque, IA: William C. Brown.

American College of Sports Medicine. (1978). Position statement on the recommended quantity and quality of exercise for developing and maintaining fitness in healthy adults. *Sports Medicine Bulletin, 13*, 1.

Cooper, K. (1977). *The aerobics way: New data on world's most popular exercise program*. New York: M. Evans.

deVries, H. (1980). *Physiology of exercise for physical education and athletics*. Dubuque, IA: William C. Brown.

Fox, E. (1984). *Sport physiology*. New York: CBS College Publishing.

Fox, E., & Mathews, D. (1981). *The physiological basis of physical education and athletics* (2nd ed.). Philadelphia: W.B. Saunders.

Hockey, R. (1985). *Physical Fitness: the pathway to healthful living* (5th ed.). St. Louis: Times Mirror/Mosby College Publishing.

Jensen, C., & Fisher, G. (1979). *Scientific basis of athletic conditioning*. Philadelphia: Lea & Febiger.

McArdle, W. & others. (1981). *Exercise physiology, energy, nutrition, and human performance*. Philadelphia: Lea & Febiger.

Roy, S. & Irvin, R. (1983). *Sports medicine: Prevention, evaluation, management and rehabilitation*. Englewood Cliffs, N.J.: Prentice-Hall.

Strauss, R. (1984). *Sports medicine*. Philadelphia: W.B. Saunders.

Wilmore, J. (1982). *Training for sport and activity: The physiological basis of the conditioning process* (2nd ed.). Boston: Allyn & Bacon.

3

CARDIORESPIRATORY

ENDURANCE

After completing this chapter, you will be able to:

- Describe the oxygen transport system and the concept of maximal rate of oxygen utilization.
- Explain the relationships between heart rate, stroke volume, cardiac output, and rate of oxygen utilization.
- Describe the function of the heart, blood, vessels, and lungs in oxygen transport.
- Describe the principles of continuous, interval, fartlek, and circuit training and the potential of each technique for improving cardiorespiratory endurance.

- Describe the differences between aerobic and anaerobic activity.
- Identify the risk factors associated with cardiovascular heart disease.
- Identify methods for assessment of cardiorespiratory endurance.

Of all the components of physical fitness listed in Chapter 2, none is more important to the college-age student than cardiorespiratory endurance. By definition, cardiorespiratory endurance is the ability to perform whole-body activities for extended periods of time. The cardiorespiratory system provides a means by which oxygen is supplied to the various tissues of the body. Without oxygen, the cells within the human body cannot possibly function, and ultimately death will occur.

Transport and Utilization of Oxygen

Basically, transport of oxygen throughout the body involves the coordinated function of four components: (1) the heart, (2) the lungs, (3) the blood vessels, and (4) the blood. The improvement of cardiorespiratory endurance through

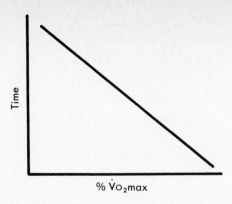

FIGURE 3-1

The higher % $\dot{V}O_2$max, the less time an activity can be performed.

training occurs because of increased efficiency of each of these four elements in providing necessary oxygen to the working tissues. The greatest rate at which oxygen can be taken in and utilized during exercise is referred to as *maximal oxygen consumption ($\dot{V}O_2$max)*. The performance of any activity requires a certain rate of oxygen consumption that is about the same for all persons, depending on the present level of fitness. Generally, the greater the rate or more intense the performance of an activity, the greater will be the oxygen consumption. Each person has his or her own maximal rate of oxygen consumption. That person's ability to perform an activity (or to fatigue) is closely related to the amount of oxygen required by that activity and is limited by the maximal rate of oxygen consumption of which the person is capable. It should be apparent that the higher the percentage of maximal oxygen consumption required during the activity, the lower will be the time that an activity can be performed (Figure 3-1).

The maximal rate at which oxygen can be utilized is a genetically determined characteristic; we inherit a certain range of $\dot{V}O_2$ max, and the more active we are, the higher the existing $\dot{V}O_2$ max will be in that range. A training program is capable of increasing $\dot{V}O_2$ max to its highest limit within our range. $\dot{V}O_2$ max is most often presented in terms of the volume of oxygen used relative to body weight per unit of time (ml/kg/min). A normal $\dot{V}O_2$ max for most college-age men and women would fall somewhere in the range of 38 to 46 ml/kg/min.[1] A world-class male marathon runner may have a $\dot{V}O_2$ max in the 70 to 80 ml/kg/min range.

There are three factors that determine the maximal rate at which oxygen can be utilized: (1) external respiration, involving the ventilatory process, or pulmonary function, (2) gas transport, which is accomplished by the cardiovascular system (that is, the heart, blood vessels, and blood), and (3) internal respiration, which involves the use of oxygen by the cells to produce energy. Of these three factors, the most limiting is generally the ability to transport oxygen through the system; thus the cardiovascular system limits the overall rate of oxygen con-

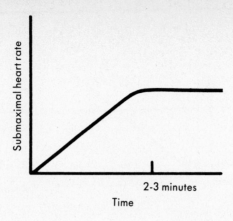

FIGURE 3-2

Two to three minutes are required for heart rate (HR) to plateau at a given workload.

sumption. A high $\dot{V}O_2$max within a person's inherited range indicates that all three systems are working well.

It is well beyond the scope of this text to discuss the detailed anatomy and physiology involved in the cardiorespiratory system. However, a basic discussion of the training effects and response to exercise that occur in the heart, blood vessels, blood, and lungs should make it easier to understand why the training techniques to be discussed later are so effective in improving cardiorespiratory endurance.

Effects on the Heart

The heart is the main pumping mechanism and circulates oxygenated blood throughout the body to the working tissues. The heart receives deoxygenated blood from the venous system and then pumps the blood through the pulmonary vessels to the lung, where carbon dioxide is exchanged for oxygen. The oxygenated blood then returns to the heart, from which it exits through the aorta to the arterial system and is circulated throughout the body, supplying oxygen to the tissues.

As the body begins to exercise, the muscles utilize the oxygen at a much higher rate, and the heart must pump more oxygenated blood to meet this increased demand. The heart is capable of adapting to this increased demand through several mechanisms. *Heart rate* shows a gradual adaptation to an increased workload by increasing proportionally to the intensity of the exercise and will plateau at a given level after about 2 to 3 minutes (Figure 3-2). The heart rate will continue to increase linearly with the workload until it reaches some maximal rate. Maximal heart rate is age related and decreases with age.

Maximal heart rate is achieved simultaneously with maximal oxygen con-

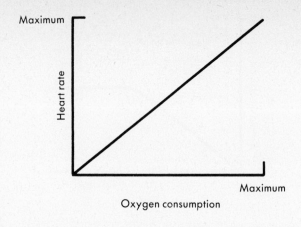

FIGURE 3-3

Maximal HR is achieved at about the same time as $\dot{V}O_2$max.

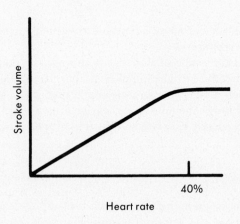

FIGURE 3-4

Stroke volume plateaus at 40% of maximal HR.

sumption (Figure 3-3). Thus, oxygen consumption also increases with increasing intensity of the work. Because of these direct linear relationships, it should become apparent that the rate of oxygen consumption can be estimated by taking the heart rate.

A second mechanism by which the heart is able to adapt to increased demands during exercise is to increase the volume of blood being pumped out with each beat. This is referred to as the *stroke volume*. The heart pumps out approximately 70 ml of blood per beat. Stroke volume can continue to increase only to the point at which there is simply not enough time between beats for the heart to fill up. This occurs at about 40% of maximal heart rate, and above this level

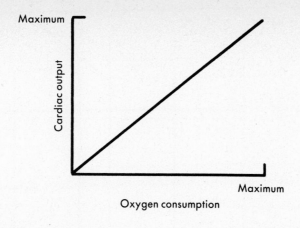

FIGURE 3-5

Cardiac output limits $\dot{V}O_2$max.

increases in the volume of blood being pumped out per unit of time must be caused entirely by increases in heart rate (Figure 3-4).

Stroke volume and heart rate together determine the volume of blood being pumped through the heart in a given unit of time. Approximately 5 L of blood are pumped through the heart during each minute at rest. This is referred to as the *cardiac output*, which indicates how much blood the heart is capable of pumping in exactly 1 minute. Thus cardiac output is the primary determinant of the maximal rate of oxygen consumption possible (Figure 3-5).

A training effect that occurs on the heart is that the stroke volume increases while exercise heart rate is reduced at a given standard exercise load. The heart becomes more efficient because it is capable of pumping more blood with each stroke. Because the heart is a muscle, it will hypertrophy to some extent, but this is in no way a negative effect of training.

Blood Vessels

The amount of blood flowing to the various organs increases during exercise. However, there is a change in overall distribution of cardiac output; the percentage of total cardiac output to the nonessential organs is decreased, whereas it is increased to active skeletal muscle. Volume of blood flow to the *myocardium* increases substantially during exercise, even though the percentage of total cardiac output supplying the heart muscle remains unchanged. In skeletal muscle there is increased capillarization, although it is not clear whether new ones form or dormant ones become patent.

Blood pressure in the arterial system is determined by the cardiac output in relation to total peripheral resistance to blood flow. Overall there is a decrease in total peripheral resistance and an increase in cardiac output.

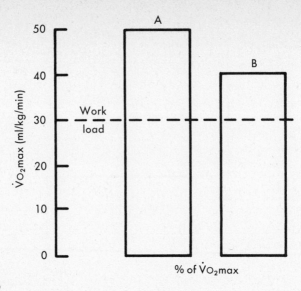

FIGURE 3-6

Student *A* should be able to work longer than student *B* as a result of lower utilization of % $\dot{V}O_2$max.

Blood

Blood transports oxygen throughout the system by binding it with *hemoglobin.* Hemoglobin is an iron-containing protein that has the capability of easily accepting or giving up molecules of oxygen as needed. Training for improvement of cardiorespiratory endurance produces an increase in total blood volume, with a corresponding increase in the amount of hemoglobin. The concentration of hemoglobin, or the hematocrit, of circulating blood increases with both brief and sustained periods of exercise.

Lungs

As a result of training, there are some changes in lung volumes and capacities. The volume of air that can be inspired in a single maximal ventilation is increased. The diffusing capacity of the lungs is also increased, facilitating the exchange of oxygen and carbon dioxide. Pulmonary resistance to air flow is also decreased.

Effects on Work Ability

Cardiorespiratory endurance plays a critical role in our ability to carry out normal daily activities. Fatigue is closely related to the percentage of $\dot{V}O_2$max that a particular workload demands. For example, Figure 3-6 presents two persons, *A* and B. A has a $\dot{V}O_2max$ of 50 ml/kg/min, whereas B has a $\dot{V}O_2max$ of only 40 ml/kg/min. If both A and B are exercising at the same intensity, then A will be working at a much lower percentage of $\dot{V}O_2max$ than B. Consequently, A should be able to sustain his or her activity over a much longer period of time. Everyday activities may be impaired if your ability to utilize oxygen efficiently is impaired. Thus improvement of cardiorespiratory endurance should be an essential component of any training program.

Regardless of the training technique used for the improvement of cardiorespiratory endurance, one principal goal remains the same. You are trying to increase the efficiency with which your cardiorespiratory system is able to supply a sufficient amount of oxygen to the working muscles. Without oxygen, the body is incapable of producing energy for an extended time.

THE ENERGY SYSTEMS

Various sports activities involve specific demands for energy. For example, sprinting and jumping are high-energy output activities, requiring a relatively large production of energy for a short time. Long-distance running and swimming, on the other hand, are mostly low-energy output activities per unit of time, requiring energy production for a prolonged time. Other sports activities demand a blend of both high- and low-energy output. These various energy demands can be met by the different processes in which energy can be supplied to the skeletal muscles.

ATP—The Immediate Energy Source

Adenosine triphosphate (ATP) is the ultimate, usable form of energy for muscular activity. ATP is produced in the muscle tissue from blood glucose or glycogen. Glucose is derived from the breakdown of dietary carbohydrates. Fats and proteins can also be metabolized to generate ATP. Glucose not needed immediately is stored as *glycogen* in the resting muscle and liver. Stored glycogen in the liver can later be converted back to glucose and transferred to the blood to meet the body's energy needs.

Once much of the muscle and liver glycogen is depleted, the body relies more heavily on fats stored in adipose tissue to meet its energy needs. The longer the duration of an activity, the greater the amount of fat being used, especially during the later stages of endurance events. During rest and submaximal exertion, both fat and carbohydrate are utilized as energy substrate in approximately a 60%:40% ratio.

Regardless of the nutrient source that produces ATP, it is always available in the cell as an immediate energy source. When all available sources of ATP are utilized, more must be regenerated for muscular contraction to continue.

TABLE 3-1 Energy Systems Used According to Length of Time and Type at Activity

Energy System	Length of Time	Type of Activity
Anaerobic	0-90 seconds	Any type of spring (Running, swimming, cycling) Short duration explosive activities
Combined systems	90 seconds-4 minutes	Medium distance activities ($1/2$ mile-1 mile run) Intermittent sport activities
Aerobic	Longer than 4 minutes	Long distance events Long duration intermittent activities

AEROBIC vs. ANAEROBIC METABOLISM

Two major energy systems function in muscle tissue: anaerobic and aerobic metabolism. Each of these systems generates ATP.

During sudden outbursts of activity in intensive, short-term exercise, ATP can be rapidly metabolized to meet energy needs. After a few seconds of intensive exercise, however, the small stores of ATP are used up. The body then turns to glycogen as an energy source. Glycogen can be metabolized within the muscle cells to generate ATP for muscle contractions.

Both ATP and muscle glycogen can be metabolized without the need for oxygen. Thus this energy system involves *anaerobic metabolism* (occurring in the absence of oxygen).

As exercise continues, the body has to rely on the metabolism of carbohydrates (more specifically, glucose) and fats to generate ATP. This second energy system requires oxygen and is therefore referred to as *aerobic metabolism* (occurring in the presence of oxygen).

The degree to which the two major energy systems are involved is determined by the intensity and duration of the activity. For example, short bursts of muscle contraction, as in running or swimming sprints, utilize predominantly the anaerobic system. However, endurance events depend a great deal on the aerobic system. Most sports use a combination of both anaerobic and aerobic metabolism. Table 3-1 illustrates the predominant energy systems used in various activities.

TRAINING TECHNIQUES FOR IMPROVING CARDIORESPIRATORY ENDURANCE

There are a number of different methods through which cardiorespiratory endurance may be improved, including (1) continuous or sustained training, (2) interval training, (3) circuit training, and (4) fartlek.

Continuous Training

Continuous training involves four considerations:
1. The *mode* or type of activity
2. The *frequency* of the activity
3. The *duration* of the activity
4. The *intensity* of the activity

Mode. The type of activity used in continuous training must be aerobic. At this point it is necessary to differentiate aerobic from anaerobic activity. Basically, an aerobic activity is one in which the amount of oxygen being supplied is sufficient to meet the demands of the working tissues. Conversely, an anaerobic activity is one in which the intensity of the activity is too high for the system to keep up with oxygen demands; consequently an "oxygen debt" is incurred that must be "paid back" during a recovery period. Aerobic activities are any type that elevate the heart rate and maintain it at that level for an extended time. Aerobic activities generally involve repetitive, whole body, large-muscle movements that are performed over an extended time. Examples of aerobic activities are running, jogging, walking, cycling, swimming, rope skipping, and cross-country skiing. The advantage of these aerobic activities as opposed to more intermittent activities, such as racquetball, squash, basketball, or tennis, is that aerobic activities are easy to regulate by either speeding up or slowing down the pace. Because we already know that the given intensity of the workload elicits a given heart rate, these aerobic activities allow us to maintain heart rate at a specified or target level. Intermittent activities involve variable speeds and intensities that cause the heart rate to fluctuate considerably. Although these intermittent activities will improve cardiorespiratory endurance, they are much more difficult to monitor in terms of intensity.

Again, the fact that you enjoy a specific type of activity should be an important criterion in the selection of a particular aerobic activity.

Frequency. To see at least minimal improvement in cardiorespiratory endurance, it is necessary to engage in no less than three sessions per week. However, you should aim for 4 or 5 sessions per week. A competitive athlete should be prepared to train as often as six times per week. Everyone should take off at least 1 day per week to give damaged tissues a chance to repair themselves.

Duration. For minimal improvement to occur, you must participate in at least 20 minutes of continuous activity with the heart rate elevated to its working level. Generally, the greater the duration of the workout, the greater the improvement in cardiorespiratory endurance. The competitive athlete should train for at least 45 minutes.

Intensity. Of the four factors we are considering with continuous training, the most critical factor is the intensity of training, even though recommendations regarding training intensities vary. This is particularly true in the early stages of training, when the body is forced to make a lot of adjustments to increased workload demands.

Because heart rate is linearly related to the intensity of the exercise as well as to the rate of oxygen consumption, it becomes a relatively simple process to identify a specific workload (pace) that will make the heart rate plateau at the desired level. By monitoring heart rate, we know whether the pace is too fast or too slow to get heart rate into a target range.

Monitoring Heart Rate

There are several points at which heart rate is easily measured. The most reliable is the radial artery located on the thumb side of the wrist joint. By placing your index and middle fingers on the thumb side of the flexor tendon, you should be able to locate a strong pulse. Each pulse represents one heart beat. By counting the number of beats that occur in 1 minute, you will get an accurate heart rate. Because the heart rate will slow down during a 1-minute period, you should monitor your heart rate for 10 seconds and then multiply by 6 to give you the number of beats per minute. A second area in which the pulse is easily located is the carotid artery in the neck. Again using your index and middle fingers, locate the Adam's apple and then slide your fingers into the groove on either side. The carotid artery is extremely simple to find, especially during exercise. However, there are pressure receptors located in the carotid artery that, if subjected to hard pressure from the two fingers, will slow down the heart rate, giving

---

Worksheet For Calculation of Training Heart Rate

Estimation of Maximal Heart Rate	Example
220	220
− Age	− 20
Predicted maximal heart rate	200
× % Intensity	× 0.7
Training heart rate	140 beats/min
Karvonen Equation	Example
Maximal heart rate	200
− Resting heart rate	− 70
	130
× % Intensity	× 0.6
	78
+ Resting heart rate	+ 70
Training heart rate	148 beats/min

a false indication of exactly what the heart rate really is. Thus the pulse at the radial artery provides the most accurate measure of heart rate.

Another factor must be considered when measuring heart rate during exercise. You are trying to elevate your heart rate to a specified target rate and maintain it at that level during your entire workout. Heart rate can be increased or decreased by speeding up or slowing down your pace. It has already been indicated that heart rate increases proportionately with the intensity of the workload and will plateau after 2 to 3 minutes of activity. Thus you should be actively engaged in the workout for 2 to 3 minutes before measuring your pulse.

There are several formulas that will easily allow you to identify a *target training heart rate*. This target zone is generally between 60% and 90% of maximal heart rate. It was stated previously that maximal heart rate is age related. Maximal heart rate is thought to be about 220 beats per minute. Thus a relatively simple estimate of your maximal heart rate (HR) would be Maximal HR = 220 − Age. For a 20-year-old college student, maximal heart rate would be about 200 beats per minute (220 − 20 = 200). If you are interested in working at 70% of your maximal rate, the target heart rate can be calculated by multiplying 0.7 × (220 − Age). Again using a 20-year-old student as an example, target heart rate would be 140 beats per minute (0.7 × [220 − 20] = 140).

Another commonly used formula that takes into account your current level of fitness is the Karvonen equation[3]:

Target training heart rate = Resting HR + (0.6 [Maximum HR − Resting HR]).

A 20-year-old person with a resting pulse of 70 beats per minute, according to the Karvonen equation, would have a target training heart rate of 148 beats per minute (70 + 0.6 [200 − 70] = 148).

A third formula for establishing a target training heart rate is to simply double your resting heart rate. A person with a resting heart rate of 72 beats per minute would have a target training heart rate of 144 beats per minute.

Regardless of the formula you use, it should be clear that to see minimal improvement in cardiorespiratory endurance, you must train with the heart rate elevated to at least 60% of its maximal rate. Most authorities would agree that for the college-age student it is more desirable to train at around 85% of maximal rate, although there is no conclusive research to support this 85% maximal intensity.

In summary, when using the continuous training method, the activity selected must be aerobic and should be enjoyable. To see minimal improvement in cardiorespiratory endurance, training must be done for a period of 20 minutes three times per week with the heart rate elevated to an intensity of no less than 60% of its maximal rate.

Guidelines for Continuous Training

As mentioned in Chapter 2, each training program should be designed to meet individual needs and abilities. Everyone should begin slowly with the idea that

TABLE 3-2 Guidelines for Continuous Training

Training Level	Frequency (Sessions per Week)	Duration (Minutes)*	Intensity of Training Heart Rate (% Maximal Heart Rate)†
Beginner	3	20	60%
Intermediate	4-5	30-45	70%
Advanced	5-6	45-60	75%-80%

*The heart rate should be elevated to training levels during this entire period.
†Maximal heart rate = 220 − your age.

they will progress as quickly as possible at their own rate. Beginning at too high a level will probably produce various musculoskeletal injuries that will often result in setbacks in a training program.

All training programs are based on monitoring heart rate during some type of aerobic activity. Heart rate can be increased or decreased by altering the pace. The following rough guidelines can be applied to beginning, intermediate, and advanced levels (Table 3-2).

Interval Training

Unlike continuous training, *interval training* involves activities that are more intermittent. Interval training consists of alternating periods of relatively intense work and active recovery. It allows for performance of much more work at a more intense workload over a longer period of time than if working continuously.

We have stated that it is most desirable in continuous training to work at an intensity of about 85% of maximal heart rate. Obviously, sustaining activity at this high intensity over a 20-minute period would be extremely difficult. The advantage of interval training is that it allows work at this 85% or higher level for a short period of time followed by an active period of recovery during which you may only be working at 30% to 45% of maximal heart rate.[2] Thus the intensity of the workout and its' duration can be greater than with continuous training.

Most sports are anaerobic, involving short bursts of intense activity followed by a sort of active recovery period (for example, football, basketball, soccer, or tennis). Training with the interval technique allows you to be more sport-specific during the workout. With interval training, you can apply the overload principle by making the training period much more intense.

There are several important considerations with interval training. The work period is the amount of time that continuous activity is actually being performed, and the rest period is the time between work periods. A set is a group of combined work and rest periods, and a repetition is the number of work periods per set. Training time or distance refers to the rate or distance of the work period. The work/rest ratio indicates a time ratio for work vs. rest.

TABLE 3-3   Recommended Interval Training Workouts

Level	Intensity During Training Period	Intensity During Recovery Period	Duration
Beginner	70%-75% of maximal HR	30%-35% of maximal HR	20 min
Intermediate	75%-85% of maximal HR	35%-40% of maximal HR	30-40 min
Advanced	85%-95% of maximal HR	40%-45% of maximal HR	40-60 min

Table 3-3 indicates recommended training intervals in terms of both time and distance and may be used as a guide for establishing an interval workout.

An example of interval training would be a soccer player running wind sprints. An interval workout would involve running two sets of four 440-yard dashes in under 70 seconds, with a 2-minute 20-second walking recovery period between each dash. During this training session, the soccer player's heart rate would probably increase to 85% to 90% of maximal level during the dash and should probably fall to the 30% to 45% level during the recovery period.

Circuit Training

There is some controversy as to whether circuit training should be included as a technique for improving cardiorespiratory endurance. *Circuit training* employs a series of exercise stations that consist of weight training, flexibility, calisthenics and brief aerobic exercises. With circuit training, you move rapidly from one station to the next and perform whatever exercise is to be done at that station within a specified time period. A typical circuit would consist of 8 to 12 stations, and the entire circuit would be repeated three times.

The primary reason that circuit training is often not considered an acceptable technique for improving cardiorespiratory endurance is that recovery periods tend to be too long between stations to keep the heart rate elevated to at least 60% of maximal level. Circuit training is most definitely an effective technique for improving strength and flexibility. Certainly if the pace or the time interval between stations is rapid and if workload is maintained at a high level of intensity, the cardiorespiratory system may benefit from this circuit. However, there is no research evidence that shows that circuit training is very effective in improving cardiorespiratory endurance. It should be and is most often used as a technique for developing and improving muscular strength and endurance. The box on p. 60 indicates a simple circuit training setup that can be easily completed by normal college students.

If a circuit training routine is performed according to the above guidelines, some improvement of cardiorespiratory endurance will occur.

Fartlek Training

Fartlek is a training technique that is a type of cross-country running originated in Sweden. Fartlek literally means "speed play." It is similar to interval training

Circuit Training Setup

Station 1 Push-ups—30 repetitions
Station 2 Hamstring—Low back stretching
Station 3 Bent-knee sit-ups (25 repetitions)
Station 4 Bench press (10 repetitions at 75% maximal heart rate)
Station 5 Rope skipping (100 repetitions)
Station 6 Knee extensions (15 repetitions at 80% maximal heart rate)
Station 7 Shoulder adduction (15 repetitions)
Station 8 Knee flexions (15 repetitions at 80% maximal heart rate)
There would be 60 seconds to complete each station, and the entire circuit would
be repeated three times in succession.

in that you must run for a specified period of time; however, specific pace and
speed are not identified. It is recommended that the course for a fartlek workout
be some type of varied terrain with some level running, some uphill and downhill
running, and some running through obstacles such as trees or rocks. The object
is to put surges into a running workout, varying the length of the surges according
to individual purposes.

One big advantage of fartlek training is that because the terrain is always
changing, the run may prevent boredom and may actually turn out to be relaxing.

Again, if fartlek training is going to improve cardiorespiratory endurance, it
must elevate the heart rate to at least minimal training levels. Fartlek may best
be utilized as an off-season conditioning activity or as a change of pace activity
to counteract the boredom of training using the same activity day after day.

Prevention of Cardiovascular Disease

Half of all people who die in the United States each year die of coronary heart
disease (CHD). There is no question that the cardiovascular system has not been
designed to handle many of the stresses placed on it. American adults form many
habits during the college-age years, such as eating, drinking, and levels of
physical exercise, that carry over for the rest of their lives. The life-style you
choose plays a major role in determining whether or not you develop CHD.

Coronary heart disease (CHD) results from the accumulation of fatty deposits
(atherosclerotic plaque) within the coronary arteries. The coronary arteries supply
blood to the heart muscle, which functions properly only when provided with a
steady blood supply. The deposition of fatty plaque often begins early in life,
and the continued, gradual deposition of plaque can lead to a significant narrowing of the coronary arteries, or *atherosclerosis*. The partial or complete
occlusion of one or more of the major coronary arteries can lead to a condition
called myocardial ischemia, in which the heart muscle fails to receive an adequate

supply of oxygen. This can produce symptoms such as chest pain (angina pectoris) and, if sufficiently severe, can precipitate a heart attack.

Coronary heart disease is related to certain personal health habits known as risk factors. Risk factors also include age, sex, and family history, over which we have little control. These risk factors cannot be called causes but are instead characteristics that increase the probability of having CHD. The following risk factors have been identified:

Primary Risk Factors
    Cigarette smoking
    Hypertension
    Elevated blood lipids
Secondary Risk Factors
    Obesity
    Pulmonary function abnormalities
    Diabetes
    High uric acid levels
    Sedentary life-style
    Electrocardiographic (ECG) abnormalities during exercise
    Family history (heredity)
    High-stress life-style
    Personality and behavior patterns
    Age
    Sex

The three primary CHD risk factors are cigarette smoking, high blood pressure, and elevated serum cholesterol. Each of these factors is related to CHD in an additive fashion; that is, the higher the risk factor score, the greater the chances of developing the disease. Also, each of these factors is, at least in part, a function of individual behavior. This observation holds out hope that it may be possible to prevent premature CHD through the modification of risk factors.

Following is a brief discussion of the three primary risk factors.

Blood Pressure

Blood pressure is the pressure that the blood exerts against the iı er wall of the arteries. Normal blood pressure is considered to be 120/80 in uⱥult Americans. The systolic blood pressure (the larger of the two numbers) represents the pressure in the artery at the time when the heart beats. Diastolic blood pressure is recorded during the resting phase of the heart.

High blood pressure, or hypertension, may develop as a condition secondary to another disease. However, the causes of the most common form of hypertension are not fully understood. Fortunately, in most instances high blood pressure can be effectively treated through medication. Weight reduction, cessation of smoking, decreased psychologic stress, and increased exercise also produce beneficial effects in some cases of hypertension.

It should be noted that blood pressure varies from minute to minute, going up with excitement or exertion and down with rest and relaxation. Thus a single measurement of your blood pressure may differ somewhat from your "normal" blood pressure.

Hyperlipidemia

Cholesterol is a fatty substance that is manufactured by the body and is also found in some of the foods we eat. It is either synthesized by cells in the body or consumed in the diet. Cholesterol is transported in the bloodstream and, if present in excessive amounts, adheres to the walls of the arteries. This contributes to the deposition of atherosclerotic plaque.

Cholesterol is transmitted through the cardiovascular system in the form of *lipoprotein* of either high-density of low-density varieties. Low-density lipoprotein (LDL) is that which adheres to the arterial wall, whereas high-density lipoprotein (HDL) seems to be able to break cholesterol deposited by LDL away from the arterial walls. Thus the more HDL present, the better off you are, because it appears to be somewhat of an antirisk factor. Physically active persons have a far more desirable HDL/LDL ratio than those who are inactive. An excess of these lipoproteins is referred to as *hyperlipidemia*.

Serum cholesterol concentration is related to the dietary intake of cholesterol and saturated fats. Cholesterol and saturated fats are found in especially large quantities in egg yolks, organ meats (such as liver or kidney), red meats, and shellfish. A reduction of the dietary intake of cholesterol and saturated fats usually results in a decrease in the serum cholesterol concentration.

It should be noted that Americans represent a high-risk population that tends to exhibit rather high serum cholesterol values. Many other societies around the world, in which the typical diet is lower in cholesterol and saturated fats, show lower average cholesterol levels. Not coincidentally, these societies also tend to show lower rates of death from CHD.

Cholesterol is directly related to the incidence of CHD; that is, the higher the cholesterol, the greater the risk of CHD. Thus it is not possible to designate a specific cholesterol concentration that is safe or optimal. However, it is generally true that values below 200 mg/dl are associated with relatively low CHD risk.

Cigarette Smoking

As with the other primary CHD risk factors, cigarette smoking is related to CHD risk in a graded fashion: the more you smoke, the greater the risk. Smokers of low-tar, low-nicotine cigarettes are probably at a similar risk of smokers of cigarettes with higher tar and nicotine contents.[4] It should be noted that *all* cigarette smokers are at a much higher risk than nonsmokers. Cigarette smokers have roughly twice the risk of death from CHD of nonsmokers.

Cessation of smoking is associated with a reduction of CHD risk. Within 2 years after smoking cessation, overall mortality risk returns to only slightly higher than that of a nonsmoker.

Among middle-aged adults, cigarette smokers are a declining minority. The rate of smoking cessation has been greatest among middle-aged men, who constitute the group at highest CHD risk.[4]

Effects of Exercise on CHD

There is evidence that physical activity does in fact aid in the reduction of CHD. Physical activity tends to increase:
  Coronary collateral vascularity
  Efficiency of the myocardium
  Efficiency of peripheral blood distribution
  Blood volume and concentration of red blood cells
  Tolerance to stress
  Prudent living habits
Physical activity tends to decrease:
  Serum lipid levels
  Arterial blood pressure
  Strain associated with psychologic stress

Assessment of Cardiorespiratory Endurance

How fit is your cardiorespiratory system? Numerous tests have been developed to evaluate fitness levels. Most of these tests are based on the idea that cardiorespiratory endurance capacity is best indicated by the maximal capacity of the working tissues to utilize oxygen ($\dot{V}O_2$ max). We know from an earlier discussion that $\dot{V}O_2$max can be predicted or estimated by measuring heart rates at varying workloads. You can easily perform the following tests so that specific levels of cardiorespiratory endurance may be identified. It must be remembered that each of the tests described below are based to a large extent on two factors: (1) the motivation of the person and (2) the minimal level of cardiovascular endurance.

Test A—The Harvard Step Test (see Figure 3-7)
  Purpose
  To determine the state of physical fitness of a subject.
  Equipment
  1. 20-inch step bench
  2. Metronome
  3. Stopwatch
  4. Towel
  Procedures
  1. Have the subject stand in front of the step bench.
  2. Set the metronome cadence at 120 so that the subject steps up and down 30 times per minute, or once every 2 seconds.
  3. The stepping rhythm is "up-up-down-down" and so forth.
     a. One foot is placed on the bench with the first metronome beat, and the other foot is brought up and set next to the first foot on the second beat.

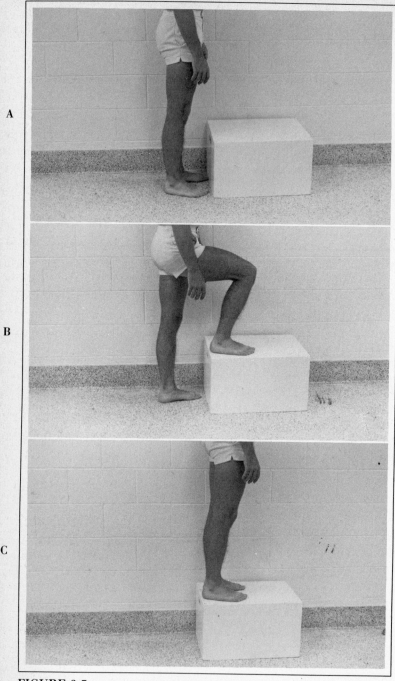

FIGURE 3-7

Harvard Step Test.

Sample Worksheet For Harvard Step Test

	Example
1. Look up the "Duration of effort" _____	1. 3½
2. Find the "Total heart beats" for 60 to 90 seconds following cessation of exercise _____	2. 60-64
3. Intersect the "Duration of effort" row with the score column _____	3. 57
4. Determine the fitness level _____	4. Average

---

    b. The back should be erect and the legs straightened with each step.

    c. When the third metronome beat occurs, the first foot should be placed back on the floor and the second foot placed next to the first foot when the fourth beat occurs.

    d. The hands should not be used for leverage in stepping.

4. The subject should lead off each cycle with the same foot. However, one to two lead changes can be made during the test as long as cadence is not broken.

5. Begin timing the test for 5 full minutes when the subject begins his or her first step.

6. If the subject's cadence falls behind the metronome pace, stop after he or she has been unable to keep up the pace for 20 seconds. Be sure to record the duration of the subject's work period to the nearest second if the test has to be terminated early.

7. At the end of the 5 minutes, stop the subject and have him or her sit down.

    a. Have the subject sit quietly.

    b. Immediately start timing the recovery period.

8. Time the recovery period and determine the heart rate by palpating the carotid artery.

    a. Begin counting the heart rate exactly 1 minute after work cessation.

    b. Record the number of beats that occur during next *30 seconds* from 1 minute to 1 minute 30 seconds after the cessation of exercise.

Determine the arbitrary fitness score of the subject by consulting Table 3-4. Arbitrary scores are roughly interpreted as follows:

Poor—50 or below

Average—50 to 80

Good—80 and above

Test B—Åstrand Rhyming Nomogram for Estimation of Physical Fitness (see Figure 3-8)

   Purpose

To determine the physical fitness of a subject based on cardiac and oxygen transport changes that occur during a 6-minute bicycle ergometer test.

TABLE 3-4   Scoring for the Harvard Step Test

Duration of Effort (Minutes)	Total Heart Beats 1 to 1½ Minutes in Recovery											
	40-44	45-49	50-54	55-59	60-64	65-69	70-74	75-79	80-84	85-89	90-94	95-99
0-½	6	6	5	5	4	4	4	4	3	3	3	3
½-1	19	17	16	14	13	12	11	11	10	9	9	8
1-1½	32	29	26	24	22	20	19	18	17	16	15	14
1½-2	45	41	38	34	31	29	27	25	23	22	21	20
2-2½	58	52	47	43	40	36	34	32	30	28	27	25
2½-3	71	64	58	53	48	45	42	39	37	34	33	31
3-3½	84	75	68	62	57	53	49	46	43	41	39	37
3½-4	97	87	79	72	66	61	57	53	50	47	45	42
4-4½	110	98	89	82	75	70	65	61	57	54	51	48
4½-5	123	110	100	91	84	77	72	68	63	60	57	54
5	129	116	105	96	88	82	76	71	67	63	60	56

From Conzolazio, C.F., Johnson, R.E., & Pecora, L.J. (1963). *Physiological measurements of metabolic function in man*. New York: McGraw-Hill. Used by permission of McGraw-Hill Book Company.

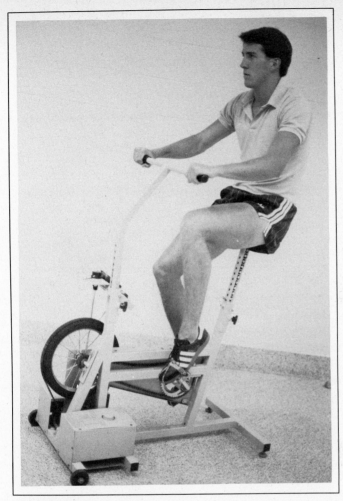

FIGURE 3-8

Bicycle ergometer used in Åstrand Rhyming Nomogram Test.

Equipment
1. Monarch bicycle ergometer
2. Metronome
3. Stopwatch
4. Towel

Pretest Procedures
1. Record the resting heart rate of the subject after a 5-minute rest period.
2. Adjust the saddle height of the ergometer for the subject.
   a. With the front part of the foot on the pedal, there should be a slight bend in the knee joint.

Sample Worksheet For Åstrand Rhyming Nomogram Test

		Example
1. Count heart rate at end		
Of minute 5 _____ HR		168
Of minute 6 + _____ HR		164
_____ Total		272
÷ 2		÷ 2
= Mean HR		166
2. Note workload setting on ergometer _____		1200 kp/min
3. Find points on nomogram under "Pulse rate" and "Workload" columns and connect them with a straight line.		
4. Predicted $\dot{V}O_2$max _____		3.6 L/min

b. The pedal should be at its lowest point.
3. Set the metronome to produce 100 beats per minute.
   a. The setting is equal to 50 complete pedal turns per minute. Each time the metronome clicks, one foot should reach the bottom of a pedal revolution.
   b. Both the light and sound stimuli are switched to the "on" position.
4. Work is started with a slack brake belt.
   a. The subject should begin pedaling 15 seconds before the timed work period begins.
   b. Tighten the brake belt with the handwheel until the red pointer is on 1, 2, or 3 kp (kilopounds).
   c. A suitable beginning workload for women is 2 kp (600 kp/min).
   d. A suitable beginning workload for men is 3 kp (900 kp/min).

Test Procedures
1. Begin timing the work period, which is 6 minutes long.
2. Count the heart rate at the end of the fifth and sixth minutes during the last 30 seconds of each minute.
3. Utilizing the average heart rate of the last 2 minutes of exercise, cross-reference it with the workload level (kp/min) for men or women.
4. The mean value of the heart rate at the end of the fifth and sixth minutes is designated as the "working pulse" for the load being used. If the difference between the last two readings is five beats or more, the test should be continued another minute or more until a steady-state heart rate occurs.
5. Consult the Åstrand-Rhyming Nomogram and follow the directions to calculate maximal oxygen uptake (Figure 3-9).

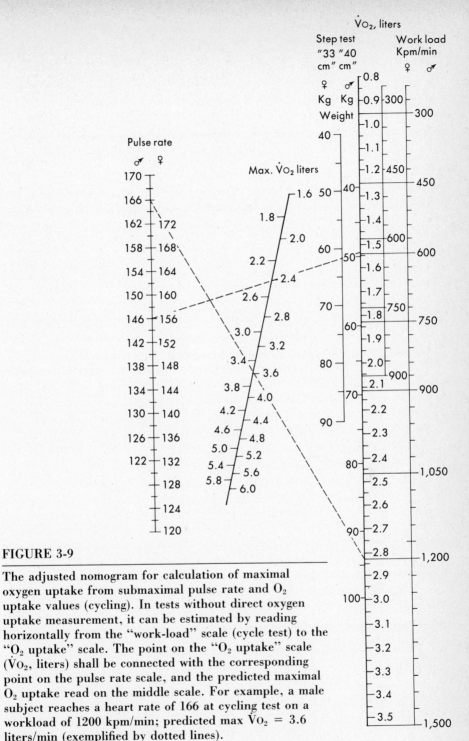

FIGURE 3-9

The adjusted nomogram for calculation of maximal oxygen uptake from submaximal pulse rate and O_2 uptake values (cycling). In tests without direct oxygen uptake measurement, it can be estimated by reading horizontally from the "work-load" scale (cycle test) to the "O_2 uptake" scale. The point on the "O_2 uptake" scale ($\dot{V}O_2$, liters) shall be connected with the corresponding point on the pulse rate scale, and the predicted maximal O_2 uptake read on the middle scale. For example, a male subject reaches a heart rate of 166 at cycling test on a workload of 1200 kpm/min; predicted max $\dot{V}O_2$ = 3.6 liters/min (exemplified by dotted lines).

From Åstrand, P.O., and Rodahl, K. (1977). *Textbook of work physiology*. New York: McGraw-Hill. (Reproduced with permission of McGraw-Hill.)

TABLE 3-5   12-Minute Walking/Running Test

Fitness Category		Distance (Miles) Covered in 12 Minutes — Age (Years)					
		13-19	20-29	30-39	40-49	50-59	60+
I. Very poor	(men)	<1.30*	<1.22	<1.18	<1.14	<1.03	<.87
	(women)	<1.0	<.96	<.94	<.88	<.84	<.78
II. Poor	(men)	1.30-1.37	1.22-1.31	1.18-1.30	1.14-1.24	1.03-1.16	.87-1.02
	(women)	1.00-1.18	.96-1.11	.95-1.05	.88-.98	.84-.93	.78-.86
III. Fair	(men)	1.38-1.56	1.32-1.49	1.31-1.45	1.25-1.39	1.17-1.30	1.03-1.20
	(women)	1.19-1.29	1.12-1.22	1.06-1.18	.99-1.11	.94-1.05	.87-.98
IV. Good	(men)	1.57-1.72	1.50-1.64	1.46-1.56	1.40-1.53	1.31-1.44	1.21-1.32
	(women)	1.30-1.43	1.23-1.34	1.19-1.29	1.12-1.24	1.06-1.18	.99-1.09
V. Excellent	(men)	1.73-1.86	1.65-1.76	1.57-1.69	1.54-1.65	1.45-1.58	1.33-1.55
	(women)	1.44-1.51	1.35-1.45	1.30-1.39	1.25-1.34	1.19-1.30	1.10-1.18
VI. Superior	(men)	>1.87	>1.77	>1.70	>1.66	>1.59	>1.56
	(women)	>1.52	>1.46	>1.40	>1.35	>1.31	>1.19

From the Aerobics Program for Total Well-Being by Dr. Kenneth H. Cooper. Copyright © 1982 by Kenneth H. Cooper. Reprinted by permission of the publisher, M. Evans & Co., Inc., New York, NY 10017.
*<Means "less than"; >means "more than."

Sample Worksheet For Cooper's 12-Minute Walking/Running Test

	Example
1. Measure distance covered and round off to nearest ⅛ mile _____	1. 1.50
2. Locate this distance in appropriate "Age" column _____	2. Age 20
3. Determine fitness level _____	3. Good

Test C—Cooper's 12-Minute Walking/Running Test
  Purpose
  To determine the level of cardiorespiratory endurance of college students during a 12-minute running or walking activity.
  Equipment
  1. Measured running course, preferably a track
  2. Stopwatch
  Procedures
  1. During a 12-minute period the subject attempts to cover as much distance as possible by either running or walking.
  Treatment of Data
  1. Distance covered should be rounded off to the nearest ⅛ mile.
  2. Consult Table 3-5. Locate the distance covered for either men or women under the appropriate age classification and determine the level of fitness.

SUMMARY

- Cardiorespiratory endurance involves the coordinated function of the heart, lungs, blood, and blood vessels to supply sufficient amounts of oxygen to the working tissues.
- The best indicator of how efficiently the cardiorespiratory system functions is the maximal rate at which oxygen can be utilized by the tissues.
- Heart rate is directly related to the rate of oxygen consumption. It is therefore possible to predict the intensity of the work in terms of a rate of oxygen utilization by monitoring heart rate.
- Aerobic exercise involves a sufficient amount of oxygen available to supply the demands of the working tissues. An anaerobic activity is one in which oxygen is being utilized more quickly than it can be supplied; thus an oxygen debt is incurred that must be repaid before working tissue can return to its normal resting state.
- Continuous or sustained training for improvement of cardiorespiratory endurance involves selecting an activity that is aerobic in nature, and training at least 3 times per week for a time period of no less than 20 minutes with the heart rate elevated to at least 60% of maximal rate.
- Interval training involves alternating periods of relatively intense work followed by

active recovery periods. Interval training allows performance of more work at a relatively higher workload than continuous training.

- Circuit training involves a series of exercise stations consisting of weight training, flexibility, and calisthenic exercises in which you move rapidly from one station to the next.
- Coronary heart disease (CHD) accounts for half of all deaths in the United States each year. CHD results from an accumulation of fatty deposits within the coronary arteries.
- The primary risk factors that predispose a person to CHD are cigarette smoking, hypertension, and elevated serum cholesterol.

GLOSSARY

aerobic metabolism The process of energy production in which oxygen supply is sufficient to meet the demand

anaerobic metabolism The process of energy production in which oxygen supply cannot keep pace with the tissue demands

atherosclerosis A disease of the coronary arteries of the heart that involves deposition of fatty plaques and narrowing of the arteries

adenosine triphosphate (ATP) The ultimate usable form of energy for muscular activity

blood pressure The pressure that the blood exerts against the internal wall of the arteries

cardiac output The amount of blood pumped by the heart during a 1-minute period; it is a product of stroke volume multiplied by heart rate

circuit training A series of exercise stations for strength training, flexibility, and calisthenics

continuous training Aerobic activities that involve repetitive, whole-body large muscle movements performed repeatedly over an extended period of time

Fartlek A training technique involving running on varied terrain at varying speeds

glycogen The form in which carbohydrates are stored in the muscle and liver

heart rate (HR) The number of beats of the heart in 1 minute

hemoglobin An iron-containing protein that binds with and transports oxygen molecules throughout the circulatory system

hyperlipidemia An excess of fatty substances in the blood

interval training Alternating periods of relatively intense work followed by an active recovery period

lipoprotein Primary transporting mechanism for fat (or cholesterol) in the blood system

maximal oxygen consumption ($\dot{V}O_2max$) The greatest rate at which oxygen can be taken in and utilized during exercise

myocardium The heart muscle

stroke volume The volume of blood ejected from the heart during a single contraction

REFERENCES

1. Åstrand, P.O. (1954). Rhyming nomogram for calculation of aerobic capacity from pulse rate during submaximal work. *Journal of Applied Physiology*, 7,218.
2. Fox, E., & Mathews, D. (1976). *The physiological basis of physical education and athletics*. Philadelphia: W.B. Saunders.
3. Karvonen, M.J., & others. (1957). The effects of training on heart rate. A longitudinal study. *Annals of Medicine and Experimental Biology*, 35,305.
4. McCardle, W., Katch, F., & Katch, V. (1981). *Exercise physiology, energy, nutrition, and human performance*. Philadelphia: Lea & Febiger.

SUGGESTED READINGS

American College of Sports Medicine. (1978). Position statement on the recommended quantity and quality of exercise for developing and maintaining fitness in healthy adults. *Sports Medicine Bulletin*, 13,1.

Åstrand, P.O., & Rodahl, K. (1977). *Textbook of work physiology*. New York: McGraw-Hill.

Corbin, C., Linus, D., Lindsey, R., & Tolson, H. (1981). *Concepts in physical education with laboratories and experiments*. Dubuque, IA: William C. Brown.

deVries, H. (1980). *Physiology of exercise for physical education and athletics*. Dubuque, IA: William C. Brown.

Fox, E. (1984). *Sport physiology*. New York: CBS College Publishing.

Getchell, B. (1983). *Physical fitness: A way of life*. New York: John Wiley & Sons.

Hockey, R. *Physical Fitness: the pathway to healthful living* (5th ed.). St. Louis: Times Mirror/ Mosby College Publishing.

Jensen, C., & Fisher, G. (1979). *Scientific basis of athletic conditioning*. Philadelphia: Lea & Febiger.

McCardle, W., Katch, F., & Katch, V. (1981). *Exercise physiology, energy, nutrition, and human performance*. Philadelphia; Lea & Febiger.

Miller, D., & Allen, E. (1982). *Fitness: A lifetime concept*. Minneapolis: Burgess.

Stokes, R., & Farls, D. (1983). *Fitness everyone!* Winston-Salem, NC: Hunter Textbooks.

Wilmore, J. (1982). *Training for sport and activity: The physiological basis of the conditioning process* (2nd ed.). Boston: Allyn & Bacon.

4

IMPROVEMENT OF STRENGTH
THROUGH WEIGHT TRAINING

After completing this chapter, you will be able to:

- Define strength and indicate its significance to health and skill of performance.

- Discuss the anatomy and physiology of skeletal muscle.

- Discuss the physiology of strength development and factors that determine strength.

- Describe specific techniques for improving muscular strength.

- Differentiate between muscle strength and muscle endurance.

- Identify strength-training exercises for developing specific muscle groups.

The development of muscular strength is an essential component of fitness for anyone involved in a physical activity program. By definition, *strength* is the maximal force that can be applied by a muscle during a single maximal contraction. If a large amount of force is generated very quickly, the movement can be referred to as a *power* movement. Most movements in sport are explosive and must include elements of both strength and speed if they are to be effective. Without the ability to generate power, an athlete will be limited in his or her performance capabilities.

The development of muscular strength may best be considered as both a skill-related and a health-related component of physical fitness. Maintenance of at least a normal level of strength in a given muscle or muscle group is important for normal healthy living. Muscle weakness or imbalance can result in abnormal movement or gait and can impair normal functional movement. One of the most common health ailments in the United States is lower back pain, which is related in the large majority of cases to lack of muscular fitness, especially lack of muscular strength in the abdominals and loss of flexibility of the hamstrings. Thus strength training may play a critical role not only in training programs but also in injury rehabilitation.

Muscular strength is also related to agility, or the ability of the body to change direction rapidly in a coordinated manner. Agility not only enhances athletic

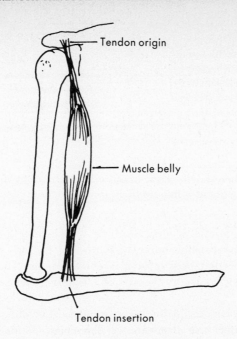

FIGURE 4-1

The musculotendinous unit consists of the muscle belly and its tendon, which attaches the contractile portion of the muscle to bone.

performance but also may allow the performer to avoid potentially injurious situations.

Muscular strength is very closely related to muscular endurance. *Muscular endurance* is the ability to perform repetitive muscular contractions against some resistance. As we will see later, as muscular strength increases, there tends to be a corresponding increase in endurance. For example, a person can lift a weight 25 times. If muscular strength is increased by 10% through weight training, it is very likely that the maximal number of repetitions would be increased because it is easier for the person to lift the weight.

ANATOMY AND PHYSIOLOGY OF SKELETAL MUSCLE CONTRACTION

Skeletal muscle consists of two portions, (1) the muscle belly and (2) its tendons, which are collectively referred to as a *musculotendinous unit* (Figure 4-1). The muscle belly is composed of separate, parallel elastic fibers. Muscle fibers are composed of thousands of small protein fibers, called **myofilaments**, as well as a substantial amount of connective tissue that hold the fibers together. The skeletal musculotendinous unit attaches two bones across a joint, and when a

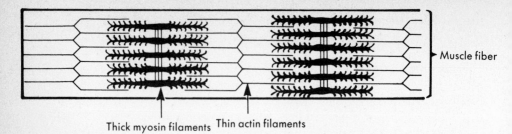

Thick myosin filaments Thin actin filaments

FIGURE 4-2

Muscles contract when an electrical impulse from the central nervous system causes the myofilaments in a muscle fiber to move closer together.

contraction of that muscle occurs, the bony attachments are pulled closer together, producing movement around the joint.

The muscle tendon attaches muscle directly to bone. The muscle tendon is composed primarily of connective tissue and is relatively inelastic when compared with muscle fibers.

All skeletal muscles exhibit three characteristics: (1) the ability to change in length or stretch, which is elasticity, (2) the ability to shorten and return to normal length, which is extensibility, and (3) the ability to respond to stimulation from the nervous system, which is excitability.

Skeletal muscles show considerable variation in size and shape. Large muscles generally produce gross motor movements at large joints, such as knee flexion produced by contraction of the large, bulky hamstring muscles. Smaller skeletal muscles, such as the long flexors of the fingers, produce fine motor movements. Muscles producing movements that are powerful in nature are usually thicker and long, whereas those producing finger movements requiring coordination are thin and relatively shorter. Other muscles may be flat, round, or fan-shaped.

Muscles may be connected to bone by a single tendon or by two or three separate tendons at either end. Those muscles that have two separate muscle and tendon attachments are called biceps, and those with three separate muscle and tendon attachments are called triceps.

Muscles contract in response to stimulation by the central nervous system. An electrical impulse transmitted from the central nervous system to a *motor unit* connecting with a group of muscle fibers causes a depolarization of those fibers. When the muscle depolarizes, the small contractile elements, or myofilaments, are stimulated to move closer together, thus producing a shortening of the muscle and movement at the joint which that muscle crosses (Fig. 4-2).

Fast-Twitch vs. Slow-Twitch Fibers

All fibers in a particular motor unit are either *slow-twitch* or *fast-twitch fibers*, each of which have distinctive metabolic as well as contractile capabilities. Slow-twitch fibers are reddish. They are more resistant to fatigue than are fast-twitch fibers; however, the time required to generate force is much greater in slow-twitch fibers.

Fast-twitch fibers are white. They are capable of producing very quick, forceful contractions but have a tendency to fatigue more rapidly than slow-twitch fibers. Fast-twitch fibers are capable of producing powerful contractions, whereas slow-twitch fibers produce a long endurance type of force.

Within a particular muscle there are both types of fibers, and the ratio varies with each person. The average is about 50% slow-twitch and 50% fast-twitch fibers. However, tremendous variations have been demonstrated in various athletes.[5]

Because this ratio is genetically determined, it may play a large role in determining athletic ability for a given sport. Sprinters, for example, have a large percentage of fast-twitch fibers in relation to slow-twitch fibers.[2] One study has shown that they may have as much as 95% fast-twitch fibers. Conversely, marathon runners generally have a higher percentage of slow-twitch fibers. Alberto Salazar, one of the great marathon runners in the world, is reported to possess as high as 97% slow-twitch muscle fibers in certain muscles.

FACTORS THAT DETERMINE MUSCULAR STRENGTH

Muscular strength is very closely related to the cross-sectional diameter of a muscle. The bigger a particular muscle is, the stronger it is and thus the more force it is capable of generating. The size of a muscle tends to increase in cross-sectional diameter with weight training. This increase in muscle size is referred to as *hypertrophy*.

Strength is a function of the number and diameter of muscle fibers composing a given muscle. The number of fibers is an inherited characteristic; thus a person with a large number of muscle fibers to begin with has the potential to hypertrophy to a much greater degree than does someone with relatively fewer fibers.

Strength in a given muscle is determined not only by the physical properties of the muscle itself but also by mechanical factors that dictate how much force can be generated through a system of levers to an external object.

If we think of the elbow joint as one of these lever systems, we would have the biceps muscle producing flexion of this joint (Figure 4-3). The position of attachment of the biceps muscle on the lever arm, in this case the forearm, will largely determine how much force this muscle is capable of generating. If there are two persons, A and B, and A has a biceps attachment that is closer to the fulcrum (the elbow joint) than B, then A must produce a greater force with the biceps muscle to hold the weight at a right angle because the length of the lever arm will be greater than with B.

When the weight is held at an angle of 45° (Figure 4-4, A) or 150° (Figure 4-4, C) the contracting force of the biceps muscle required to hold the weight stationary is considerably less than it would be at 90°. Thus if we move this weight through a full range of motion from extension to flexion, the amount of

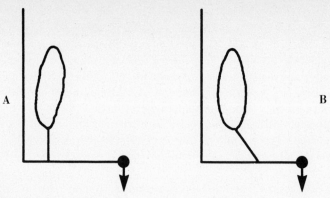

FIGURE 4-3

The position of attachment of the muscle tendon on the lever arm can affect the ability of that muscle to generate force. *B* should be able to generate greater force than *A* because the tendon attachment on the lever arm is closer to the resistance.

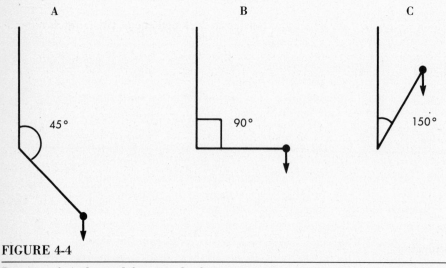

FIGURE 4-4

Because of mechanical factors, the force necessary to overcome a resistance changes at different joint angles.

strength, or force, required to move the weight varies at different angles, forming a strength curve for that movement (Figure 4-5).

A third critical factor in determining muscle strength is muscle length. A muscle is capable of generating its maximal force when it is in its fully stretched or extended position. If the muscle is stretched beyond its normal length, it may be incapable of producing any muscular force, and it is likely that injury will occur. In fact, the initial stretch of a muscle will evoke a reflex called the stretch

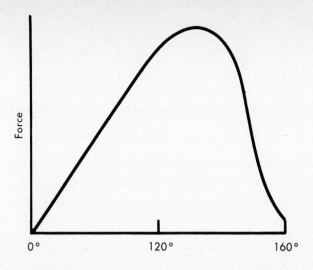

FIGURE 4-5

Strength curve indicating changes in force through a full range of motion.

reflex, which will not allow the muscle to be lengthened. This stretch reflex is discussed in detail in Chapter 5.

The shorter a muscle becomes, the less force it is capable of generating. A muscle that is fully contracted is incapable of producing any additional muscular force past this point.

The ability to generate muscular force is also related to age. Both men and women seem to be able to increase strength throughout puberty and adolescence, reaching a peak age 20-25 years, at which time this ability begins to level off and in some cases decline. After about age 25 years a person generally loses an average of 1% of his maximal remaining strength each year. Thus at age 65 a person would have only about 60% of the strength he or she had at age 25.[6]

This loss in muscle strength is definitely related to individual levels of physical activity. Those people who are more active or perhaps those who continue to strength train considerably decrease this tendency toward declining muscle strength.

PHYSIOLOGY OF STRENGTH DEVELOPMENT

There is no question that weight training to improve muscular strength results in an increased size, or hypertrophy, of a muscle. What causes a muscle to hypertrophy? There have been a number of theories proposed as possible explanations for this increase in muscle size.

At one time it was thought that the number of muscle fibers increased as a result of strength training. However, we now know that the number of muscle fibers a person has is genetically determined and cannot be altered.

TABLE 4-1   Methods for Improving Muscular Strength

Method	Action	Equipment
Isometric	Force develops while muscle length remains constant	Any immovable resistance
Isotonic	Force develops while muscle length either increases or decreases	Free weights, Universal, Nautilus
Isokinetic	Force develops while muscle is contracting at a constant velocity	Cybex, Orthotron, Minigym

It was also hypothesized that because the muscle was working harder in weight training, more blood was required to supply that muscle with oxygen and other nutrients. Thus it was thought that the number of capillaries was increased. This hypothesis was only partially correct; no new capillaries are formed during strength training; however, a number of dormant capillaries may well become patent to meet this increased demand for blood supply.

A third theory to explain this increase in muscle size seems the most credible. It was mentioned earlier that muscle fibers are composed primarily of small protein filaments, called *myofilaments*, which are the contractile elements in muscle. These myofilaments increase in both size and number as a result of strength training, causing the individual muscle fibers themselves to increase in cross-sectional diameter.[7] This is particularly true in men, although women will also see some increase in muscle size.

METHODS OF IMPROVING STRENGTH

There are three different methods of training for strength improvement: isometric training, isotonic training, and isokinetic training. Regardless of which of these three methods is used, one basic principle of training is extremely important. For a muscle to improve in strength, it must be forced to work at a higher level than that to which it is accustomed. In other words, the muscle must be *overloaded*. Without overload, the muscle will be able to maintain strength as long as training is continued against a resistance the muscle is accustomed to. However, no additional strength gains will be realized. Weight training requires a consistent, increasing effort against progressively increasing resistance. If this principle of overload is applied, all three training methods will produce improvement of muscular strength over a period of time. Figure 4-6 summarizes the three different methods for improving muscular strength.

Isometric Exercise

An *isometric exercise* involves a muscle contraction in which the length of the muscle remains constant while tension develops toward a maximal force against

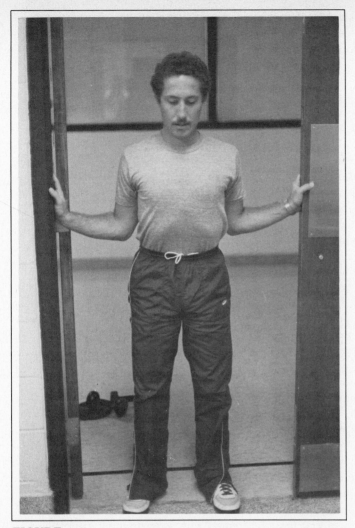

FIGURE 4-6

Isometric exercises involve contraction against some immovable resistance.

an immovable resistance. The muscle should generate a maximal force for 5 seconds at a time, and this contraction should be repeated 5 to 10 times per day.

Isometric exercises were very popular in the late 1960s and early 1970s. Several books were published that discussed a series of isometric exercises that could be done while sitting at a desk. The exercises included techniques such as putting your arms underneath the middle desk drawer and pushing up as hard as you can, or pushing out on the inside of the chair space with your knees. It was claimed that these brief maximal isometric contractions were capable of producing some rather dramatic increases in muscular strength. And indeed these isometric exercises are capable of increasing muscular strength; unfortunately, strength gains are specific to the joint angle at which training is performed. At other angles, the strength curve drops off dramatically because of a lack of motor activity at that angle. Thus arm strength is increased at the specific angle pressed against the desk drawer, but there is no corresponding increase in strength at other positions in the range of motion.

Another major disadvantage of these isometric "sit at your desk" exercises is that they tend to produce a spike in blood pressure that can result in potentially life-threatening cardiovascular accidents.[4] This sharp increase in blood pressure results from holding your breath and increasing intrathoracic pressure. Consequently, the blood pressure experienced by the heart is increased significantly. This has been referred to as the Valsalva effect. To avoid or minimize this effect, it is recommended that breathing be done during the maximal contraction to prevent this increase in pressure.

We do not mean to imply that isometric exercises have no place in a training program. There are certain instances in which an isometric contraction can greatly enhance a particular movement. For example, one of the exercises in power weight-lifting is a squat. A squat is an exercise in which the weight is supported on the shoulders in a standing position. The knees are then flexed and the weight is lowered to a three-quarter squat position, from which the lifter must stand completely straight once again.

It is not uncommon for there to be one particular angle in the range of motion at which smooth movement through that specific angle is difficult because of insufficient strength. This joint angle is referred to as a "sticking point." A power lifter will typically employ an isometric contraction against some immovable resistance to increase strength at this sticking point. If strength can be improved at this joint angle, than a smooth, coordinated power lift can be performed through a full range of movement.

A more common use for isometric exercises would be for injury rehabilitation or reconditioning. There are a number of conditions or ailments resulting either from trauma or overuse that must be treated with strengthening exercises. Unfortunately, these problems may be exacerbated with full range-of-motion strengthening exercises. It may be more desirable to make use of isometric exercises until the injury has healed to the point at which you are able to perform full-range activities.

Isotonic Exercise

A second method of weight training is more commonly used in improving muscular strength. *Isotonic exercise* involves a muscle contraction in which force is generated while the muscle is changing in length.

There are two types of isotonic contractions. Suppose you are going to perform a biceps curl (see Figure 4-18 on p. 102). To lift the weight from the starting

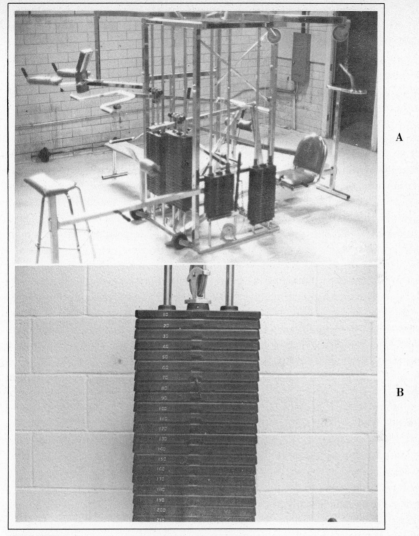

A

B

FIGURE 4-7

A, Universal equipment is isotonic; **B,** resistance may be easily changed by changing the key in the stack of weights.

position, the biceps muscle must contract and shorten in length. This shortening contraction is referred to as a *concentric (positive) contraction.* If the biceps muscle does not remain contracted when the weight is being lowered, gravity would cause this weight to simply fall back to the starting position. Thus to control the weight as it is being lowered the biceps muscle must continue to contract while at the same time gradually lengthening. A contraction in which the muscle is lengthening while still applying force is called an *eccentric (negative) contraction.*

It is essential when training isotonically to utilize both concentric and eccentric contractions. Research has clearly demonstrated the muscle must be overloaded and fatigued both concentrically and eccentrically for the greatest strength improvement to occur. Both types of contractions can be done using any type of isotonic equipment.

Various devices and machines exist that can be classified as isotonic devices. Free weights, barbells, and dumbbells are the most common forms of isotonic equipment. Universal and Nautilus machines are also considered to be isotonic machines. Free weights and barbells require the use of iron plates of varying weights that can be easily changed by adding or subtracting equal amounts of weight to both sides of the bar. The Universal and Nautilus machines both have a stack of weights that are lifted through a series of levers or pulleys. The stack of weights slides up and down on a pair of bars that restrict the movement to only one plane. Weight can be increased or decreased simply by changing the position of a weight key (Figure 4-7, *B*).

There are advantages and disadvantages to each type of isotonic device. The Nautilus and Universal machines are both relatively safe to use in comparison to free weights. For example, if you are doing a bench press with free weights, it is essential to have someone to "spot" you, to help you lift the weights back onto the support racks if you don't have enough strength to complete the lift; otherwise you may end up dropping the weight on your chest. With the Nautilus and Universal equipment, you can easily and safely drop the weight without fear of injury.

It is also a simple process to increase or decrease the weight by moving a single weight key with Nautilus and Universal equipment, although changes can generally only be made in increments of 10 or 15 pounds. With free weights, iron plates must be added or removed from each side of the barbell.

Regardless of which type of equipment is used, the same principles of isotonic training may be applied.

When training specifically for the development of muscular strength, the concentric, or positive, contraction should be an explosive power movement, with the weight being lifted against gravity at maximal speed and force. Conversely, when lowering the weight, the eccentric contraction should be relatively slow and gradual. Physiologically the muscle will fatigue much more rapidly concentrically than eccentrically. Arthur Jones, the inventor of the Nautilus equipment, stresses the use of these positive and negative contractions in his training program, although this principle should be applied regardless of which brand of equipment is being used.

Persons who have strength-trained using both free weights and either the Nautilus or Universal machine realize the difference in the amount of weight that can be lifted. Unlike the machines, free weights have no restricted motion and can thus move in many different directions, depending on the forces applied. With free weights, an element of muscular control on the part of the lifter to

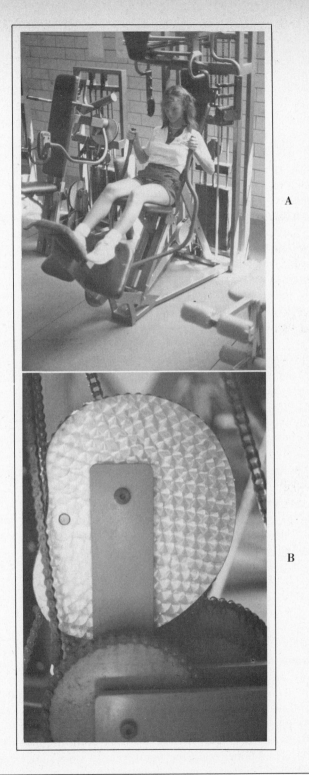

FIGURE 4-8

A, Nautilus bench press machine; **B,** the cam on Nautilus is designed to equalize resistance throughout the full range of motion.

prevent the weight from moving in any other direction other than vertical will usually decrease the amount of weight that can be lifted.

One problem often mentioned in relation to isotonic training involves changes that occur in the muscles' capabilities of moving the resistance throughout the range of motion. In discussing mechanical factors that determine levels of strength, it was indicated that the amount of force necessary to move a weight through a range of motion changes according to the joint angle and is greatest when the joint angle is approximately 90° (Figure 4-4, *B*). In addition, once the inertia of the weight has been overcome and momentum has been established, the force required to move the resistance varies according to the force that muscle can produce through the range of motion. Thus it has been argued that a disadvantage of any type of isotonic equipment is that force required to move the resistance is constantly changing throughout the range of movement.

Nautilus has attempted to alleviate this problem of changing force capabilities by making use of a cam in its pulley system (Figure 4-8, *B*). The cam has been individually designed for each piece of equipment so that the resistance is variable throughout the movement. It attempts to increase resistance where the muscle can handle a greater load, but at the points where the joint angle or muscle length is mechanically disadvantageous, it reduces the resistance to muscle movement. Whether this design does what it claims is debatable.

Isokinetic Exercise

The third method of strength training takes a little different approach to the problem of changing force capabilities. An *isokinetic exercise* is one in which the length of the muscle is changing while the contraction is performed at a constant velocity. In theory, maximal resistance is provided throughout the range of motion.

Several isokinetic devices are available commercially, Cybex, Orthotron, and Mini-gym are three of the more common isokinetic devices. In general, they rely on hydraulic, pneumatic, and mechanical pressure systems to produce this constant velocity of motion.

A major disadvantage of the Cybex and Orthotron units is their cost. The Cybex comes with a computer and printing device and along with the Orthotron is used primarily as a diagnostic and rehabilitative tool in the treatment of various injuries.

Isokinetic devices are designed so that regardless of the amount of force applied against a resistance, it can only be moved at a certain speed. That speed will be the same whether maximal force or only half the maximal force is applied. Consequently, when training isokinetically, it is absolutely necessary to exert as much force against the resistance as possible (maximal effort) for maximal strength gains to occur. This is one of the major problems with an isokinetic strength-training program.

Anyone who has been involved in a weight-training program knows that on some days it is difficult to find the motivation to work out. Because isokinetic

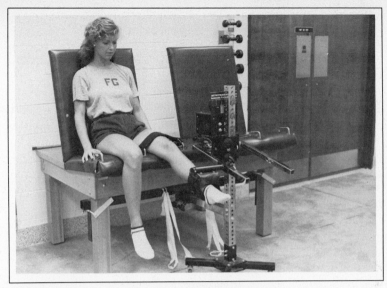

FIGURE 4-9

The Orthotron is an isokinetic device that provides resistance at a constant velocity.

training requires a maximal effort, it is very easy to "cheat" and not go through the workout at a high level of intensity. In an isotonic program, you know how much weight has to be lifted with how many repetitions. Thus isokinetic training is often more effective if a partner system is used primarily as a means of motivation toward a maximal effort.

When isokinetic training is done properly with a maximal effort, it is theoretically possible that maximal strength gains are best achieved through the isokinetic training method in which the velocity and force of the resistance is equal throughout the range of motion.

Whether this changing force capability is in fact a deterrent to improving the ability to generate force against some resistance is debatable. It must be remembered that in real life it doesn't matter whether the resistance is changing; what is important is that you develop enough strength to move objects from one place to another. The amount of strength necessary for each person is largely dependent on his or her life-style and occupation.

Specific Techniques of Strength Training

There are probably as many fallacies and misconceptions associated with weight training as with any other component of fitness. It seems that everyone has their own ideas about the best techniques for increasing muscular strength. A considerable amount of research has been done in the area of weight training to

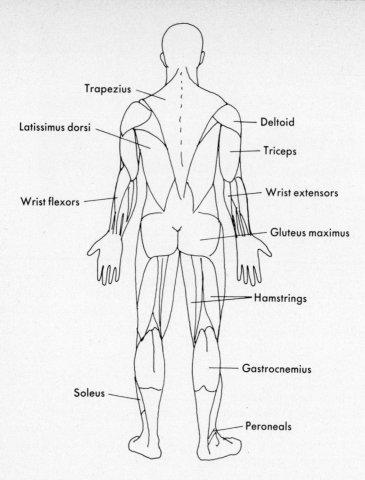

Posterior view

FIGURE 4-10

Major muscles of the body.

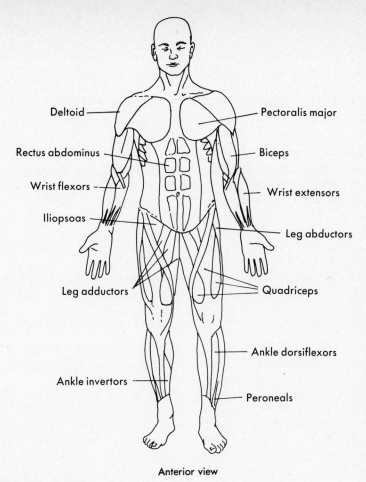

Anterior view

FIGURE 4-10, cont'd

Major muscles of the body.

determine optimal techniques in terms of (1) the amount of weight to be used, (2) the number of *repetitions*, (3) the number of *sets*, and (4) the frequency of training.

The following recommendations are based on this research and are principles that seem to be most widely accepted by strength training experts. However, it is important to realize that there are other effective techniques and training regimens that weight lifters and body builders can use. It may be obvious from looking at the size of a muscle or seeing the amount of weight these persons are able to lift that they are doing something right even though the training regimens they use do not follow the recommendations of researchers.

Regardless of specific techniques used, it is certain that to improve strength the muscle must be overloaded. The amount of weight used and the number of repetitions must be enough to make the muscle work at a higher intensity than it is used to. This is the single most critical factor in any strength-training program. It is also essential to design the strength training program to meet the specific needs of a person whether he or she is a competitive athlete or a recreational athlete.

One of the first widely accepted strength development programs was developed by DeLorme and was based on a *repetition maximum* of 10 (10 RM).[7] The amount of weight used is that which can be lifted exactly 10 times. DeLorme's program is as follows:

Set	Amount of Weight	Repetitions
1	50% of 10 RM	10
2	75% of 10 RM	10
3	100% of 10 RM	10

DeLorme's technique of three sets of 10 repetitions was a standard for many years, until Dr. Richard Berger,[1] considered by many to be the foremost expert in strength training, proposed modifications. His research suggests that optimal training involves selecting an amount of weight sufficient to allow 6 to 8 repetitions in each of the three sets. If at least 3 sets of 6 repetitions cannot be completed, the weight is too heavy and should be reduced. If it is possible to do more than 3 sets of 8 repetitions, the weight is too light and should be increased.[4]

Dr. Berger also indicates that a particular muscle or muscle group should be exercised consistently every other day. Thus weight training should be done at least three times per week but no more than four times per week. It is common for serious weight trainers to lift every day; however, they exercise different muscle groups on successive days. For example, Monday, Wednesday, and Friday may be used for upper body muscles, whereas Tuesday, Thursday, and Saturday are used for lower body muscles.

Arthur Jones, inventor of the Nautilus machine, has suggested that if training is done properly with the Nautilus equipment (that is, using both positive and negative contractions), it is necessary to strength-train only twice each week, although this has not been sufficiently documented experimentally.

Strength Training Worksheet I

Upper Body Exercises

Exercise	Reps	Sets		Date and Weight
Bench press	6-8	3	Date / Weight	
Military press	6-8	3	Date / Weight	
Lateral pulls	6-8	3	Date / Weight	
Flys	6-8	3	Date / Weight	
Reverse flys	6-8	3	Date / Weight	
Medial rotation	6-8	3	Date / Weight	
Lateral rotation	6-8	3	Date / Weight	
Bicep curls	6-8	3	Date / Weight	
Tricep extensions	6-8	3	Date / Weight	
Wrist curls	6-8	3	Date / Weight	
Wrist extensions	6-8	3	Date / Weight	

Strength Training Worksheet II

Lower Body Exercises

Date and Weight

Exercise	Reps	Sets		
Hip adduction	6-8	3	Date	
			Weight	
Hip abduction	6-8	3	Date	
			Weight	
Hip flexion	6-8	3	Date	
			Weight	
Hip extension	6-8	3	Date	
			Weight	
Hip internal rotation	6-8	3	Date	
			Weight	
Hip lateral rotation	6-8	3	Date	
			Weight	
Quadricep extensions	6-8	3	Date	
			Weight	
Hamstring flexions	6-8	3	Date	
			Weight	
Toe raises	6-8	3	Date	
			Weight	
Ankle inversion	6-8	3	Date	
			Weight	
Ankle eversion	6-8	3	Date	
			Weight	
Ankle dorsiflexion	6-8	3	Date	
			Weight	

Training for Muscular Strength vs. Muscular Endurance

Muscular endurance was defined as the ability to perform repeated muscle contractions against resistance. Most weight-training experts believe that muscular strength and muscular endurance are closely related to one another. As one improves, there is a tendency for the other to improve also.

It is generally accepted that when weight training for strength, heavier weights with a lower number of repetitions should be used. Conversely, endurance training uses relatively lighter weights with a greater number of repetitions.

It has been suggested that endurance training should consist of 3 sets of 10 to 12 repetitions; thus suggested training regimens for both muscular strength and endurance are very similar in terms of sets and numbers of repetitions. Persons who possess great levels of strength tend to also exhibit greater muscular endurance when asked to perform repeated contractions against resistance.

Strength Training for Women

Perhaps the most critical difference between men and women regarding physical performance is the ratio of strength to weight. The reduced strength/body weight ratio in women is the result of a higher percentage of body fat than in men.

Strength is just as important to women as to men; unfortunately, many women are reluctant to engage in a weight-training program because of the fear of developing bulky muscles, which are still regarded as unfeminine. This fear is unfounded; the average woman will not build little significant muscle bulk through weight training. Significant muscle hypertrophy is dependent on the presence of an anabolic steroidal hormone known as testosterone. Testosterone is considered a male hormone, although all women possess some testosterone in their systems. Women with higher testosterone levels tend to have more masculine characteristics such as increased facial and body hair, a deeper voice, and the potential to develop a little more muscle bulk.[19]

For the average college-age woman there is no need to worry about developing large bulky muscles with strength training. What does happen is that muscle tone is improved. Muscle tone basically refers to the firmness, or tension, of the muscle during a resting state. For example, doing sit-ups increases the firmness of the abdominal muscles and makes them more resistant to fatigue. All of us would agree that a person who has a firm, well-toned body is physically attractive.

A woman in weight training will probably see some remarkable gains in strength initially, even though muscle bulk does not increase. How is this possible?

For a muscle to contract, an impulse must be transmitted from the nervous system to the muscle. Each muscle fiber is innervated by a specific motor unit. By overloading a particular muscle, as in weight training, the muscle is forced to work more efficiently. Efficiency is achieved by getting more motor units to fire, causing a stronger contraction of the muscle. Consequently, it is not uncommon for a woman to see extremely rapid gains in strength when a weight-training program is first begun. These tremendous initial strength gains, which can be attributed to improved neuromuscular system efficiency, tend to plateau, and minimal improvement in muscular strength will be realized during a continuing strength-training program. It must be added, however, that these initial neuromuscular strength gains will also be seen in men, although strength will continue to increase with appropriate training.

It must be reiterated that women who do possess higher testosterone levels have the potential to further increase their strength because of the development of greater muscle bulk.

The strength/body weight ratio may be significantly improved through weight training by decreasing the body fat percentage while increasing lean weight. Strength training programs for women should follow the same guidelines as those for men.

Use of Anabolic Steroids in Weight Training

Unfortunately, the use of anabolic steroids by persons attempting to develop high levels of strength is becoming commonplace. Anabolic steroids are organic compounds that contain primarily sterols and sex hormones (testosterone). These drugs are used therapeutically in the treatment of diseases in which protein synthesis is an essential component of the healing process. Athletes use the drug for increasing lean body weight, muscle mass, and strength. There has been a considerable amount of research in this area, and results have been at best conflicting. It is likely that *anabolic steroids* do increase muscle size and strength when taken in conjunction with an intense weight-training program over a period of 1 to 2 months. However, it has also been proposed that prolonged use of anabolic steroids may result in harmful side effects such as liver disfunction, reduced testicular function and loss of sexual interest, headaches, nausea, and so forth. For this reason, the use of anabolic steroids for the purpose of strength improvement cannot be recommended and has in fact been banned by the International Olympic Committee. Despite the uncertainty about the long-range effects of these drugs, anabolic steroid use is a continuing problem for many persons involved with heavy weight training at all levels. The following position statement of the American College of Sports Medicine is the result of a world-wide literature review on the effects of anabolic steroids.

> The administration of anabolic-androgenic steroids to healthy humans below age 50 in medically approved therapeutic doses often does not of itself bring about any significant improvements in strength, aerobic endurance, lean body mass, or body weight.
>
> There is no conclusive scientific evidence that extremely large doses of anabolic-androgenic steroids either aid or hinder athletic performance.
>
> The prolonged use of oral anabolic-androgenic steroids has resulted in liver disorders in some persons. Some of these disorders are apparently reversible with the cessation of drug usage, but others are not.

The administration of anabolic-androgenic steroids to male humans may result in a decrease in testicular size and function and a decrease in sperm production. Although these effects appear to be reversible when small doses of steroids are used for short periods of time, the reversibility of the effects of large doses over extended periods of time is unclear.

Serious and continuing efforts should be made to educate male and female athletes, coaches, physical educators, physicians, trainers, and the general public regarding the inconsistent effects of anabolic-androgenic steroids on improvement of human physical performance and the potential dangers of taking certain forms of these substances, especially in large doses, for prolonged periods.

Specific Strength-Training Exercises

To say that a person is strong is probably incorrect. We should instead refer to a specific muscle, muscle group, or movement as being strong because increases in strength occur only in muscles that are regularly subjected to overload.

Because muscle contractions result in joint movement, the goal of the serious weight trainer should be to increase strength in every movement possible about a given joint. Exercises must be designd to place stress on those groups of muscles collectively to produce a specific joint movement.

For this reason, our approach to specific strength-training exercises deviates from the traditional approach. The following program is organized to include all motions about a particular joint rather than discussing exercises for each specific muscle.

Figures 4-11 to 4-33 describe exercises for strength improvement of shoulder, hip, knee, and ankle joint movements.

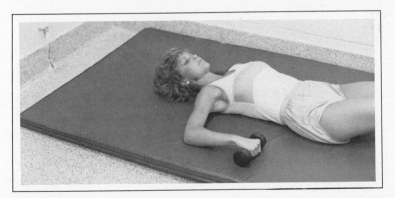

FIGURE 4-11

Lateral rotation.
Joint affected: shoulder.
Movement: External rotation.
Position: Supine, shoulder abducted and elbow flexed.
Primary muscles: Infraspinatus, teres minor.

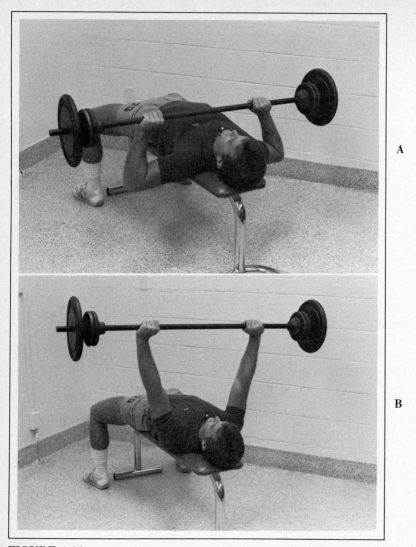

A

B

FIGURE 4-12

Bench press.
Joint affected: Shoulder.
Movement: Pushing away.
Position: Supine, feet flat on floor, back flat on bench.
Primary muscles: Pectoralis major tricep.

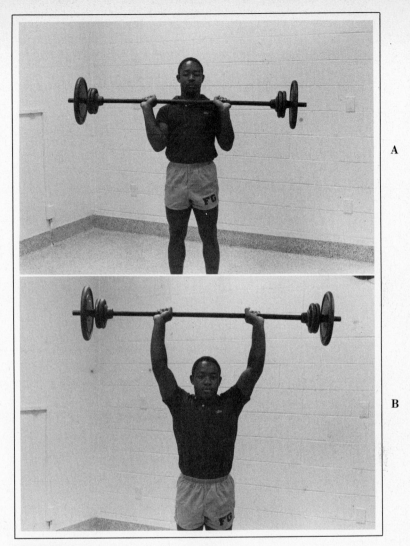

FIGURE 4-13

Military press.
Joint affected: Shoulder and elbow.
Movement: Abduction and extension.
Position: Standing, back straight.
Primary muscles: Deltoid, trapezius, triceps.

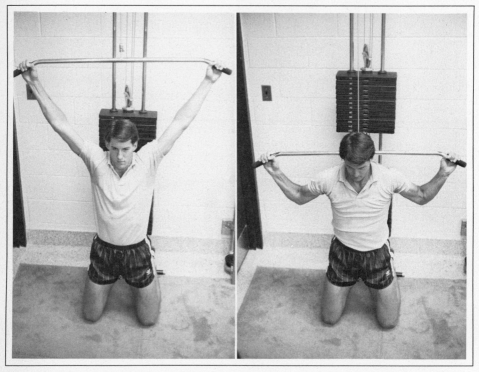

FIGURE 4-14

Lateral pulls.
Joint affected: Shoulder and elbow.
Movement: Adduction and flexion.
Position: Kneeling, back straight, head up.
Primary muscles: Latissimus dorsi, biceps.

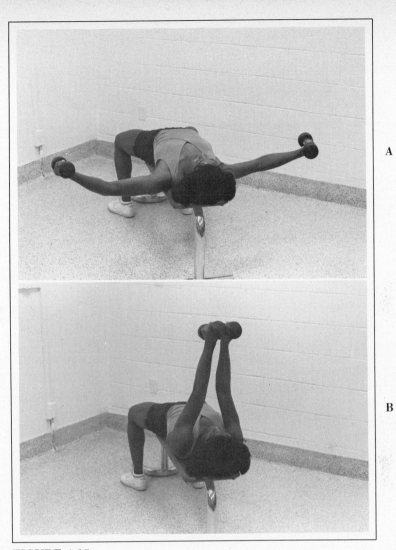

A

B

FIGURE 4-15

Flys.
Joint affected: Shoulder.
Movement: Horizontal flexion.
Position: Supine, feet flat on floor, back flat on bench.
Primary muscles: Deltoid, pectoralis major.

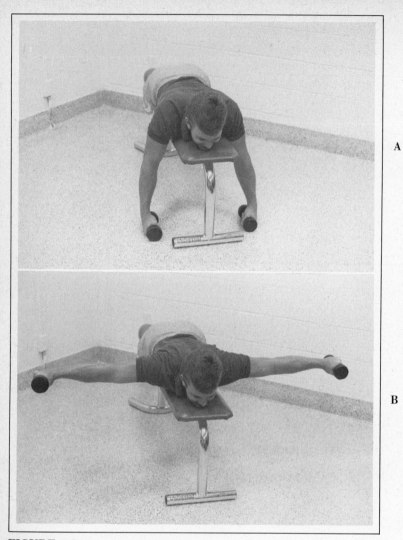

A

B

FIGURE 4-16

Reverse flys.
Joint affected: Shoulder.
Movement: Horizontal extension.
Position: Prone, feet on floor.
Primary muscles: Deltoid, trapezius.

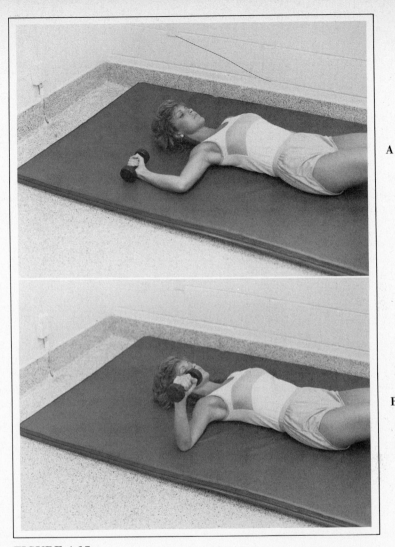

FIGURE 4-17

Medial rotation.
Joint affected: Shoulder.
Movement: Internal rotation.
Position: Supine, shoulder abducted and elbow flexed.
Primary muscles: Subscapularis.

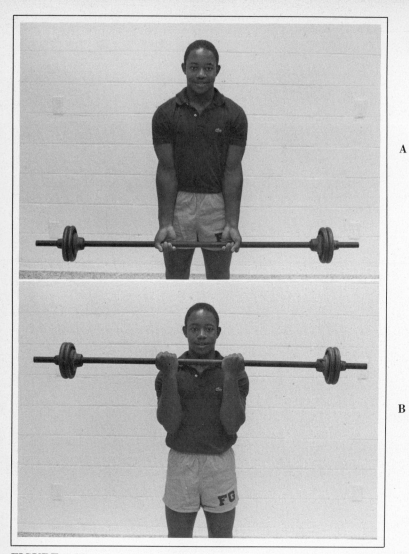

A

B

FIGURE 4-18

Bicep curl.
Joint affected: elbow.
Movement: Elbow flexion.
Position: Standing, back straight, arms extended.
Primary muscles: Biceps.

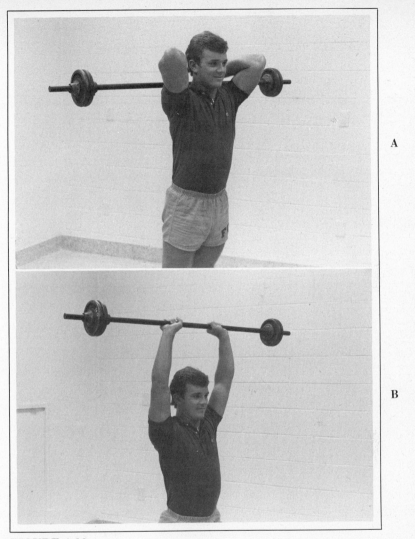

A

B

FIGURE 4-19

Tricep extension.
Joint affected: Elbow.
Movement: Elbow extension.
Position: Standing, elbows pointing directly toward ceiling beside ears.
Primary muscles: Triceps.

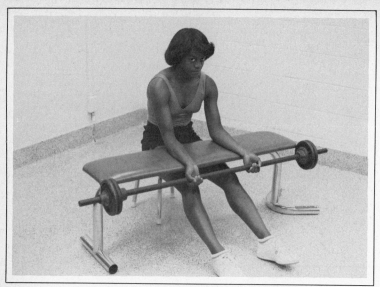

FIGURE 4-20

Wrist curls.
Joint affected: Wrist.
Movement: Wrist flexion.
Position: Seated, forearms on table, palms up.
Primary muscles: Long flexors of forearm.

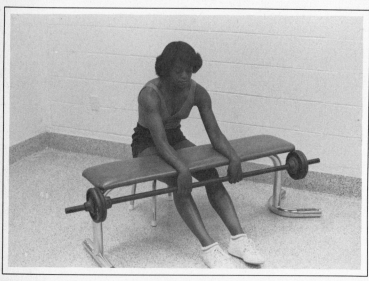

FIGURE 4-21

Wrist extension.
Joint affected: Wrist.
Movement: Extension
Position: Seated, forearms on table, palms down.
Primary muscles: Long extensors of forearm.

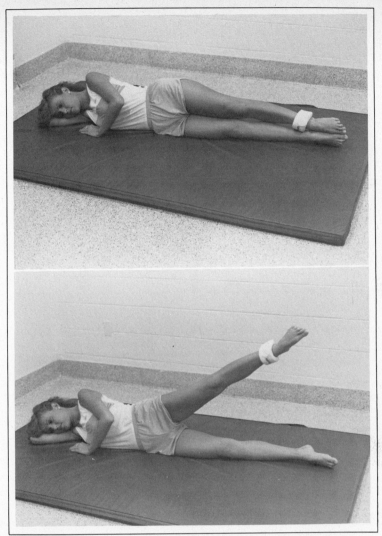

FIGURE 4-22

Leg raises.
Joint affected: Hip.
Movement: Hip abduction.
Position: Sidelying.
Primary muscles: Hip abductors.

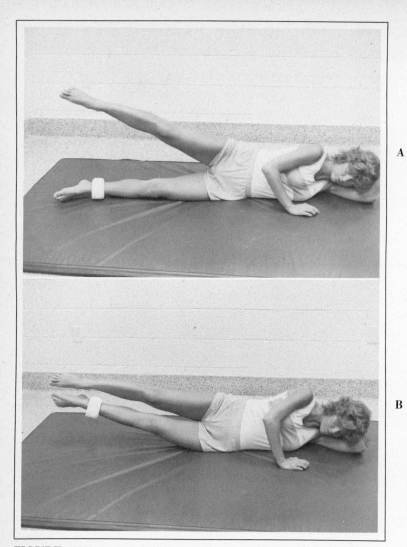

A

B

FIGURE 4-23

Leg to leg raises.
Joint affected: Hip.
Movement: Hip adduction.
Position: Sidelying, one leg abducted.
Primary muscles: Hip adductors.

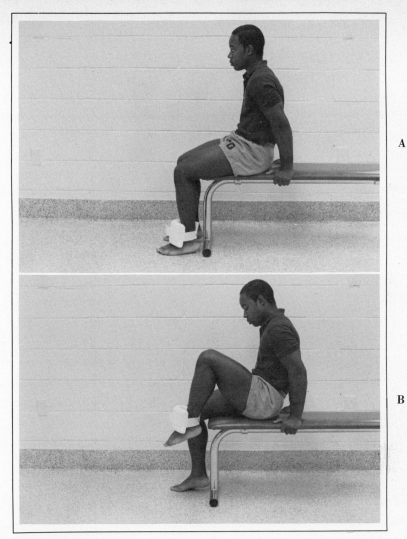

FIGURE 4-24

Bent knee leg lifts.
Joint affected: Hip.
Movement: Hip flexion.
Position: Sitting, knee flexed, weight around ankle.
Primary muscles: Iliopsoas.

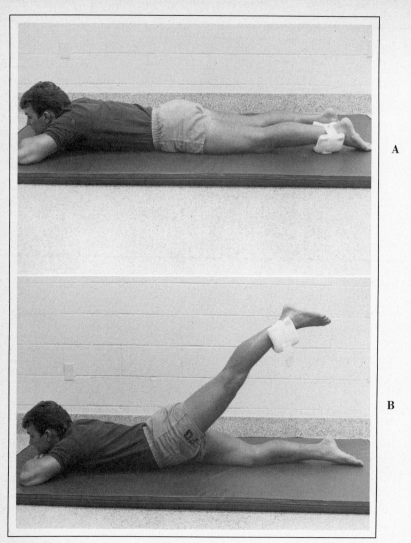

A

B

FIGURE 4-25

Reverse leg lifts.
Joint affected: Hip.
Movement: Hip extension.
Position: Prone, knee extended.
Primary muscles: Gluteus maximus, hamstrings.

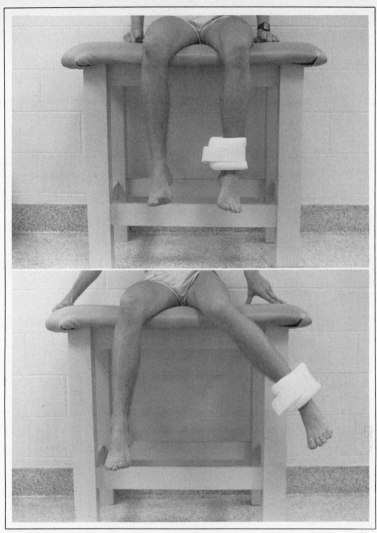

A

B

FIGURE 4-26

Hip medial rotation.
Joint affected: Hip.
Movement: Internal rotation.
Position: Sitting, knee flexed, weight on ankle.
Primary muscles: Medial rotators.

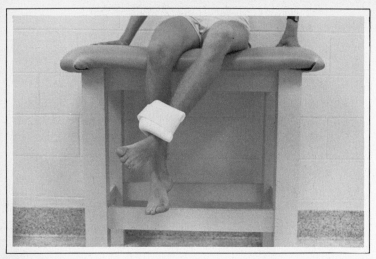

FIGURE 4-27

Hip lateral rotation.
Joint affected: Hip.
Movement: External rotation.
Position: Sitting, knee flexed, weight on ankle.
Primary muscles: Gluteus medius.

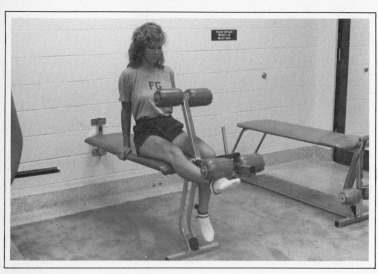

FIGURE 4-28

Quadriceps extensions.
Joint affected: Knee.
Movement: Extension.
Position: Sitting, on knee machine.
Primary muscles: Quadriceps group.

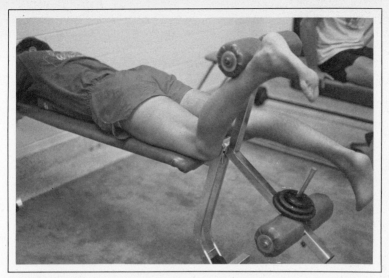

FIGURE 4-29

Hamstring curls.
Joint affected: Knee.
Movement: Flexion.
Position: Prone, on knee machine.
Primary muscles: Hamstring group.

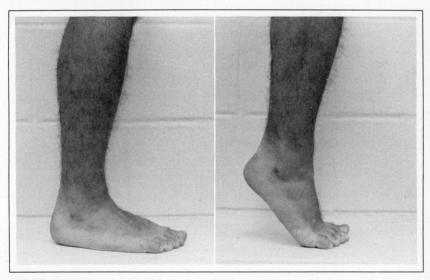

FIGURE 4-30

Toe raises.
Joint affected: Ankle.
Movement: Plantar flexion.
Position: Standing on one leg and lifting body weight.
Primary muscles: Gastrocnemius and soleus.

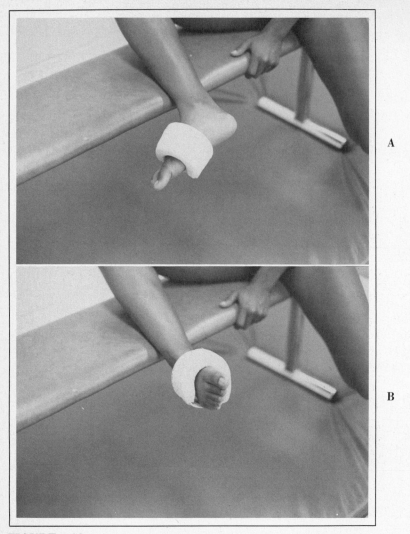

FIGURE 4-31

Ankle inversion.
Joint affected: Ankle.
Movement: Inversion.
Position: Sitting, knee flexed, instep up, weight on foot.
Primary muscles: Anterior tibialis.

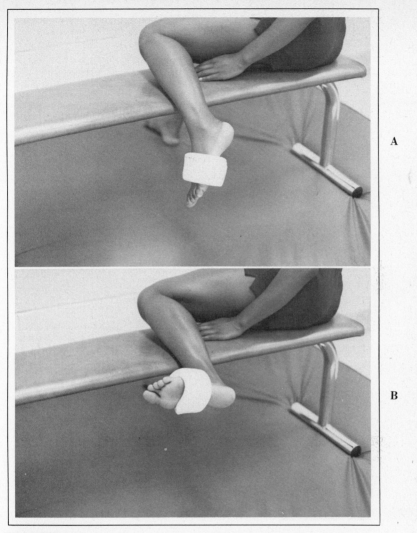

FIGURE 4-32

Ankle eversion.
Joint affected: Ankle.
Movement: Eversion.
Position: Sitting, knee flexed, instep down, weight on foot.
Primary muscles: Peroneals.

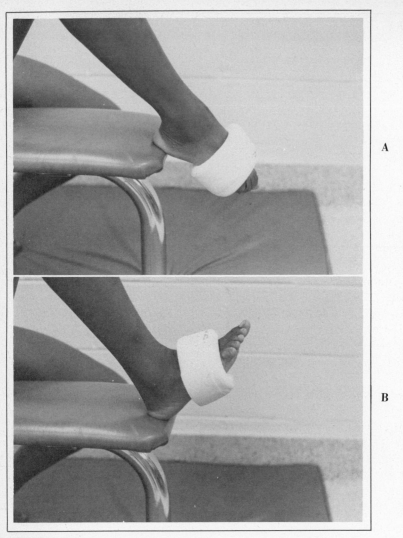

A

B

FIGURE 4-33

Ankle dorsiflexion.
Joint affected: Ankle.
Movement: Dorsiflexion.
Position: Sitting, knee flexed, heel on edge of table, weight on foot.
Primary muscles: Dorsiflexors in shin.

SUMMARY

- Strength is an essential component of physical fitness for anyone involved in a physical activity program. Strength may be defined as the maximal force that can be generated by a muscle during a single maximal contraction.
- The ability to generate force is dependent of the physical properties of the muscle itself as well as the mechanical factors that dictate how much force can be generated through the lever system to an external object.
- Muscular power involves the speed with which a forceful muscle contraction is performed.
- Hypertrophy of a muscle is caused by increases in the size of the protein myofilaments, which result in an increased cross-sectional diameter of the muscle.
- The key to improving strength through weight training is utilizing the principle of overload.
- There are three training techniques that can improve muscular strength; isometric training, isotonic training, and isokinetic training.
- In an isometric contraction, the muscle increases its tension while the length remains constant.
- In an isotonic contraction, the muscle generates force while changing in length.
- An isokinetic movement is one in which the length of the muscle is changing but the contraction is performed at a constant velocity.
- Research has indicated that the best training technique for improving strength involves 3 sets of 6 to 8 repetitions done every other day.
- Muscular endurance is the ability to perform repeated isotonic or isokinetic muscle contractions or to sustain an isometric contraction. Muscular endurance tends to improve with muscular strength; thus training techniques for these two components are similar.
- The use of anabolic steroids has many negative physiologic side effects and cannot be recommended for the purpose of increasin muscular size and stength.
- Women generally will not build large muscle bulk as a result of strength training because of a relative lack of the hormone testosterone.

GLOSSARY

anabolic steroids Organic compounds that contain sterols and sex hormones—used to increase muscle mass and strength

concentric (positive) contraction An isotonic contraction in which the muscle is shortening while contracting

eccentric (negative) contraction An isotonic contraction in which the muscle is lengthening while contracting

fast-twitch fibers Muscle fibers that are white and can produce very quick contractions

hypertrophy An increase in the size and cross-sectional diameter of the muscle that results from strength training *isokinetic exercise* An exercise in which the length of the muscle changes although the contraction is performed at a constant velocity against resistance

isometric exercise An exercise that involves a muscle contraction in which the length of the muscle remains constant while tension develops toward a maximal force against an immovable resistance

isotonic exercise An exercise that involves a muscle contraction in which force is being generated while the muscle is changing in length

motor unit A group of muscle fibers innervated by a single nerve fiber

muscular endurance The ability to perform repetitive muscle contractions against a resistance

musculotendinous unit A term that refers to the contractile elements of the muscle belly and its relatively inelastic tendon

myofilaments Thousands of small protein fibers that compose the belly of the muscle

power The ability to generate a large amount of force very quickly

repetition maximum The maximal number of repetitions a person is capable of performing in a single set

set The number of repetitions performed between rest intervals

slow-twitch fibers Muscle fibers that are reddish and are more resistant to fatigue than are fast-twitch fibers

strength The maximal force that can be applied by a muscle during a single maximal contraction

REFERENCES

1. Berger, R. (1962). Effect of varied weight training programs on strength. *Research Quarterly, 33,*168.
2. Costill, D., & others. (1976). Skeletal muscle enzymes and fiber compositions in male and female track athletes. *Journal of Applied Physiology, 40,*149-154.
3. DeLorme, T., & Wilkens, A. (1951). *Progressive resistance exercise.* New York: Appleton-Century-Crofts.
4. Donald, K., & others. (1967). Cardiovascular responses to sustained (static) contractions. In *Physiology of muscular exercise.* American Heart Association Monograph, Nov. 15, 15-30.
5. Gollnick, P., & Sembrowich, W. (1977). Adaptations in human skeletal muscle as a result of training, in E.A. Amsterdam (Ed.), *Exercise in cardiovascular health and disease.* New York: York Medical Books.
6. Jensen, C., & Fisher, G. (1979). *Scientific basis of athletic conditioning.* Philadelphia: Lea & Febiger.
7. McCardle, W., Katch, F., & Katch, V. (1981). *Exercise physiology, energy, nutrition, and human performance.* Philadelphia: Lea & Febiger.

SUGGESTED READINGS

Allsen, P., Harrison, J., & Vance, B. (1984). *Fitness for life: An individualized approach.* Dubuque, IA: William C. Brown.

Åstrand, P.O., & Rodahl, K. (1977). *Textbook of work physiology.* New York: McGraw-Hill.

Bell, R. (1977). Muscle fiber types and morphometric analysis of skeletal muscle in six-year-old children, *Med. Science Sports. 12,*28.

Corbin, C., Linus, D., Lindsey, R., & Tolson, H. (1981). *Concepts in physical education with laboratories and experiments.* Dubuque, Iowa: William C. Brown.

deVries, H. (1980). *Physiology of exercise for physical education and athletics.* Dubuque, IA: William C. Brown.

Fox, E. (1984). *Sport physiology*. New York: CBS College Publishing.

Getchell, B. (1983). *Physical fitness: A way of life*. New York: John Wiley & Sons.

Hockey, R.V. (1985). *Physical fitness—The pathway to healthful living*. St. Louis: Times Mirror/ Mosby College Publishing.

Miller, D., & Allen, E. (1982). *Fitness—A lifetime concept*. Minneapolis: Burgess.

Riley, D. (1977). *Strength training by the experts*. West Point, NY: Leisure Press.

Stokes, R., & Farls, D. (1983). *Fitness everyone!* Winston-Salem, NC: Hunter Textbooks.

Wilmore, J. (1979). Alterations in strength body composition and anthoropometric measurement consequent to a 10-Week weight training program. *Medicine and Science in Sports, 6*, 133.

Wilmore, J. (1982). Training for sport and activity: *The physiological basis of the conditioning process*, (2nd ed.). Boston: Allyn & Bacon.

5

THE DEVELOPMENT
OF FLEXIBILITY
THROUGH STRETCHING

After completing this chapter, you will be able to:

- Define flexibility and describe its importance as a health-related component of fitness.
- Identify factors that limit flexibility.
- Differentiate between static and dynamic flexibility.
- Explain the difference between ballistic, static, and PNF stretching.

- Discuss the neurophysiologic principles of stretching.
- Describe stretching exercises that may be used to improve flexibility at specific joints throughout the body.

Flexibility was defined earlier as a health-related as opposed to skill-related component of fitness, although for most of us it may be considered important for both. The ability to move a joint smoothly throughout a full range of motion is certainly essential to healthy living. The arthritic patient who suffers from degeneration in one or more joints loses the capacity of painless, nonrestricted motion and is thus hampered in the performance of daily acts of healthful living. Likewise, the athlete who has a restricted range of motion will probably realize a decrease in performance capabilities. For example, a sprinter with tight, inelastic hamstring muscles probably loses some speed because the hamstring muscles restrict the ability to flex the hip joint, thus shortening stride length.

Lack of flexibility may result in uncoordinated or awkward movements and probably predisposes a person to muscle strain.

Most activities we engage in require relatively "normal" amounts of flexibility. However, some activities, such as gymnastics, ballet, diving, karate, and yoga require increased flexibility for superior performance (Figure 5-1). Experts in the field of training and the development of physical fitness would all agree that good flexibility is essential to successful physical performance, although their ideas are based primarily on observation rather than scientific research.

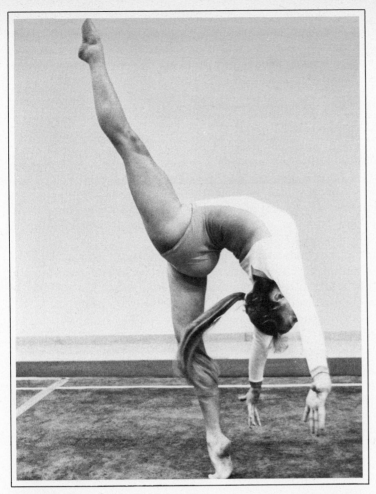

FIGURE 5-1

Certain sport activities require extreme flexibility for successful performance.

Most athletic trainers and therapists believe that maintaining good flexibility is important in prevention of injury to the musculotendinous unit. Thus coaches will generally insist that stretching exercises be included as part of the warm-up before engaging in strenuous activity.

Flexibility may best be defined as the range of motion possible about a given joint or series of joints. Flexibility can be discussed in relation to movement that may involve only one joint, such as in the knees, or movement that might involve a whole series of joints, such as the spinal vertebral joints, which must all move together to allow smooth bending, or rotation, of the trunk.

You may often hear someone say that "Joe has good flexibility." It is really incorrect to talk about the entire person as being flexible; flexibility is specific to a given joint or movement. A person may have good range of motion in an ankle, knee, hip, back and one shoulder joint. However, if the other shoulder joint lacks normal movement, then a problem exists that needs to be corrected before that person can function normally.

FACTORS THAT LIMIT FLEXIBILITY

There are a number of factors that may limit the ability of a joint to move through a full, unrestricted range of motion. The structure of the skeletal system may restrict the endpoint in the range. An elbow that has been fractured through the joint may lay down excess calcium in the joint space, and the joint may lose its ability to fully extend. However, in many instances we rely on bony prominences to stop movements at normal endpoints in the range.

Fat may also limit the ability to move through a full range of motion. A person who has a large amount of fat on the abdomen may be severely restricted in trunk flexion when asked to bend forward and touch the toes. The fat may act as a wedge between two lever arms, restricting movement wherever it is found.

Skin might also be responsible for limiting movement. For example, a person who has had some type of injury or surgery involving a tearing incision or laceration of the skin, particularly over a joint, will have inelastic scar tissue formed at that site. This scar tissue is incapable of stretching with joint movement.

Connective tissue surrounding the joint, such as ligaments on the joint capsule may be subject to contractures. Ligaments and joint capsules do have some elasticity; however, if a joint is immobilized for a period of time, these structures tend to lose some elasticity and actually shorten in length. This condition is most commonly seen after surgical repair of an unstable joint but it can also result from long periods of inactivity.

It is also possible for a person to have ligaments and joint capsules that are relatively slack. These people are generally referred to as being *loose-jointed*. Examples of this would be an elbow or knee that hyperextends beyond 180° (Figure 5-2). Frequently there is instability associated with loose-jointedness that may present as great a problem in movement as ligamentous or capsular contractures.

Muscles and their tendons, along with the fascial sheaths that surround them, are most often responsible for limiting range of motion. When performing stretching exercises for the purpose of improving flexibility about a particular joint, you are attempting to take advantage of the highly elastic properties of a muscle. Over time it is possible to increase the elasticity, or the length that a given muscle can be stretched. Persons who have a good deal of movement at a particular joint tend to have highly elastic and flexible muscles.

With the exception of bony structure, all of the other factors that limit flexibility may be altered to increase range of joint motion. Fat loss is possible through weight reduction, which removes a physical obstruction to movement.

Skin contractures caused by scarring, ligaments, joint capsules, and mus-

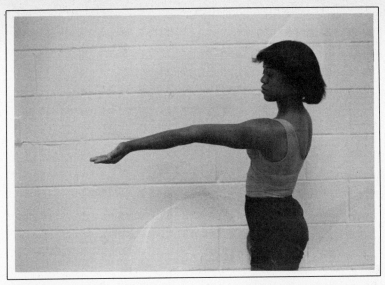

FIGURE 5-2

Excessive joint movement, such as in a hyperextended elbow, can predispose a joint to injury.

Other Factors Affecting Flexibility	
Age	For the average person, flexibility tends to decrease through early childhood until the age of 10 to 12 years, after which it steadily improves through the college-age years. From about age 20, flexibility gradually declines with age.
Sex	It appears that women generally tend to be more flexible than men. However, this factor may possibly be related to the fact women tend to spend more time on activities such as dance and gymnastics in which flexibility is essential to performance.
Activity	Those persons who are physically active and remain so throughout life seem to exhibit better flexibility than sedentary persons.

culotendinous units are each capable of improving elasticity to varying degrees through stretching over time.

STATIC AND DYNAMIC FLEXIBILITY

There are two different types of flexibility: static and dynamic.[2] *Static flexibility* refers to the degree to which a joint may be passively moved to the endpoints

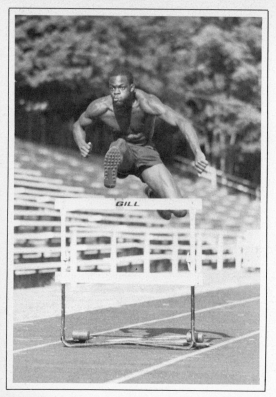

FIGURE 5-3

Flexibility is an essential component of many sport-related activities.

in the range of motion. No muscle contraction is involved with static flexibility.

Dynamic flexibility refers to the degree which a joint can be moved as a result of a muscle contraction, usually through the midrange of movement. Dynamic flexibility is not necessarily a good indicator of the stiffness or looseness of a joint because it applies to the ability to move a joint quickly with little resistance to motion.

When a muscle contracts, it produces a joint movement through a specific range of motion. However, if passive pressure is applied to an extremity, it is capable of moving further in the range of motion.

Dynamic flexibility is important in athletic performance. It is essential in sport activities that an extremity be capable of moving through a nonrestricted range of motion. For example, a sprinter who cannot fully extend the knee joint in a normal stride is at considerable disadvantage because stride length and thus speed will be significantly reduced (Figure 5-3).

Static flexibility is important for injury prevention. There are many situations

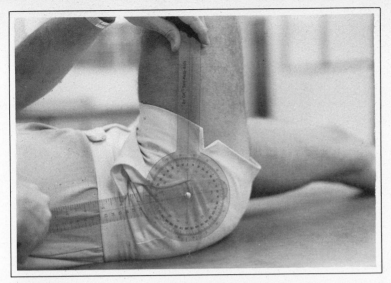

FIGURE 5-4

Goniometric measurement of hip joint flexion.

in sport in which a muscle is forced to stretch beyond its normal active limits. If the muscle does not have enough elasticity to compensate for this additional stretch, it is likely that injury will occur to the musculotendinous unit.

In most physical activities the ability to achieve flexibility of motion seems to be more important than the ability to reach extreme degrees of motions. Possible exceptions to this would be activities such as gymnastics, dance, and karate.

ASSESSMENT OF FLEXIBILITY

The accurate measurement of range of joint motion is difficult. Various devices have been designed to accomodate variations in the sizes of the joints as well as the complexity of movements in articulations that involve more than one joint. Of these devices, the simplest and most widely used is the *goniometer* (Figure 5-4).

A goniometer is a large protractor with measurements in degrees. By aligning the two arms parallel to the longitudinal axis of the two segments involved in motion about a specific joint, it is possible to obtain relatively accurate measures of range of movement. The goniometer has its place in a rehabilitation setting, where it is essential to assess improvement in joint flexibility for the purpose of modifying injury rehabilitation programs.

Because it is most appropriate to talk about flexibility as being specific to a given joint or movement, there is no doubt that the most accurate method for assessing joint movement is through the use of a goniometer. However, for the

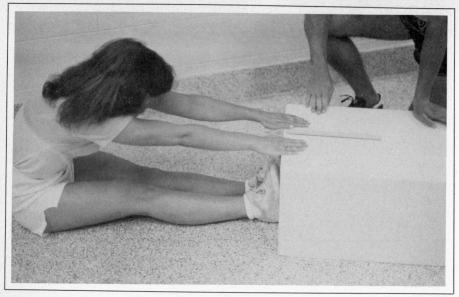

FIGURE 5-5

Trunk flexion test.

TABLE 5-1   Flexibility in Trunk Flexion (Sit and Reach)

Classification	Men	Women
Poor	0 in	0 in
Average	1-3 in	2-4 in
Good	4-6 in	5-7 in
Excellent	7 in	8 in

average college student, it is not practical to assess joint movement using goniometry. Therefore the following three tests allow at best a gross indication of the ability to stretch.

1. Trunk flexion (Figure 5-5)

    This test measures the flexibility of the lower back muscles and the hip extensors (that is, the hamstrings and gluteals).

    Technique is to sit with the legs together, knees flat on the floor, and feet flat against some vertical surface. Bend forward at the waist and reach as far forward as possible with the fingers.

    Your score is determined by measuring the number of inches you can reach either in front of or beyond the vertical surface.

    To determine your classification, see Table 5-1.

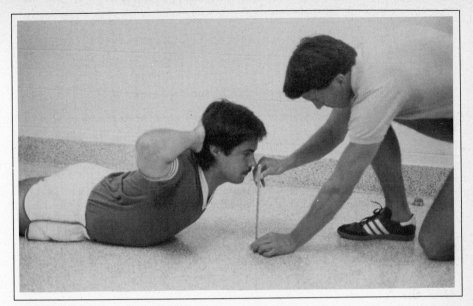

FIGURE 5-6

Trunk extension test.

TABLE 5-2   Flexibility in Trunk Extension

Classification	Men	Women
Poor	16 in	17 in
Average	17-18 in	18-19 in
Good	19-21 in	20-22 in
Excellent	22 in	24 in

2. *Trunk extension* (Figure 5-6)
   This test measures the flexibility of the abdominal and hip flexor muscles.
   Technique is to lie in a prone position on the floor. Have a partner sit on
   your legs and hold the legs and buttocks to the ground. Grasp your hands
   behind the neck and raise the upper trunk as high off the ground as
   possible and hold.
   Your score is determined by measuring the distance from the chin to the
   ground.
   To determine your classification, see Table 5-2.
3. *Shoulder lift test* (Figure 5-7)
   This test measures the flexibility of the shoulder flexors.
   Technique is to lie prone on the floor with arms extended over the head
   while holding a stick in the hands. The stick should be raised as high

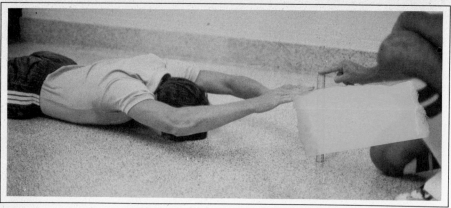

FIGURE 5-7

Shoulder lift test.

TABLE 5-3   Flexibility of the Shoulder Joint

Classification	Men	Women
Poor	0-19 in	0-20 in
Average	20-22 in	21-23 in
Good	23-25 in	24-25 in
Excellent	26 in	27 in

as possible, with the face and chest kept flat on the floor. This position should be held.

Your score is determined by measuring the distance from the ruler to the ground.

To determine your classification, see Table 5-3.

STRETCHING TECHNIQUES

Flexibility has been defined as the range of motion possible about a single joint or through a series of articulations. The maintenance of a full, nonrestricted range of motion has long been recognized as an essential component of physical fitness. Flexibility is important not only for successful physical performance but also in the prevention of injury.

The goal of any effective flexibility program should be to improve the range of motion at a given articulation by altering the extensibility of the musculotendinous units that produce movement at that joint. It is well documented that exercises that stretch these musculotendinous units over a period of time will increase the range of movement possible about a given joint.[5]

Stretching techniques for improving flexibility have evolved over the years. The oldest technique for stretching is the so-called *ballistic stretching*, which makes use of repetitive bouncing motions.

A second technique, known as *static stretching*, involves stretching a muscle to the point of discomfort and then holding it at that point for an extended time. This technique has been used for many years. Recently, another group of stretching techniques known collectively as *proprioceptive neuromuscular facilitation (PNF)*, involving alternating contractions and stretches, have also been recommended.[3]

There has been considerable discussion among researchers as to which of these techniques is most effective for improving range of motion.

Checklist For Individualized Stretching Program

Exercise	Hold Time (sec)	Repetitions	Day 1 2 3 4 5 6 7 8 9 10 11 12 13 14
Arm hang	30	5	
Shoulder towel stretch	10	5	
Upper trunk stretch	30	3	
Lower trunk stretch	30	3	
Upper back and neck	30	3	
Lower back stretch	30*	3	
Lower back twister	30	3	
Pelvic thrust	30	3	
Quadriceps stretch	30	3	
Hamstring stretch	30	3	
Hurdlers stretch	30	3	
Groin stretch	30	3	
Achilles heel cord stretch	30	3*	
Toe pointer	30	3	

*In each position.

Agonist vs. Antagonist Muscles

Before discussing the three different stretching techniques, it is essential to define the terms *agonist* and *antagonist*.

Most joints in the body are capable of more than one movement. The knee joint, for example, is capable of flexion and extension. The quadriceps group of muscles on the front of the thigh, when contracted, cause knee extension, whereas contraction of the hamstring muscles on the back of the thigh produces knee flexion.

If the quadriceps group contracts, the hamstring muscles must relax and stretch for knee extension to occur. Muscles that work in concert with one another in this manner are called *synergistic* muscle groups. The muscle that contracts to produce a movement, in this case the quadriceps, is referred to as the *agonist* muscle. Conversely, the muscle being stretched in response to contraction of the agonist muscle is called the *antagonist* muscle. In this example of knee extension, the antagonist muscle would be the hamstring group.

An understanding of this synergistic muscle action is essential to understanding the three techniques of stretching.

Ballistic Stretching

If you were to walk out to the track on any spring or fall afternoon and watch people who are warming up to run by doing their stretching exercises, you would probably see them using bouncing movements to stretch a particular muscle. This bouncing technique is more appropriately known as ballistic stretching, in which repetitive contractions of the agonist muscle are used to produce quick stretches of the antagonist muscle. The ballistic stretching technique, although apparently effective, has been virtually abandoned by most experts in the field because of the fact that increased range of motion is achieved through a series of jerks or pulls on the resistant muscle tissue. If the forces generated by the jerks are greater than the extensibility of which the tissues are capable, injury to the muscle may result.

Static Stretching

The *static stretching* technique is still an extremely effective and popular technique of stretching. This technique involves passively stretching a given antagonist muscle by placing it in a maximal position of stretch and holding it there for an extended period of time. Recommendations for the optimal time for holding this stretched position vary, ranging from as short as 3 seconds to as long as 60 seconds.[3] Data are inconclusive at the present time; however, it appears that 30 seconds may be as good a figure as any. The static stretch of each muscle should be repeated 3 or 4 times.

Much research has been done comparing ballistic and static stretching techniques for the improvement of flexibility. It has been shown that both static and

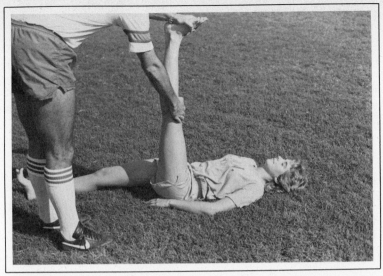

FIGURE 5-8

The slow-reversal-hold technique for stretching the hamstring muscles.

ballistic stretching are effective in increasing flexibility and that there is no significant difference between the two. However, with static stretching there is less danger of exceeding the extensibility limits of the involved joints because the stretch is more controlled. Ballistic stretching is apt to cause muscular soreness, whereas static stretching generally does not. Static stretching is commonly used in injury rehabilitation of sore or strained muscles.

PNF Techniques

PNF techniques were first used by physical therapists for treating patients who had various types of neuromuscular paralysis. Only recently have PNF stretching exercises been used as a stretching technique for increasing flexibility. A disadvantage of the PNF techniques is that they require a partner to help you stretch.

There are a number of different PNF techniques currently being used for stretching, including slow-reversal-hold, contract-relax, and hold-relax techniques. All involve some combination of alternating contraction and relaxation of both agonist and antagonist muscles. PNF techniques also involve a 10-second pushing phase followed by a 10-second relaxing phase.

Using a hamstring stretching technique as an example (Figure 5-8), the slow-reversal-hold technique would be done as follows. Lying on your back with the knee extended and the ankle flexed to 90°, a partner passively flexes your leg at the hip joint to the point at which you feel slight discomfort in the muscle.

At this point, you begin pushing against your partner's resistance by contracting the hamstring muscle. After pushing for 10 seconds, the hamstring muscles are relaxed and the agonist quadriceps muscle is contracted while your partner applies passive pressure to further stretch the antagonist quadriceps. This should move the leg so that there is increased hip joint flexion. The relaxing phase lasts for 10 seconds, at which time you again push against your partner's resistance, beginning at this new joint angle. The push-relax sequence is repeated at least 3 times.[5]

The contract-relax and hold-relax techniques are variations on the slow-reversal-hold method. In the contract-relax method, the hamstrings are isotonically contracted so that the leg actually moves toward the floor during the push phase. The hold-relax method involves an isometric hamstring contraction against immovable resistance during the push phase. During the relax phase, both techniques involve relaxation of hamstrings and quadriceps while the hamstrings are passively stretched. This same basic PNF technique can be used to stretch any muscle in the body.

NEUROPHYSIOLOGIC BASIS OF STRETCHING

All three stretching techniques are based on a neurophysiologic phenomenon involving the *stretch reflex* (Figure 5-9). Every muscle in the body contains various types of receptors that when stimulated inform the central nervous system of what is happening with that muscle. Two of these receptors are important in the stretch reflex; the *muscle spindle* and the *Golgi tendon organ*. Both types of receptors are sensitive to changes in muscle length. The Golgi tendon organs are also affected by changes in muscle tension.

When a muscle is stretched, the muscle spindles are also stretched, sending a volley of sensory impulses to the spinal cord that inform the central nervous system that the muscle is being stretched. Impulses return to the muscle from the spinal cord, which causes the muscle to reflexly contract, thus resisting the stretch.

If the stretch of the muscle continues for an extended period of time (at least 6 seconds), the Golgi tendon organs respond to the change in length and the increase in tension by firing off sensory impulses of their own to the spinal cord. The impulses from the Golgi tendon organs, unlike the signals from the muscle spindle, cause a reflexive relaxation of the antagonist muscle. This reflex relaxation serves as a protective mechanism that will allow the muscle to stretch through relaxation before the extensibility limits are exceeded, causing damage to the muscle fibers.

With the jerking, bouncing motion of ballistic stretching, the muscle spindles are being repetitively stretched; thus there is continuous resistance by the muscle to further stretch. The ballistic stretch is not continued long enough to allow the Golgi tendon organs to have any relaxing effect.

The static stretch allows a continuous sustained stretch lasting anywhere from

FIGURE 5-9

The stretch reflex.

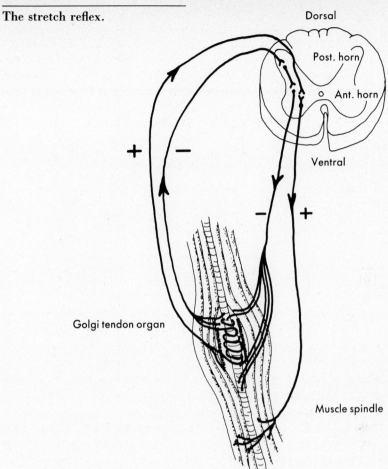

6 to 60 seconds, which is sufficient time for the Golgi tendon organs to begin responding to the increase in tension. The impulses from the Golgi tendon organs have the ability to override the impulses coming from the muscle spindles, allowing the muscle to reflexly relax after the initial reflexive resistance to the change in length. Thus lengthening the muscle and allowing it to remain in a stretched position for an extended period of time is unlikely to produce any injury to the muscle.

The effectiveness of the PNF techniques may be attributed in part to these same neurophysiologic principles. The slow-reversal-hold technique discussed previously takes advantage of two additional neurophysiologic phenomena.

The maximal isometric contraction of the antagonist muscle during the 10-second "push" phase again causes an increase in tension, which stimulates the Golgi tendon organs to effect a reflex relaxation of the antagonist even before

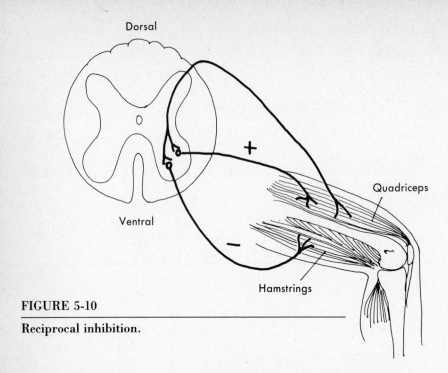

Dorsal

Ventral

Quadriceps

Hamstrings

FIGURE 5-10

Reciprocal inhibition.

the muscle is placed in a position of stretch. This relaxation of the antagonist muscle during contractions is referred to as autogenic inhibition.

During the relaxing phase the antagonist is relaxed and passively stretched while there is a maximal isotonic contraction of the agonist muscle pulling the extremity further into the agonist pattern. In any synergistic muscle group, a contraction of the agonist causes a reflex relaxation in the antagonist muscle, allowing it to stretch and protecting it from injury. This phenomenon is referred to as *reciprocal inhibition* (Figure 5-10).

Thus with the PNF techniques the additive effects of autogenic inhibition and reciprocal inhibition should theoretically allow the muscle to be stretched to a greater degree than is possible with either the static stretching technique or the ballistic technique.

PRACTICAL APPLICATION

Although all three stretching techniques have been demonstrated to effectively improve flexibility, there is still considerable debate as to which technique produces the greatest increases in range of movement. The ballistic technique is seldom recommended because of the potential for causing muscle soreness, whereas static stretching is perhaps the most widely used technique. It is a simple technique and does not require a partner. A fully nonrestricted range of motion can be attained through static stretching over a period of time.

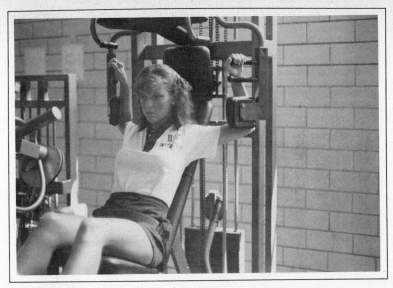

FIGURE 5-11

Strength training through a full range of movement will not impair flexibility.

PNF stretching techniques are capable of producing dramatic increases in range of motion during one stretching session. Studies comparing static and PNF stretching suggest that PNF stretching is capable of producing greater improvement in flexibility over an extended training period.[4] The major disadvantage of PNF stretching is that a partner is required to help you stretch, although stretching with a partner may have some motivational advantages. More and more college athletic teams seem to be adopting the PNF techniques as the method of choice for improving flexibility.

THE RELATIONSHIP OF STRENGTH AND FLEXIBILITY

We often hear about the negative effects that strength training has on flexibility. For example, someone who develops large bulk through strength training is often referred to as "muscle bound." The term *muscle bound* has negative connotations in terms of the ability of that person to move. We tend to think of people who are highly developed muscularly as having lost much of their ability to move freely through a full range of motion.

Occasionally a person develops so much bulk that the physical size of the muscle prevents a normal range of motion. It is certainly true that strength training that is not properly done can impair movement; however, there is no reason to believe that weight training, if done properly through a full range of motion, will impair flexibility. Proper strength training probably improves dynamic flexibility and, if combined with a rigorous stretching program, can greatly enhance powerful and coordinated movements that are essential for success in many athletic activities (Figure 5-11).

SPECIFIC STRETCHING EXERCISES

Figures 5-12 to 5-25 illustrate stretching exercises that may be used to improve flexibility at specific joints throughout the body. The exercises described may be done statically or with slight modification; they may also be done with a partner using a PNF technique.

There are many possible variations to each of these exercises. The exercises selected are those that seem to be the most effective for stretching of various muscle groups. *Text continued on p. 144.*

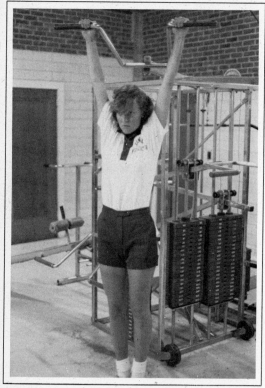

FIGURE 5-12

Exercise: Arm hang.
Muscles stretched: Entire shoulder girdle complex.
Instructions: Using a chinning bar, simply hang with shoulders and arms fully extended for 30 seconds. Repeat 5 times.

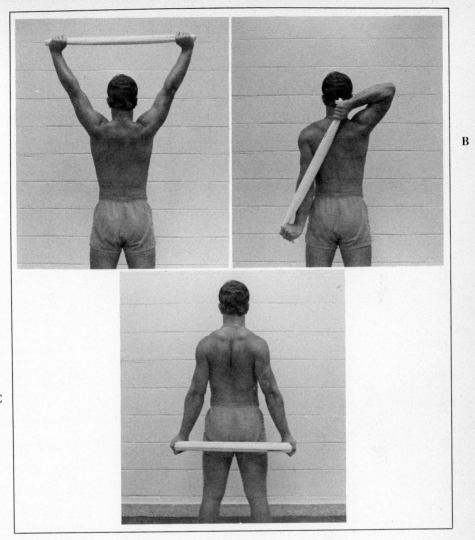

FIGURE 5-13

Exercise: Shoulder towel stretch.
Muscles stretched: Internal and external rotators.
Instructions: Begin by holding towel above head shoulder width apart (**A**). Try to pull towel down behind back first with left hand then right (**B** and **C**); you should end up in position **D**. Reverse order to get back to position **A**. Repeat 5 times.

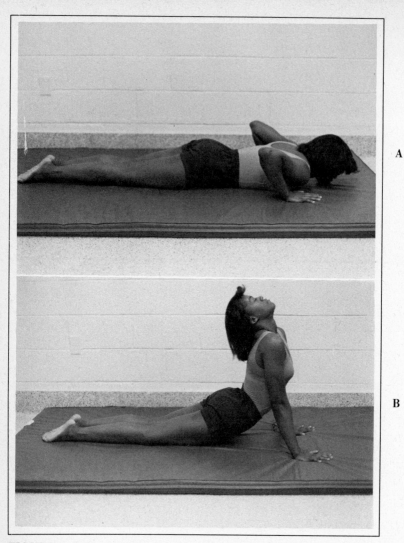

A

B

FIGURE 5-14

Exercise: Upper trunk stretch.
Muscles stretched: Muscles of respiration in thorax.
Instructions: Begin in push-up position. Extend upper trunk, keeping pelvis on the ground. Repeat 3 times, hold for 30 seconds. (Precaution: lower back pain.)

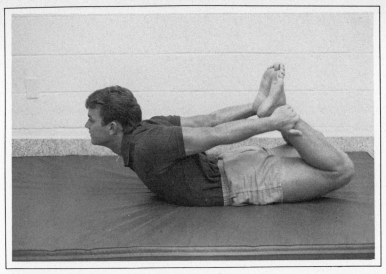

FIGURE 5-15

Exercise: Lower trunk stretcher.
Muscles stretched: Abdominals.
Instructions: Lift head up. Grab ankles from behind and pull. Repeat 3 times, hold for 30 seconds. (Precaution: lower back pain.)

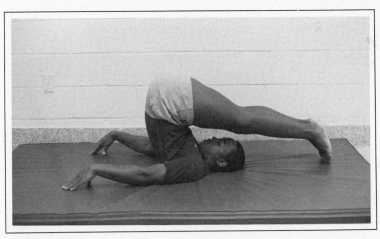

FIGURE 5-16

Exercise: Upper back and neck stretch
Muscles stretched: Extensors of cervical and thoracic vertebrae
Instructions: Lying on back, bring feet up over the head (it may help the stretch to bend your knees). Repeat 3 times, hold for 30 seconds.

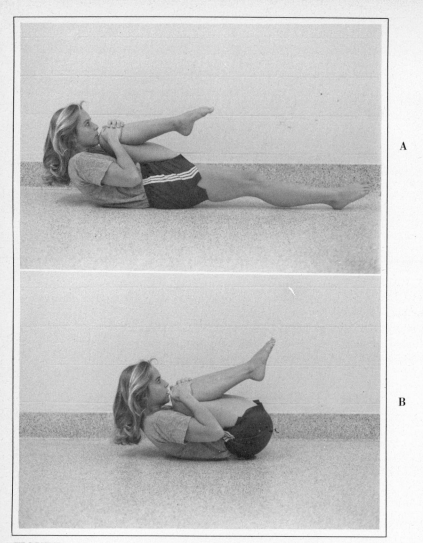

A

B

FIGURE 5-17

Williams flexion exercises. **A,** Touch chin to right knee and hold, then to left knee and hold. **B,** Touch chin to both knees and hold.

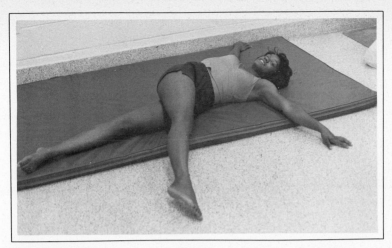

FIGURE 5-18

Exercise: Lower back twister.
Muscles stretched: Rotators of lower back and sacrum and hip abductors.
Instructions: Lying on back on edge of bed or table. Keep shoulders and arms flat on surface. Cross leg furthest from edge over the top and let it hang off the side of bed keeping knee straight; repeat with other leg. Repeat 3 times with each leg, hold for 30 seconds.

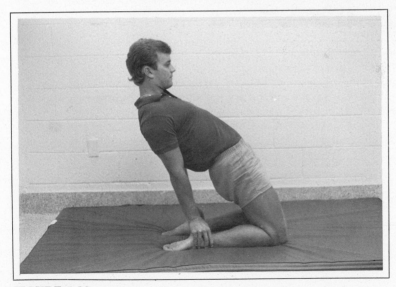

FIGURE 5-19

Exercise: Pelvic thrust.
Muscles stretched: Hip flexors.
Instructions: In a kneeling position, grasp ankles with hands. Thrust pelvis forward. Repeat 3 times, hold for 30 seconds.

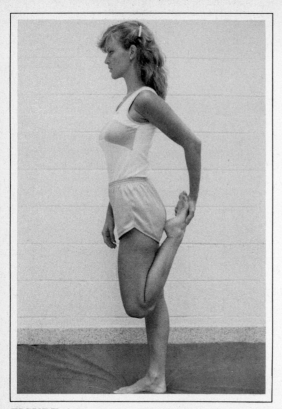

FIGURE 5-20

Exercise: Quadriceps stretch.
Muscles stretched: Knee extensors.
Instructions: In standing position, flex one leg behind you, grab ankle with
hand, and pull the foot up toward buttocks. Repeat with opposite leg. Repeat 3
times with each leg, hold for 30 seconds.

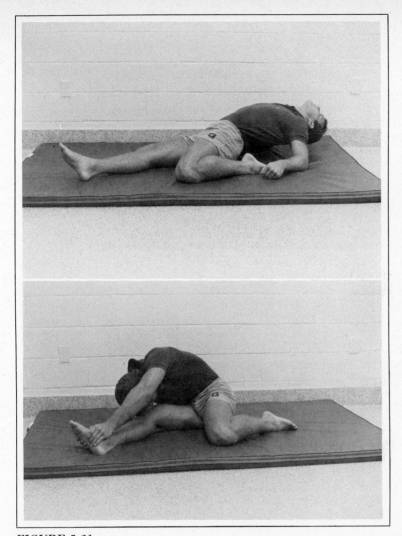

FIGURE 5-21

Exercise: Hurdler's stretch.
Muscles stretched: Hip extensors, knee flexors, and knee extensors.
Instructions: Sitting with one knee extended and the other flexed and to the side, lean forward, trying to touch head to knee. Lie back, trying to get flat on floor. Switch leg positions and repeat. Repeat entire sequence 3 times, hold for 30 seconds.

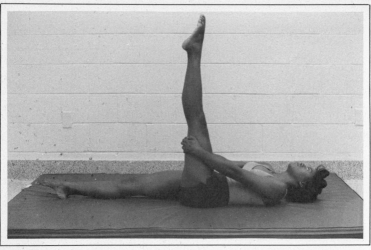

FIGURE 5-22

Exercise: Hamstring stretch.
Muscles stretched: Hip extensors and knee flexors.
Instructions: Lie flat on back. Raise one leg straight up with knee extended and
ankle flexed to 90°. Grab leg around calf and pull toward head; repeat with
opposite leg. Repeat 3 times with each leg, hold for 30 seconds.

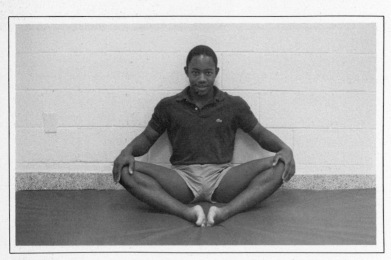

FIGURE 5-23

Exercise: Groin stretch.
Muscles stretched: Hip adductors in groin.
Instructions: Sit with knees flexed and soles of feet together. Try to press knees
flat on the floor; if they are flat to begin with, try to touch face to floor. Repeat
3 times, hold for 30 seconds.

A   B

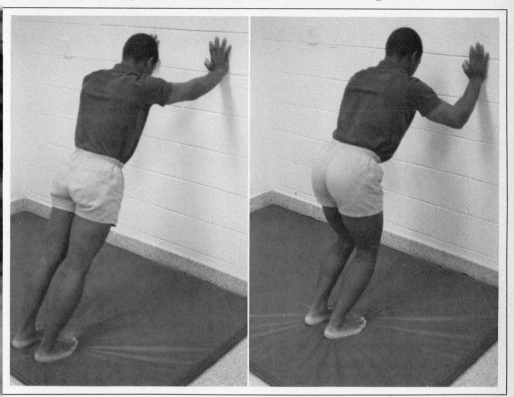

FIGURE 5-24

Exercise: Achilles heel cord stretch.
Muscles stretched: Foot plantar flexors; (A) Gastrocnemius, (B) soleus.
Instructions: **A,** Stand facing wall with toes pointing straight ahead and knees *straight*. Lean forward toward wall, keeping heels flat on floor. You should feel stretching high in calf. **B,** Stand facing wall with toes pointing straight ahead and knees *flexed*. Lean forward toward wall, keeping heels flat on floor. You should feel stretching low in calf. Repeat each position 3 times, hold each for 30 seconds.

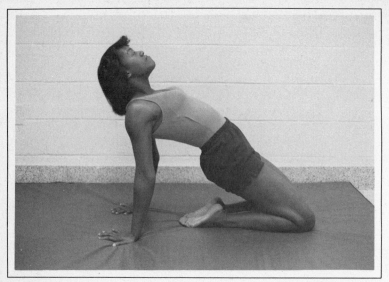

FIGURE 5-25

Exercise: Toe pointer.
Muscles stretched: Foot dorsiflexors.
Instructions: Sitting with knees flexed and feet directly under buttocks, lean backwards and take weight on hands. Repeat 3 times, hold for 30 seconds.

SUMMARY

- Flexibility is defined as the ability to move a joint or a series of joints smoothly through a full range of motion.
- Flexibility is specific to a given joint, and the term *good flexibility* implies that there are no joint abnormalities restricting movement.
- Flexibility may be limited by bone structure, fat, skin, connective tissue, ligaments, and muscles and tendons.
- Static flexibility refers to the degree to which a joint may be passively moved to the end points in the range of motion, whereas dynamic flexibility refers to movement through the midrange of motion resulting from active contraction.
- Measurement of joint flexibility is accomplished through the use of a goniometer.
- An agonist muscle is one that contracts to produce joint motion; the antagonist muscle is stretched with contraction of the agonist.
- Ballistic, static, and propriceptive neuromuscular facilitation (PNF) techniques have all been used as stretching techniques for improving flexibility.

- Each of these stretching techniques are based on the neurophysiologic phenomena involving the muscle spindles and Golgi tendon organs.
- PNF techniques appear to be the most effective in producing increases in flexibility.
- Stretching should be included as part of the warm-up as well as the cool-down periods for the purpose of preparing the muscles for what they are going to be asked to do and to prevent injury.
- Strength training, if done correctly through a full range of motion, will probably improve flexibility.

GLOSSARY

agonist muscle The muscle that contracts to produce a specific movement

antagonist muscle The muscle that stretches in response to contraction of the agonist muscle

autogenic inhibition A relaxation of the antagonist muscle mediated by the Golgi tendon organ

ballistic stretching Repetitive contractions of the agonist muscle used to produce quick bouncing stretches of the antagonist muscle

dynamic flexibility The degree to which a joint can be moved as a result of a muscle contraction, usually through the midrange of motion

flexibility The range of movement possible about a given joint or through a series of articulations

Golgi tendon organ A receptor important in the stretch reflex and sensitive to a change in muscle tension

goniometer A device used for measuring joint angles and range of motion

loose-jointed Descriptive term for a person whose joints have relatively slack ligaments and joint capsules, allowing excessive motion

muscle spindle A receptor important in the stretch reflex and sensitive to a change in muscle length

proprioceptive neuromuscular facilitation (PNF) A group of stretching techniques involving alternating contractions and relaxations of the antagonist muscle

reciprocal inhibition A condition in which contraction of the agonist causes a reflex relaxation in the antagonist muscle, allowing it to stretch and thus protecting it from injury

static flexibility The degree to which a joint may be passively moved to the endpoints in the range of motion

static stretching Passively stretching the antagonist muscle by placing it in a position of stretch and holding it for an extended period of time

stretch reflex Automatic response to stretch that involves a reflexive contraction of the muscle being stretched

synergistic muscles A group of muscles that work together to produce smooth, coordinated movement

REFERENCES

1. Basmajian, J. (1978). *Therapeutic exercise*. Baltimore: Williams & Wilkins.
2. Jensen, C., & Fisher, G. (1979). *Scientific basis of athletic conditioning*. Philadelphia: Lea & Febiger.
3. Knott, M., & Voss, P. (1965). *Proprioceptive neuromuscular facilitation*. New York: Harper & Row.
4. Miller, D., & Allen, E. (1982). *Fitness: A lifetime concept*. Minneapolis: Burgess.
5. Prentice, W. (1983). A comparison of static and PNF stretching for improvement of hip joint flexibility. *Athletic Training, 18*(1), 56-59.

SUGGESTED READINGS

Allsen, P., Harrison, J., & Vance, B. (1984). *Fitness for life: An individualized approach*. Dubuque, IA: William C. Brown.

Åstrand, P.O., & Rodahl, K. (1977). *Textbook of work physiology*. New York: McGraw-Hill.

Corbin, C., Linus, D., Lindsey, R., & Tolson, H. (1981). *Concepts in physical education with laboratories and experiments*. Dubuque, IA: William C. Brown.

deVries, H. (1980). *Physiology of exercise for physical education and athletics*. Dubuque, IA: William C. Brown.

Johnson, P., Updike, W., Schaefer, M., & Stolberg, D. (1975). *Sport, exercise and you*. New York: Holt, Rinehart, & Winston.

Miller, D., & Allen, E. (1982). *Fitness: A lifetime concept*. Minneapolis: Burgess.

Rasch, P., & Burke, R. (1974). *Kinesiology and applied anatomy*. Philadelphia: Lea & Febiger.

WEIGHT CONTROL

AND MAINTENANCE

OF BODY COMPOSITION

After completing this chapter, you will be able to:

- Discuss the problem of obesity in American society.
- Discuss the distinction between body weight and body composition.
- Discuss the principle of caloric balance and how to assess it.

- Discuss various methods for weight loss.
- Discuss the importance of life-style modification in weight loss.
- Discuss methods for losing and gaining weight.

It is safe to assume everyone in America has at one time or another been conscious of and concerned about their body weight. We have all spent a couple of extra minutes looking in a mirror at the "roll" that seems to be spreading around the midsection or at the extra layer of fat that seems to have suddenly appeared on the back of the thigh.

The battle by the American public against excess body fat has turned into a multibillion dollar industry whose products include highly specialized diet plans, exercise studios, and countless thousands of gimmicks and gadgets guaranteed to help you lose those extra pounds and inches.

It has been estimated that about 50 million adult men and 60 million adult women are overweight and need to do something to get rid of the excess weight.[1] The problem of *obesity* is truly epidemic.

Obesity has been attributed to several factors, including heredity, environment, and social influence. But the simple truth is that we all have a tendency to overeat. Perhaps it is more accurate to attribute the reasons for overeating to heredity, environment, and social influence.

For most of us, eating to the point of gorging ourselves has become a social event. It is virtually impossible to do anything socially with a group of people and not have something to eat or drink. Overeating easily tends to become a way of life. It doesn't take too long to realize that weight gain is a real problem. Too often the question changes from "am I gaining weight?" to "how overweight am I?"

How is ideal body weight determined? It is usually done by consulting age-related height and weight charts such as those published by life insurance companies. Unfortunately, these charts are inaccurate because they involve broad ranges and often fail to take individual body types into account. Because they are based solely on gross body weight, their accuracy is questionable. Thus health and performance may best be related to body composition rather than body weight.

BODY COMPOSITION

Body composition indicates the percentage of total body weight that is composed of fat tissue in relation to lean tissue. Assessment of body composition is perhaps a bit more difficult than simply stepping on a scale and measuring actual weight. However, body composition measurements are more accurate in attempting to determine precisely how much weight a person is capable of gaining or losing.

There are two factors that determine the amount of fat in the body: (1) the number of fat or *adipose* cells and (2) the size of the adipose cell. Proliferation of adipose cells begins at birth and continues to puberty. It is thought that after early adulthood the number of fat cells remains fixed, although there is some recent evidence to suggest that the number of cells is not necessarily fixed. Thus those adolescents who tend to be overweight develop a considerably greater number of adipose cells than those who have a somewhat normal body weight. In addition, adipose cell size also increases gradually to early adulthood and can increase or decrease as a function of caloric balance. In adults, weight loss or gain is primarily a function of the change in cell size, not cell number.

The adipose cell stores *triglyceride* (a form of liquid fat). This liquid fat moves in and out of the cell according to the energy needs of the body. The greater the amount of triglyceride contained in the adipose cell, the greater the amount of total body weight composed of fat. One pound of body fat is made up of approximately 3500 *calories* stored as triglyceride within the adipose cell. changes in body weight are almost entirely the result of changes in caloric balance.

Caloric balance = Number of calories taken − Number of calories expended
                         into the body in
                         the food

Calories may be expended by three different processes: (1) basal metabolism, (2) work (work may be defined as any activity which requires more energy than sleeping), and (3) excretion. Very simply, if more calories are taken in than burned off, there is a positive caloric balance resulting in weight gain. Conversely, weight loss results from a negative caloric balance in which more calories are burned off than are consumed.

Caloric balance is a function of the number of calories taken in regardless of whether the calories are contained in *fat, carbohydrate*, or *protein*. The *total* caloric value of the food is all that really matters. There are differences in the caloric content of these three foodstuffs. Proteins and carbohydrates each deliver four calories of energy per gram. One gram of fat delivers nine calories of energy. Therefore 1 pound of fat will contain a lot more calories than 1 pound of either protein or carbohydrate. Thus it becomes extremely important to consider the implications of caloric values when considering programs for weight loss or gain.

In behavioral terms, the number of calories in food ingested and the number of calories expended may both be modified. In general the problem is that caloric expenditure as a result of work decreases with age, although intake remains the same. Most people who gain weight are not very far off caloric balance, but over a period of months, or perhaps years, this adds up.

Weight increases frequently begin with a drop in physical activity that in many cases is associated with the end of formal schooling during the college years. Patterns of weight gain and loss established in childhood carry over into adulthood. Thus the old adage that "a fat baby is a healthy baby" is a misconception. Sometimes a fat baby grows up to be a fat adult.

The percentage of the total body weight that is fat is highly related to the level of physical activity. Persons who are fat tend to be most sedentary and to have a positive caloric balance.

Calculating Desirable Body Weight

1. Present weight	170	lbs
2. Present percent body fat (as was determined in previous activity)	16.19	%
3. Desired body fat	10	%
4. Percent body fat to be lost	6.19	% (no. 2 − No. 3)
5. Pounds to be lost	9.9	lbs (no. 4 × no. 1)
6. Desired weight	155.1	lbs (no. 1 − no. 5)

Alternative Method

$$\text{Desired body weight} = \frac{\text{Lean body weight}}{1 - \frac{\text{Percent body fat desired}}{100}}$$

Calculated desirable weight will often need to be increased by 3 to 5 pounds if either of the following stiuations is present: (1) If the person has been sedentary, or is involved in training to build muscle mass (therefore an allowance must be made for an increase in muscle mass) and (2) an allowance must be made if the person is growing.

What percentage of body fat is considered normal? The average college-age woman has between 20% and 25% of her total body weight made up of fat. The average college-age man has between 10% and 15% body fat. However, it must be indicated that persons who engage in strenuous physical activities on a regular basis tend to have a lower percent body fat. Male endurance athletes may get their fat percentage as low as 8% to 12%, and female endurance athletes may reach 10% to 15%. It is recommended that body fat percentage not go below 3% in men and 12% in women because below these percentages the internal organs tend to lose their protective padding of fat, potentially subjecting them to injury.[4]

ASSESSMENT OF BODY COMPOSITION

There are three ways to assess body composition: (1) underwater weighing, (2) measurement of body volume, and (3) measurement of skinfold thickness. The first two techniques require placing the subject in an underwater tank to determine the specific gravity of the body. These techniques are extremely accurate provided they are done properly. Unfortunately, the necessary equipment is expensive and generally not available to the coach or physical educator.

The third technique is based on the idea that about 50% of fat in the body is contained in the subcutaneous fat layers and is closely related to total fat. The remainder of fat in the body is found around organs and vessels and serves a shock-absorptive function. It involves measurement of the thickness of this subcutaneous fat layer using a skinfold caliper. The skinfold technique is probably the least accurate of the three methods; however, expertise in measurement is easily developed, and the time required for this technique is considerably less. It has been estimated that error in skinfold measurement is ±3% to 5%.[6] Men and women tend to develop fat in different areas of the body, and measurements must be taken in these areas at specified points. A number of different methods have been described for measuring body composition using the skinfold technique. However, to demonstrate a technique for measuring percent body fat, a technique proposed by McCardle and Katch,[6] which measures the triceps skinfold and the subscapular skinfold, will be used.

Calculating Percentage of Body Fat Using Skinfold Measurements

The triceps skinfold is measured over the right arm triceps muscle (back of the upper arm) halfway between the elbow and the tip of the shoulder (see Fig. 6-1).
1. Instruct the subject to let the arm hang limply at the side.
   Grasp the skinfold parallel to the vertical axis of the arm.
   Lift the skinfold away from the arm and make sure that no muscle tissue is caught in the fold.
2. Place the contact surfaces of the calipers ½ inch below the fingers. Release the lever arm on the caliper and allow pressure from the instrument to

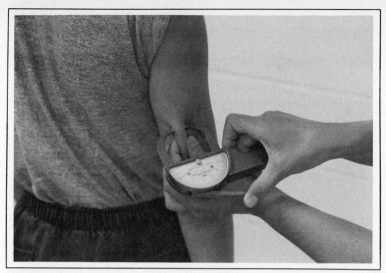

FIGURE 6-1

Measurement of triceps skinfold with a caliper.

bring the two sides together. The caliper pointer then indicates the skinfold thickness in millimeters (mm). Repeat and record the measurement two or three times; then record the average of these measurements.

The subscapular (below the shoulder blade) measurement site is approximately ½ inch below the inferior angle of the scapula in line with the natural cleavage lines of the skin (see Fig. 6-2).

1. Have the subject stand erect with shoulders thrust backward, arms at side. The point of the scapula (shoulder blade) located toward the spine should be obvious. Mark this point and then measure ½ inch below it and place a mark that will be the measurement site.
2. Standing behind the subject, use the thumb and index fingers and grasp the skinfold in the natural cleavage line (along imaginary diagonal line from elbow to neck). Lift the skinfold away from the scapula and shake it to make sure no muscle tissue is caught in the fold.
3. Use the caliper to measure as described previously.

Now that the measurements for the triceps and the subscapular skinfolds are known, percent body fat can be easily calculated using the following equations[3]:

Women: Percent body fat = $0.55(A) + 0.31(B) + 6.13$
$\qquad$ Where A = Triceps skinfold (mm)
$\qquad\qquad$ B = Subscapular skinfold (mm)

Men: Percent body fat = 0.43
$\qquad\qquad$ $(A) + 0.58(B) + 1.47$
$\qquad$ Where A = Triceps skinfold (mm)
$\qquad\qquad$ B = Subscapular skinfold (mm)

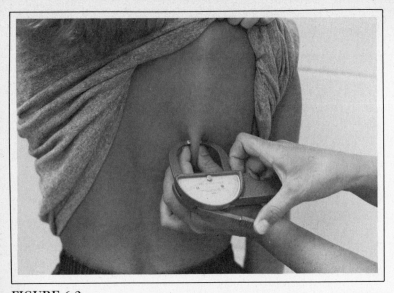

FIGURE 6-2

Measurement of subscapular skinfold with a caliper.

Some Common Sources of Error in Taking Skinfold Measurements

1. Midpoint incorrectly marked or measured
2. Arm not loose at side during measurement
3. Caliper placement too deep (muscle is involved)
4. Caliper placement too shallow (only skin grasped)
5. Caliper reading taken without marks in proper alignment
6. Skinfold grasp not maintained at time of caliper reading

Example: 20-year-old man: Triceps skinfold (A) = 14 mm
Subscapular skinfold (B) = 15 mm

Percent body fat = (0.43 × 14) + (0.58 × 15) + 1.4
Percent body fat = 6.02 + 8.7 + 1.47
Percent body fat = 16.19%

Once the percent of body fat has been calculated, it becomes relatively simple to determine a desired body weight. The example below is for a person who wanted to reach a 10% body fat level.

Worksheet For Calculating Percent Body Fat
From Skinfold Measurements

1. Triceps skinfold thickness _____ mm
2. Subscapular skinfold thickness _____ mm

Calculation of Percent Body Fat

Men

___ % Body fat = (0.43) × _____ + (0.58) × _____ + 1.47
                   Triceps skinfold   Subscapular skinfold

Women

___ % Body fat = (0.55) × _____ + (0.31) × _____ + 6.13
                   Triceps skinfold   Subscapular skinfold

Worksheet For Calculating Desired Body Weight

Method 1

1. _____ = _____ − _____
   % Body fat to be lost   Present % body fat   Desired % body fat

2. _____ = _____ × _____
   Pounds to be lost   % Body fat to be lost   Present body weight

3. _____ = _____ − _____
   Desired body weight   Present body weight   Pounds to be lost

Method 2

1. _____ = _____ × _____ % Body fat
   Fat weight   Present body weight   100

2. _____ = _____ − _____
   Fat-free weight   Present body weight   Fat weight

3. _____ = _____ ÷ _____
   Desired body weight   Fat-free weight   % Body fat desired

ESTIMATION OF CALORIC EXPENDITURE

Physical activity, whether it be competitive or recreational, results in an increased need for energy. The goal is to consume enough foodstuffs that contain the proper nutrients to satisfy tissue needs while also consuming sufficient caloric values of foods to meet increased metabolic energy demands. Generally, persons who participate in physical activity do not require additional nutrients other than those that may be obtained through a well-balanced diet; however, the additional calories required during physical activity should be obtained from foods that have a high nutrient value.

For persons who engage in some form of regular physical activity, the daily food consumption must match the energy expenditure or changes in body weight will occur. Thus some estimation of daily caloric expenditure is necessary to determine exact caloric needs. A reasonably accurate estimate of total energy needs may be based on determining the metabolic costs of various activities performed during the course of a day.

To do this it is first necessary to determine the energy you need to support your basal metabolism. This is the minimal level of energy required to sustain the body's vital functions, such as respiration, circulation, and maintenance of body temperature. The *basal metabolic rate (BMR)* is the rate at which kilocalories (kcal) are spent for these maintenance activities. The BMR is influenced by the following:

Age: In general, the younger the person is, the higher the BMR.

Body surface area: The greater the amount of body surface area, the higher the BMR. (It is important to note that surface area, not body weight, is the influencing factor.)

Sex: Men generally have a faster metabolic rate than women.

How to Determine Your Basal Metabolic Rate (BMR)

Fig. 6-3 should be used to determine your body surface area. Using a ruler, draw a straight line from your height to your weight. The point at which that line crosses the middle column shows your surface area in square meters (m^2). For example, for a 20-year-old man whose height is 6 feet and weight is 170 pounds (77.3 kg), his body surface area on the nomogram would be 1.99 m^2.

Next use Table 6-1 to find the factor for your sex and age, and multiply your surface area by this factor. For example, for a 20-year-old man, the factor is 39.9 kcal per square meter per hour (kcal/m^2/hr). This multiplied by 1.99 square meters equals 79.4 kcal/hr (39.9 kcal/m^2/hr $\times$ 1.99 m^2 = 79.4 kcal/hr). Now, multiply this product by 24 hours per day to find your BMR needs per day. Using our example:

$$79.4 \text{ kcal/hr} \times 24 \text{ hr/day} = 1906 \text{ kcal/day}$$

Therefore this 20-year-old man needs 1906 kcal/day to meet his basal metabolic requirements.

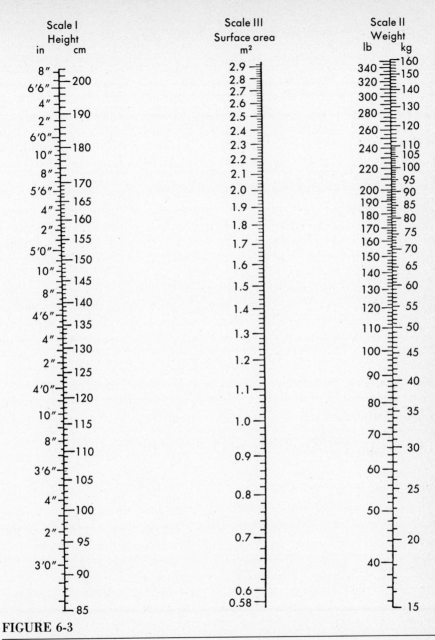

FIGURE 6-3

Estimating total body surface area. Locate your height on scale 1 and then your weight on scale 2. Using a straight edge, connect the appropriate points on scale 1 and scale 2. The intersection of this line with scale 3 is your body surface area.

TABLE 6-1   Basal Metabolic Rate According to Age and Sex

Age	BMR (kcal/m²/hr) Men	Women	Age	BMR (kcal/m²/hr) Men	Women
10	47.7	44.9	28	37.8	35.0
11	46.5	43.5	29	37.7	35.0
12	45.3	42.0	30	37.6	35.0
13	44.5	40.5	31	37.4	35.0
14	43.8	39.2	32	37.2	34.9
15	42.9	38.3	33	37.1	34.9
16	42.0	37.2	34	37.0	34.9
17	41.5	36.4	35	36.9	34.8
18	40.8	35.8	36	36.8	34.7
19	40.5	35.4	37	36.7	34.6
20	39.9	35.3	38	36.7	34.5
21	39.5	35.2	39	36.6	34.4
22	39.2	35.2	40-44	36.4	34.1
23	39.0	35.2	45-49	36.2	33.8
24	38.7	35.1	50-54	35.8	33.1
25	38.4	35.1	55-59	35.1	32.8
26	38.2	35.0	60-64	34.5	32.0
27	38.0	35.0	65-79	33.5	31.6
			70-74	32.7	31.1
			75 +	31.8	

Worksheet For Calculating Basal Metabolic Rate (BMR)

1. Estimated body surface area (see Fig. 6-3) = _____
2. BMR factor (see Table 6-1) = _____
3. _____ × _____ = _____
   Estimated body   BMR factor   BMR
   surface area
4. _____ = _____ × 24 hours
   Basal metabolic   BMR
   needs for 1 day

Once BMR has been determined, it is necessary to calculate energy requirements of all activities done in a 24-hour period.

There is a wide variation in energy output determined by the type, intensity, and duration of the physical activity. Specific energy expenditures may be determined by consulting charts that predict energy utilized in an activity based on (1) the time spent in each activity in minutes and (2) the metabolic costs of each activity in kcal/min/lb of body weight. For example, by consulting the energy expenditure chart in Table 6-3 for a 170-pound college man to play basketball for 1 hour, 642.6 (.063 kcal/min/lb × 170 lbs × 60 min) calories will be utilized. If you were to sit down and carefully calculate energy costs of all daily activities using Table 6-2 (such as sitting, walking, studying, and cooking) and add all these values together along with the BMR, the total daily caloric expenditure may be easily determined. For activities not listed in Table 6-2, use the general classifications found below.*

Activity	kcal/min/lb	Activity	kcal/min/lb
Very light (such as typing, driving)	.010	Moderate (such as dancing, bowling)	.032
Light (such as shopping)	.021	Heavy (such as football, running)	.062

Keep a 24-hour log (Table 6-3) of all activities—everything from eating breakfast to biking to school. It would be beneficial to do this for two separate days, choosing a day when the amount of physical exercise is fairly high and a day when it is fairly low. Then compare the differences in energy expenditure on those 2 days.

When recording your activities in the diary, specify the time of day, the activity, and the length of time spent in that activity. Every minute of the day should be accounted for (1440 minutes total).

Estimating Caloric Intake

A physically active person needs a sufficient number of calories to maintain body weight and composition as well as caloric balance. In general, nutritive requirements of those who are physically active correspond closely to the normal population.

It has been recommended that 15% of the total caloric intake be in the form of protein, 30% in fats, and the largest portion of the diet, 55%, should be some type of carbohydrate. The typical American diet contains far too much fat and too little carbohydrate.[5,6]

The diet should be separated into (1) the caloric requirements of normal daily activities and (2) the caloric requirements of the specific physical activities. Those calories required for normal daily activities should be acquired through

*Adapted from Food and Nutrition Board, National Research Council, (1974). *Recommended Dietary Allowances* (8th ed.). Washington, DC: National Academy of Sciences.

TABLE 6-2 Energy Expenditure in Various Activities

Activity	kcal/min/lb	Activity	kcal/min/lb
Archery	0.029	Judo	0.089
Basketball	0.063	Knitting (sewing)	0.010
Baseball	0.031	Marching, rapid	0.064
Boxing (sparring)	0.063	Painting (outside)	0.035
Canoeing (leisure)	0.020	Playing music (sitting)	0.018
Climbing hills (no load)	0.055	Racquetball	0.065
Cleaning	0.027	Running, cross-country	0.074
Cooking	0.020	Running, horizontal	0.061
Cycling		11 min 30 sec per mile	
5.5 mph	0.029	9 min per mile	0.088
9.4 mph	0.045	8 min per mile	0.094
Racing	0.077	7 min per mile	0.104
Dance (modern)	0.038	6 min per mile	0.114
Eating (sitting)	0.010	5 min 30 sec per mile	0.131
Farming		Scrubbing floors	0.050
Barn cleaning	0.061	Sailing	0.020
Driving tractor	0.017	Skiing	
Feeding animals	0.030	Snow, downhill	0.064
Forking straw bales	0.063	Water	0.052
Milking by machine	0.010	Skating (moderate)	0.038
Shoveling grain	0.039	Soccer	0.059
Field hockey	0.061	Squash	0.096
Fishing	0.028	Swimming	
Football	0.060	Backstroke	0.077
Gardening		Breast stroke	0.074
Digging	0.057	Crawl, fast	0.071
Mowing	0.051	Crawl, slow	0.058
Raking	0.024	Butterfly	0.078
Golf	0.039	Table tennis	0.031
Gymnastics	0.030	Tennis	0.050
Horseback riding		Volleyball	0.022
Galloping	0.062	Walking (normal pace)	0.036
Trotting	0.050	Wrestling	0.085
Walking	0.019	Writing (sitting)	0.013

Adapted from Bannister, W.E., & Brown, S.R. (1968). *The relative energy requirements of physical activity*. In H.B. Falls (Ed.), *Exercise physiology*. New York: Academic Press; Howley, E.T., & Glover, M.E. (1974). *Medicine in Science and Sports, 6*, 235-237; Passmore, R., & Durnin, J.V.G.A. (1955). *Physiological Reviews, 35*, 801-840.

TABLE 6-3   Daily Activities Log

Clock Time	Activity	Total Minutes Spent in Activity	kcal/min/lb per lb	Total kcal Expended
5:00-6:00	Basketball	60	.063 (per lb)	(.063 × 60 × 170) 642.6
6:00-7:00	Studying	60	.013 (per lb)	(.013 × 60 × 170) 133
7:00-7:30	Eating dinner	30	.010 (per lb)	(.010 × 30 × 170) 51
11:00-7:00	Sleeping*	8 hours	0.00 (per lb)	0.00
TOTAL		1440 min or 24 hr		

*Sleep is assumed to be at the basal level of activity; therefore it is figured into the basal metabolic caloric needs that you have already calculated in the first part of this exercise.

the specified percentages of foodstuffs. The extra calories necessary for increased physical activity should be obtained by increasing the percentage of carbohydrates consumed.

Determining precise caloric intake requires consultation of Appendix A, which indicates the nutritive value of commonly used foods. These charts identify specific foods and indicate the number of calories in a specified serving size. For example, if you consult Appendix A you will see that 1 ounce of cheddar cheese contains 115 calories.

A daily food intake log such as the one in Table 6-4 can be kept over a period of several days to let you know about how many calories are being consumed on the average each day. College students are notorious for skipping meals and eating multiple snacks. Thus it is important to record everything you consume during the entire 24-hour period. Don't neglect to record extras such as mustard and pickles that you include on a hamburger. Table 6-4 is a good example of how the daily food intake log should be filled out. Those columns that deal with hunger level and mood may help you to determine what causes you to eat when you do.

As with caloric expenditure, adding up the caloric values of all foods consumed during a 24-hour period can give you a reasonably accurate estimate of daily caloric intake.

Assessing Caloric Balance

If the daily logs for estimating caloric intake and caloric expenditure have been accurately kept, it will be relatively simple to compare the total caloric values to determine whether you are in caloric balance.

It is not easy for a college student to maintain caloric balance on a daily basis. One reason for this is that the schedule never seems to be the same from one day to the next. Eating habits are generally inconsistent, as are times spent in physical activity. Estimations of caloric intake for college students range between 1000 and 5000 calories per day. Estimations of caloric expenditure range between 2200 and 4400 calories for the average student (Table 6-5). Energy

TABLE 6-4 Daily Food Intake Log

Time	Food Eaten	Amount	No. of Calories	How Cooked	Meal or Snack	Hunger Level* (0-3)	Activity and Location While Eating	Mood† (1-3)
Breakfast 8:00 AM	Orange juice	¾ cup	80	Frozen	M	3	Talking/kitchen (home)	1
	Milk (whole)	16 oz	300		M	3	Same	1
	Cheerios	1¼ cup	30		M	3	Same	1
	Sugar	1 tsp	70		M	3	Same	1
10:30	Apple	1	90		S	2	School	2
Lunch 12:30 PM	Cheese-burger	1	580	Fried	M	3	School cafeteria	2
	French fries	1 sm	330	Fried	M	3	Same	2
	Fruit punch	16 oz	140		M	3	Same	2
Dinner 6:30 PM	Pork chop	3 oz	310	Broiled	M	1	Dining room Family talking	2
	Mashed po-tatoes	1 cup	195	Boiled	M	1	Same	2
	Butter	2 tsp	200	Buttered	M	1	Same	2
	Peas, canned	½ cup	90	Boiled	M	1	Same	2
	Milk	2 cups	300		M	1	Same	2
	Chocolate cake	1 piece (2 in)	200		M	1	Same	2
10:00 PM	Chocolate cake	1 piece (2 in)	200		S	1	My room studying	3
	Milk	8 oz	150		S	1	Same	3
		TOTAL	3265					

*Hunger: 0, none; 3, maximum.
†Mood: 1, Good, happy; 2, fair, "OK"; 3, upset.

Worksheet For Calculating Daily Energy Expenditure

| Clock Time | Daily Activities Log | | | Date: |
	Activity (see Table 6-2)	Total Minutes Spent in Activity	kcal/min/lb	Total kcal Expended

Total calories expended during activities _____

Add calories expended in basal metabolism _____

Total calories expended _____

Worksheet For Calculating Daily Calorie Intake

Daily Food Intake Log

Date:

Time	Food Eaten	Amount	No. of Calories	How Cooked	Meal or Snack	Hunger Level (0-3)	Activity and Location When Eating	Mood (1-3)

Total number of calories consumed =

TABLE 6-5   Daily Rates of Energy Expenditure by Persons with Various Occupations

Occupation	Energy Expenditure (kcal/day)		
	Mean	Minimal	Maximal
Men			
Elderly retired	2330	1750	2810
Office workers	2520	1820	3270
Laboratory technicians	2840	2240	3820
Elderly industrial workers	2840	2180	3710
University students	2930	2270	4410
Building workers	3000	2440	3730
Steel workers	3280	2600	3960
Army cadets	3490	2990	4100
Farmers	3550	2450	4670
Coal miners	3660	2970	4560
Forestry workers	3670	2860	4600
Women			
Elderly housewives	1990	1490	2410
Middle-aged housewives	2090	1760	2320
Laboratory technicians	2130	1340	2540
Assistants in department stores	2250	1820	2850
University students	2290	2090	2500
Factory workers	2320	1970	2980
Bakery workers	2510	1980	3390

Adapted from Åstrand & Rodahl, (1977). *Textbook of work physiology*. New York: McGraw-Hill.

Worksheet For Estimating Caloric Balance

_____ — _____ = _____

Number of calories   Number of calories expended   Caloric balance
consumed   during activities

If the caloric balance is positive, body weight will tend to increase.
If the caloric balance is negative, body weight will tend to decrease.

demands will be considerably higher in those who are active but particularly higher in endurance-type athletes, who may require as many as 7000 calories.

If you desire to lose weight, you must put yourself in negative caloric balance by burning off more calories than you take in. If you want to gain weight, you must consume more calories than you expend.

1800 kcal Sample Meal Pattern

Breakfast

¾ c Orange juice
¾ c Cereal
8 oz Low-fat milk
1 Slice whole wheat toast with 1 tsp margarine
Total kcal = 415

Lunch

1 Peanut butter and banana sandwich:
(2 Slices bread)
(1 Tbsp peanut butter)
(½ Banana)
5-7 Carrot sticks
1 Peach
8 oz Low-fat milk
Total kcal = 485

Dinner

1 Hamburger patty (4 oz) with 1 hamburger bun
1 c Tossed green salad with 1 Tbsp dressing
4 oz Low-fat milk
½ c Ice cream
Total kcal = 715

Total kcal for day = 1850

Snack

1 Apple
Total kcal = 80

Snack

20 Grapes
2 Graham crackers
Total kcal = 155

METHODS OF WEIGHT LOSS

There are several ways that we can go about losing weight. First, the food intake may be decreased by dieting. Secondly, the caloric expenditure may be increased by increasing the amount of physical exercise. Finally, some combination of dietary caloric restriction and increase in caloric expenditure through exercise can also be attempted.

Weight loss through dieting alone is very difficult, primarily because of the social values associated with eating. Through dieting, 35% to 45% of the weight decrease results from a loss of lean tissue. Obviously in any weight-loss program the person is interested in losing fat, not lean, tissue. The boxes above provides examples of an extremely low 1800 calorie per day diet and a moderate 2400 calorie per day diet.

The weight lost through exercise involves an 80% to 90% loss of fat tissue with almost no loss of lean tissue. Physical activity in adolescence prevents

2400 kcal Sample Meal Pattern

Breakfast

¾ c Orange juice
1 Slice toast with 1 oz. cheese
¾ c Cereal
4 oz Low-fat milk
Total kcal = 420

Snack

1 Banana
Total kcal = 100

Lunch

1 Slice cheese pizza
1 Tossed green salad with 1 Tbsp dressing
8 oz Low-fat milk
Total kcal = 425

Snack

½ c Raisin/peanut mix
½ c Apple juice
Total kcal = 360

Dinner

1 c Macaroni and cheese
½ c Lima beans
1 c Tomato and cucumber slices with 1 Tbsp dressing
1 Dinner roll with 1 tsp Margarine
8 oz Low-fat milk
Total kcal = 895

Snack

½ c Sherbet
1 Granola cookie
Total kcal = 185

Total kcal for day = 2385

---

formation of adipose tissue in both boys and girls and results in an increase in lean body weight. Physical activity in the college-age adult, particularly in the sedentary college student, may result in an initial weight gain as a result of increases in muscle tissue, which is more dense and has greater weight than fat tissue. Thus for the young adult, initial attempts at weight loss through exercise may be frustrating.

Weight loss through exercise alone is almost as difficult as losing weight through dieting. People trying to exercise solely for the purpose of losing weight will not likely stick with an exercise program for a long time. However, it is essential to realize that physical exercise will not only result in weight reduction but may also enhance cardiorespiratory endurance, improve strength, and increase flexibility. For this reason, exercise has some distinct advantages over dieting in any weight-loss program.

Undoubtedly the most efficient method of decreasing that percentage of body weight that is fat is through some combination of diet and exercise. The following section takes a look at a specific plan.

Worksheet For Monitoring Weekly Weight Loss

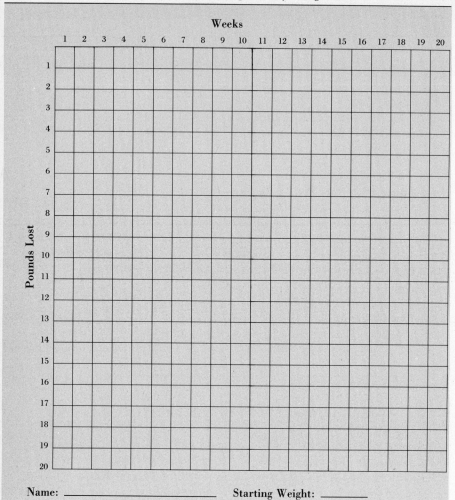

Name: _____   **Starting Weight:** _____

Life-style Modification and Weight Loss

Technology has allowed the American life-style to become increasingly sedentary. The purpose of the many devices that make work easier is to provide additional leisure time for various recreational pursuits. The problem is that there are other devices available to us that seem to be converting recreational pursuits into sedentary activities. For example, the golf cart has speeded up the game but has taken most of the physical activity out of the sport. Video games are great for improving reaction times and the powers of mental concentration, but there are few training effects from pressing a button or moving a joystick.

Most college graduates accept jobs that involve the use of the mind rather than the back. They do very little in the work environment that involves any type of physical exercise. We all try to park as close to the entrance of a building as possible so we don't waste time walking back and forth. And it is very easy to hop on an escalator or an elevator rather than walking up a flight of stairs.

Our society is also very socially oriented. Most of us enjoy eating with other people, and we frequently have lunch with coworkers or dinner with neighbors. These social eating and drinking habits make dieting extremely difficult.

Most people are concerned about controlling their weight. But because of the quality of life many of us enjoy, weight control becomes an almost impossible dream. Most people who gain weight are not far off their caloric balance, and thus gains tend to occur gradually over a period of time. All those little times we cheat on how much we eat or are a bit lazy and choose the easiest, less strenuous activity are slowly reflected as we stand assessing our form in front of a mirror.

How do you best go about controlling your weight? Most people tend to panic about their weight and either go on starvation diets or become exercise fanatics. Neither approach is particularly enjoyable or productive over a long period of time.

The key to being able to maintain your weight is to have the willpower to moderately alter your life-style so that caloric balance can be attained. Little things, no matter how insignificant they seem, add up over time. Parking the car in a lot as far away from the door as possible and walking up or down stairs instead of riding an elevator will all moderately increase caloric expenditure. Having one less roll or turning down that extra slice of meat will cause a moderate reduction in caloric intake. When these two factors are combined, weight control becomes easy.

The point is that you have to make a commitment to changing little things in your life-style that cause you to both burn off additional calories and also to consume fewer calories. The cumulative effects of these slight modifications will make weight control an integral part of your life-style rather than a deterrent to your life-style.

A moderate caloric restriction combined with a moderate increase in caloric expenditure will result in a negative caloric balance. This method is relatively fast and easy compared with either of the others because habits are being moderately changed. If caloric intake is reduced by 200 to 300 calories per day, and caloric expenditure is increased by 200 to 300 calories per day, over a 7-day period this will result in a loss of approximately 3500 calories, or 1 pound of body fat.

In any weight-loss program the "long-haul" approach must be emphasized. It generally takes a long time to put on extra weight, and there is no reason to expect that true loss of excess body fat can be accomplished in a relatively short time. Positive reinforcement is most beneficial to anyone attempting to lose weight.

Weight Loss Gimmicks

People will resort to almost anything in a desperate effort to lose weight. Each year, Americans spend billions of dollars trying to find the easiest possible way to lose weight quickly. It is easy to be lured into investing money in quick weight-loss programs that claim to require little or no effort when advertisements display physically attractive men and women claiming to have lost dozens of pounds on a particular plan.

All of us are bombarded on a daily basis with advertisements of specialized diets, diet pills, powdered drinks, rubberized suits that let you sit around and sweat off weight, electrical devices that claim to burn off calories by making the muscles contract, and mechanical devices that shake, vibrate, or roll fat off.

The fact is that there is no quick or easy method of weight loss short of starvation. It all comes down to the concept of caloric balance. To lose weight, more calories must be burned off than are taken in.

Perhaps the biggest problem with any fad or gimmick for weight loss is that sooner or later you tend to become bored and lose interest. Whatever weight may have been lost is eventually regained because you tend to return to the same life-style of eating and relatively sedentary living that caused you to gain the weight in the first place.

Guidelines for Weight Loss

The American College of Sports Medicine has made the following recommendations regarding weight loss[2]:

1. Prolonged fasting and diet programs that severely restrict caloric intake are scientifically undesirable and can be medically dangerous.
2. Fasting and diet programs that severely restrict caloric intake result in the loss of large amounts of water, electrolytes, minerals, glycogen stores, and other fat-free tissue (including proteins within fat-free tissues), with minimal amounts of fat loss.
3. Mild calorie restriction (500-1000 kcal less than the usual daily intake) results in a smaller loss of water, electrolytes, minerals, and other fat-free tissue, and is less likely to cause malnutrition.

4. Dynamic exercise of large muscles helps to maintain fat-free tissue, including muscle mass and bone density, and results in losses of body weight. Weight loss resulting from an increase in energy expenditure is primarily in the form of fat weight.

5. A nutritionally sound diet resulting in mild calorie restriction coupled with an endurance exercise program along with behavioral modification of existing eating habits is recommended for weight reduction. The rate of sustained weight loss should not exceed 1 kg (2 lb.) per week.

6. To maintain proper weight control and optimal body fat levels, a lifetime commitment to proper eating habits and regular physical activity is required.

METHODS FOR GAINING WEIGHT

The aim of a weight-gaining program should be to increase lean body mass, that is, muscle, as opposed to body fat. Muscle mass can be increased only by muscle work combined with an appropriate increase in dietary intake. It cannot be increased by the intake of any special food, vitamin, drug or hormone.

The recommended rate of weight gain is approximately 1 to 2 pounds per week. Each pound of lean body mass that is gained represents a positive caloric balance. This is an intake in excess of expenditure of approximately 2500 kcal. One pound of fat represents the equivalent of 3500 kcal; lean body tissue contains less fat, more protein and more water, and represents approximately 2500 kcal. To gain 1 pound of muscle, an excess of approximately 2500 kcal is needed; to lose 1 pound of fat, approximately 3500 kcal must be expended in activities in excess of intake. Adding 500 to 1000 kcal daily to the usual diet will provide the energy needs of gaining 1 to 2 pounds per week and fuel the increased energy expenditure of the muscle-training program. Weight training must be part of the program. Otherwise the excess intake of energy will be converted to fat.

The following suggestions are offered for the college student concerned about an appropriate weight-gaining program[2]:

1. Set a reasonable goal. An exercise program should begin in advance of the competing season. *Rapid weight gain indicates increase in fat, not muscle.*

2. Follow an exercise program prescribed by a professional and designed to develop the desired muscles (see Chapter 4).

3. Determine the usual caloric intake, then estimate the additional calories needed daily to gain weight.

   For a young active male athlete, 5000 to 7000 kcal/day may be needed to gain weight. This large intake of food is often difficult to work into the busy schedules of college students. Therefore it is important to plan both the composition and timing of meals and snacks.

   The diet should be based on the five food groups (see Chapter 7), with additional calories obtained from larger portions and from the miscella-

High-Calorie Sample Meal Pattern
(Approximately 6000 kcal)

Breakfast

¾ c Orange juice
1 c Hot cereal with 2 tsp sugar
1 Egg, fried
1 Slice whole wheat toast with:
  1 tsp Margarine
  1 tsp Jelly
8 oz Milk (whole)
Total kcal = 620

Lunch

1 Ham and cheese sandwich:
  2 Slices bread
  1 oz Cheese
  1 oz Ham
  1 Tbsp Mayonnaise
1 Serving french fries
1 c Tossed green salad with 2 Tbsp
Dressing
10 oz Chocolate milkshake
4 Oatmeal cookies

Dinner

2 Pieces baked chicken (7 oz)
1 c Rice with 1 tsp margarine
1 c Collard greens
½ c Candied sweet potatoes
2 Pieces cornbread with 1 Tbsp margarine
8 oz Milk (whole)
1 Slice apple pie
Total kcal = 1760

Total kcal for day = 5930

Snack

1 Peanut butter and jelly sandwich:
  2 Slices bread
  2 Tbsp Peanut butter
  2 tsp Jelly
½ c Raisins
1 c Apple juice
Total kcal = 680

Snack

1 Bagel with:
  2 tsp Margarine
  2 Tbsp Cream cheese
1 c Sweetened applesauce
¾ c Grape juice
Total kcal = 710

Snack

1 Banana
½ c Peanuts
1 c Chocolate milk (whole)
Total kcal = 720

neous fifth food group. (Calories obtained from the fifth food group, which includes fats and sugars, should be kept in moderation.) It is recommended that the diet contain less than 35% of calories as fat and that the fat component in the diet be low in animal fats and cholesterol. The box above is an example of a high-calorie diet.

A relatively small amount of additional protein is needed for muscular development. The daily protein intake of most athletes is more than sufficient to meet this requirement; *therefore protein supplements are not necessary*. Under unusual circumstances protein supplements may have undesirable side effects.

4. Monitor body weight weekly to assure a gradual weight gain. Measuring skinfold thickness regularly will detect any increases in body fat. An increase in the skinfold thickness indicates a need for a reduction in caloric intake or an increase in training, or both, until it is demonstrated that the percentage of body fat is not increasing.

SUMMARY

- Body composition indicates the percentage of total body weight that is composed of fat tissue vs. the percentage composed of lean tissue.
- The size and number of adipose cells determine percent body fat.
- Measurement of percent body fat can be done by measuring the thickness of the subcutaneous fat with a skinfold caliper at specific areas.
- Changes in body weight are caused almost entirely by a change in caloric balance, which is a function of the number of calories taken in and the number of calories expended.
- Caloric expenditure and caloric intake may be calculated by maintaining accurate records of the number of calories expended in activities performed during the course of a day as well as the number of calories consumed in the diet.
- Weight can be lost by either increasing caloric expenditure through exercise or by decreasing caloric intake through dieting; however, the recommended technique for losing weight involves a combination of moderate caloric restriction and a moderate increase in physical exercise during the course of each day.
- Weight loss should be accomplished over a long period of time. Realistically, no more than about 2 pounds of actual body weight should be lost during a single week.
- Weight gain may be accomplished by increasing caloric intake and engaging in a weight-training program.

GLOSSARY

adipose Another term for fat tissue

basal metabolic rate (BMR) The minimum rate of energy utilization necessary to maintain essential body functions during a resting state

body composition The percentage of total body weight composed of fat tissue vs. the percentage of total body weight composed of lean tissue

calorie A unit of measure that indicates the amount of energy production in the body

carbohydrates The primary food substance responsible for providing energy during high-intensity muscular activity

fat Another primary food substance that can provide energy during long-term endurance activities

lean body weight The amount of total body weight composed of nonfat tissue (such as bone, muscle, or viscera)

obesity An excessive amount of body fat

protein A primary food source that provides the basic building components for the cells and relatively small amounts of energy

triglyceride A form of liquid fat stored in the adipose cell

REFERENCES

1. Abraham, S., & Johnson, C. (1980). Prevalance of severe obesity in adults in the United States. *American Journal of Clinical Nutrition, 33,*364.
2. American College of Sports Medicine. (1983). Proper and improper weight loss programs. *Medicine and Science in Sports Exercise, 15,*9-13.
3. Anderson, J., Burge, J., DeWalt, J., Earey, P., Hastedt, P., & Prentice, W. (1982). *Teens, foods, fitness and sports.* Raleigh, NC: North Carolina Department of Public Instruction.
4. Behnke, R., & Wilmore, J. (1974). *Evaluation and regulation of body build and composition.* Englewood Cliffs, NJ: Prentice-Hall.
5. Brozek, J. (1965). *Human body composition approaches and applications.* Oxford:Pergamon Press.
6. Jensen, C., & Fisher, G. *Scientific basis of athletic conditioning.* Philadelphia:Lea & Febiger.

SUGGESTED READINGS

Åstrand, P.O., & Rodahl, K. (1977). *Textbook of work physiology.* New York:McGraw-Hill.

Bannister, W., & Brown, S. (1968). The relative energy requirements of physical activity. In H. B. Falls, (Ed.). *Exercise physiology.* New York:Academic Press.

deVries, H. (1980). *Physiology of exercise for physical education and athletics.* Dubuque, IA: William C. Brown.

Ferguson, J.M. (1976). *Learning to eat: Behavior modification for weight control.* Palo Alto, CA: Bull Publishing.

Fox, E. (1984). *Sport physiology.* New York:CBS College Publishing.

Getchell, B. (1983). *Physical fitness: A way of life.* New York:John Wiley & Sons.

Howley, E., & Glover, M. (1974). The caloric costs of running and walking one mile for men and women. *Medicine and Science in Sports, 6,*235-37.

McCardle, W., Katch, F., & Katch, V. (1981). *Exercise physiology, energy, nutrition, and human performance.* Philadelphia: Lea & Febiger.

Passmore, R., & Durnin, J. (1955). Human energy expenditure. *Physiological Reviews, 35,* 801-840.

Stuart, R., & Davis, B. *Slim chance in a fat world: Behavioral control of obesity.* Champaign, IL:Research Press.

BASIC NUTRITION

AND FITNESS

After completing this chapter, you will be able to:

- Describe what is meant by normal nutrition.
- Identify the function of the three basic foodstuffs: carbohydrates, fats, and proteins.
- Identify the most common vitamins and minerals and their relation to the specific body functions.
- Describe the importance of water as an essential unit.
- Explain the relationship of nutrition to physical performance.
- Discuss eating disorders.

The relation of nutrition, diet, and weight control to exercise is certainly an important aspect of any program involving physical activity. Unfortunately, all of us have been subjected to misconceptions, fads, and in many cases superstitions regarding nutrition that affect the dietary habits of the general population. There are more fallacies associated with the role of nutrition in a training program than in any other area.

Many people involved with physical activity have associated successful performance with the consumption of special foods or supplements. If a person is performing well, there may be a reluctance to change dietary habits regardless of whether the diet is physiologically beneficial to overall health. There is no question that the psychologic aspect of allowing a person to eat whatever he or she is most comfortable with can greatly affect performance. The problem is that these eating habits tend to become accepted as beneficial and may become traditional when in fact they may be physiologically detrimental to athletic performance. Thus there is a tendency for many nutrition "experts" to disseminate nutritional information based on traditional rather than experimental information.

We hope that by presenting very basic nutritional information, some of these fallacies can be dismissed.

NORMAL NUTRITION

Normal nutrition is concerned with the daily food requirements for a normal healthy person for the purpose of:
- Production of energy for muscular work
- Growth and synthesis of body material
- Providing material for tissue maintenance and repair
- Regulation of body process

A number of factors, including age, sex, physical size, growth rate, environment, pregnancy, convalescence, and physical training will likely cause variation in the food requirements and recommendations in the tables of suggested national standards.

Dietary recommendations vary from country to country because of the occurrence of deficiency diseases or malnutrition. Fortunately in the United States most persons, with limited exceptions, have an opportunity to consume a relatively well-balanced and nutritionally sound diet. Table 7-1 indicates the recommended daily allowances for nutrient consumption.

THE THREE BASIC FOODSTUFFS

The three basic foodstuffs—carbohydrates, fats, and proteins—provide the energy for muscular work.

Carbohydrates. Carbohydrates are composed of carbon, hydrogen, and oxygen. The combination of these three elements to form either sugars or starches provides a primary source of fuel for the body. Sugar products include sugars, syrups, and molasses. Starches include flour and flour products, bread, crackers, cereals, potatoes, and other starchy vegetables.

Fats. Although fats are composed of the same elements as carbohydrates, their composition is more complex. Whereas the carbohydrates are almost exclusively derived from plants, fats are the primary storage material of animals and thus are obtained to a large extent from animal products. Certain essential fatty acids are synthesized slowly or not at all in the animal body, and it is recommended that people obtain some of their fats from plant products that contain these essential substances. Three functions of fat in the diet are (1) as a highly concentrated form of fuel, (2) for flavoring of foods, and (3) as a carrier of fat-soluble vitamins. Some primary sources of fat are butter, lard, margarine, meat fats, bacon, oils, nuts, cheese, and cream, and from the plant products, whole wheat, soybeans, peanut oil, and olive oil.

TABLE 7-1 Dietary Recommendations for College Students

Nutrient	Men			Women		
	11-14	15-18	19-22	11-14	15-18	19-22

Recommended Dietary Allowances, 1980

Nutrient	11-14	15-18	19-22	11-14	15-18	19-22
Energy (kcal)*	2700	2800	2900	2200	2100	2100
Protein (gm)	45	56	56	46	46	44
Vitamin (A,RE) (IU)†	1000	1000	1000	800	800	800
	(5000)	(5000)	(5000)	(4000)	(4000)	(4000)
Vitamin D (μg)	10	10	7.5	10	10	7.5
Vitamin E (mg)	8	10	10	8	8	8
Vitamin C (mg)	50	60	60	50	60	60
Thiamine (mg)	1.4	1.4	1.5	1.1	1.1	1.1
Riboflavin (mg)	1.6	1.7	1.7	1.3	1.3	1.3
Niacin (mg)	18	18	19	15	14	14
Vitamin B_6 (mg)	1.8	2.0	2.2	1.8	2	2
Folacin (μg)	400	400	400	400	400	400
Vitamin B_{12} (μg)	3	3	3	3	3	3
Calcium (mg)	1200	1200	800	1200	1200	800
Phosphorus (mg)	1200	1200	800	1200	1200	800
Magnesium (mg)	350	400	350	300	300	300
Iron (mg)	18	18	10	18	18	18
Zinc (mg)	15	15	15	15	15	15
Iodine (μg)	150	150	150	150	150	150

Estimated Safe and Adequate Daily Dietary Intakes, Food and Nutrition Board

Nutrient	
Vitamin K (μg)	50-100
Biotin (μg)	100-200
Pantothenic acid (mg)	4-7
Copper (mg)	2-3
Manganese (mg)	2.5-5
Fluoride (mg)	1.5-2.5
Chromium (mg)	.05-.2
Selenium (mg)	.05-.2
Molybdenum (mg)	.15-.5
Sodium (mg)	900-2700
Potassium (mg)	1525-4575
Chloride (mg)	1400-4200

Adapted from Food and Nutrition Board, National Research Council. (1980). *Recommended Dietary Allowances* (9th ed.). Washington, DC: National Academy of Sciences.

*Energy recommendations represent average approximate needs; actual energy needs will vary depending on degree of physical activity.

†RE, Retinol equivalent; until recently, vitamin A content in foods has been expressed as international units (IU), one IU being equivalent to 0.3 μg of retinol or 0.6 μg B-carotene. For the purposes of this discussion, the conversion factor of 1 RE = 5 IU will be used.

Proteins. In addition to supplying carbon, hydrogen, and oxygen, the proteins also provide our only source of nitrogen and small amounts of sulfur. Some of the proteins also provide iron and phosphorus. The proteins are found in adequate amounts in both plants and animals and are essential constituents of the cells of all living tissues. Proteins are necessary for the body to build new tissues and repair old, worn-out tissues.

Proteins are not stored in the body as are the carbohydrates and fats but must be supplied regularly by eating animal or plant foods that contain them. Proteins are also needed in manufacturing regulating substances that control the complex functioning of the body. Excess amounts of protein are converted and utilized as a source of energy. Proteins are made up of substances called *amino acids*. These amino acids are needed by the body to manufacture the proteins required for growth and repair of tissues. Therefore the greatest demand for proteins comes during the periods of most rapid growth. Sources of proteins include a variety of meats, fowl, fish, soybeans, milk, eggs, cheese, legumes, bread, cereals, and nuts.

PRODUCTION OF ENERGY FROM THREE FOODSTUFFS

Every function of the human body requires energy. Consumption of fats, carbohydrates, or proteins provides the energy necessary for all types and intensities of physical activity. Therefore it is important to understand (1) how these foodstuffs are metabolized and (2) how energy is generated to meet the increased demands of exercise, depending on the particular type of activity.

The three basic foodstuffs, carbohydrates, fats, and proteins, are all large molecular complexes composed of various combinations of carbon, hydrogen, oxygen, and, in the case of protein, nitrogen. All three provide a source of energy during exercise as well as a role in the function and maintenance of body tissues. In most forms of exercise, both carbohydrates and fats contribute in varying amounts to the energy used during rest and submaximal exertion.

Carbohydrates provide the major energy source for muscular contraction. They are stored in the resting muscle and in the liver as glycogen and in the blood as glucose. Protein may be converted into glycogen and utilized to provide necessary energy to working muscle. Each gram of carbohydrate supplies 4 calories of energy. Carbohydrates are easily converted to glucose and thus are readily used in high-intensity activities. The harder the work, the greater the carbohydrate use.

Fat represents an ideal storage form for energy. Each gram of fat yields 9 calories. The longer the duration of an activity, the greater the amount of fat being used. Fat is also used more readily when the resting supply of muscle and liver glycogen is depleted.

Proteins contain the essential amino acids needed for maintenance of cell structure and the synthesis of body tissues. The exact role of proteins as an energy source at this point is unclear. It has long been accepted that protein is not used in any substantial amount as an energy source, although recent research has indicated that protein metabolism may provide greater quantities of energy in certain situations than was originally thought.[8]

The proportions of each of the three foodstuffs being utilized at any one time is a function of the type, duration, and intensity of the activity.

The energy for muscular activity is provided by a process called *glycolysis,* which involves the oxidation or breakdown of *glucose* stored in finite amounts in resting muscle. The necessary energy is delivered through either aerobic or anaerobic metabolic processes. The aerobic energy system depends on the availability of oxygen for use by the working tissues, whereas the anaerobic system does not. As long as a sufficient amount of oxygen is delivered to the tissues to meet increased demands, activity may be continued indefinitely. This form of energy supply is referred to as aerobic metabolism.

If there is not enough oxygen present, metabolism will function anaerobically and the process of glycolysis will result in the production of lactic acid. When activities that are anaerobic in nature continue for extended periods of time, enough lactic acid may be produced to inhibit muscle function, and fatigue and some muscle pain will result.

Activities that are intense but relatively short in duration, such as sprinting, are anaerobic and require a breakdown of glucose in the absence of sufficient oxygen. Because the supply of oxygen cannot keep up with demand, lactic acid is produced. Conversely, activities of long duration, such as distance running, are aerobic in nature. Large amounts of energy are required; however, oxygen supply is sufficient to meet demand. Most sports activities are intermittent in nature and involve some combination of both aerobic and anaerobic metabolic processes.

FUNCTION OF VITAMINS

Although they are required in only small amounts, *vitamins* are essential for normal growth and for regulation of body activities. Vitamins are available in varying amounts in most plants that are used for sources of food. They may also be obtained from animal foods. Persons who eat a well-rounded, substantial diet therefore usually need not take extra vitamins. The most common vitamins are thiamine, riboflavin, niacin, and ascorbic acid. The names given to the vitamins are designated by letters. Vitamins A, B, B complex, C, D, E, and K have been soundly established as contributors to the total picture of nutrition.

The word *vitamin* is applied to those substances that occur in minute quantities in food and yet produce profound and specific physiologic effects. Vitamins A, D, K, and E are the fat-soluble vitamins, which are characterized by the presence of precursors, or provitamins. These substances are not active vitamins but are converted to vitamins in the body. The water-soluble vitamins are C and the B-complex.

The fat-soluble vitamins are dissolved and then stored in fatty tissues of the body. Thus it is not essential to ingest fat-soluble vitamins on a daily basis. Deficiencies of fat-soluble vitamins appear very gradually, but excessive amounts can be harmful. Because fat-soluble vitamins are stored, toxic levels can be reached.

On the other hand, water-soluble vitamins are transported in the body fluids and, because of their water solubility, are not stored. Thus the water-soluble vitamins should be ingested daily. Table 7-2 discusses these fat-soluble vitamins in detail.

THE ESSENTIAL MINERALS

Calcium, phosphorus, sodium, potassium, chlorine, magnesium, manganese, iodine, iron, copper, sulfur, zinc, cobalt, bromine, and fluorine are the elements that compose the group of *mineral* elements of nutrition. These elements are interrelated and balance against each other in body function and thus cannot be considered as single elements with independent functions. For example, calcium, phosphorus, and fluorine have a definite relationship in the formation of bone and teeth. Calcium, potassium, and sodium are essential elements in the contraction of skeletal muscle and they also show definite relationships in the maintenance of acid-base balance. Calcium and magnesium are related in the function of soft tissues. Copper catalyzes the use of iron, and cobalt influences both in blood formation. Table 7-3 presents a detailed description of the essential minerals.

WATER AS AN ESSENTIAL NUTRIENT

Water is the most essential of all the nutrients and should be the nutrient of greatest concern to the physically active person.[2] It is the most abundant nutrient of the body, accounting for approximately 60% of the body weight. Water is essential for all of the chemical processes that occur in the body, and an adequate supply of water is necessary for energy production and normal digestion of other nutrients. It is also necessary for temperature control and for elimination of waste products of nutrient and body metabolism. Too little water leads to dehydration, and severe dehydration frequently leads to death.

The body has a number of mechanisms designed specifically to maintain body water at near-normal level. Too little water leads to accumulation of "solutes" in the blood. These signal the brain that the body is thirsty while signaling the kidney to conserve water. Excessive water dilutes these solutes. This signals the brain to stop drinking and the kidneys to get rid of the excess water.

Water is the only nutrient of greater importance to physically active persons than to those who are more sedentary, especially during prolonged exercise carried out in a hot, humid environment. These situations may cause excessive

Text continued on p. 184.

TABLE 7-2 Fat-soluble Vitamins

Vitamin	Function in Body	Sources	Deficiency	Excessive Amounts
A	Essential for maintenance and function of epithelium cells, such as skin, hair, and mucous membranes. It also aids in vision in dim light. It aids in maintaining resistance to infections, increases longevity, and delays senility. It helps in reproduction, bone growth, and tooth development.	Found in butter, fat, and egg yolk but not in lard and common vegetable fats. It is also found in fish liver oils, eggs, and butter, and green leaves and the yellow parts of plants	Deficiency can lead to night blindness and permanent blindness, rickets in children, and osteomalacia in adults. There is also a loss of tonus or skeletal muscle.	Hypervitaminosis A (too much vitamin A) can produce excessive bone fragility, enlargement of the liver and spleen, drying and peeling of skin, loss of hair, nausea, headache, menstrual irregularities, depressed serum proteins and plasma prothrombin, and elevated alkaline phosphatase.
D	Activates phosphatases from the kidneys, intestines, and bones. It enhances the net absorption of calcium and phosphorus from the intestinal tract, causes low concentration of citric acid in the blood of children with rickets to rise to normal, and increases the resorption of phosphates by the kidneys. The formation of normal bone in humans is dependent on the presence of vitamin D.	Direct sunlight is also an important facet of this vitamin. Ultraviolet treatment is used as a supplemental treatment to increased vitamin D. It is found in butter, cheese, cream, eggs, clams, and fish.	Deficiency can lead to rickets in children and osteomalacia in adults. There is also a loss of tonus of skeletal muscle.	Excessive doses of vitamin D mobilize phosphorus and calcium from the tissues; this reverses the effect of normal doses. Vitamin D poisoning may cause nausea, anorexia, diuresis, and headaches. Food intake decreases, calcium and phosphorus retention is lowered, and the rate of linear growth slows.

Continued.

TABLE 7-2 Fat-soluble Vitamins—cont'd

Vitamin	Function in Body	Sources	Deficiency	Excessive Amounts
E	Antioxidant that preserves easily oxidizable vitamins and unsaturated fatty acids in foods, mixtures, or the body. Massive doses of vitamin E have been reported to maintain normal permeability of capillaries and to protect heart muscle against degeneration. They have been used in treating cardiovascular diseases, with debatable results. Assists in formation of red blood cells and muscle tissue.	Found in wheat germ, whole grain bread and cereal, vegetable oils, green leafy vegetables, egg yolks, and liver.	Deficiency signs and symptoms include possible loss of sex interest (in men) and progressive nutritional muscular dystrophy in the musculature.	
K	Ultimately associated with normal functioning of the liver as well as the normal clotting of the blood.	Sources include green vegetables, liver, cauliflower, and cereals.	Deficiency can lead to severe bleeding.	
B_1 (Thiamine)	Aids in release of energy from carbohydrates.	Pork, heart muscle, and glandular organs. Also found in bran and whole wheat.	Deficiency can lead to edema, heart failure, and beriberi.	

B$_2$ (Riboflavin)	Aids in release of energy from the three basic foodstuffs.	Found in cheese, milk, green vegetables, cereals.	Deficiency can lead to dry skin and cracked lips
B$_3$ (Niacin)	Aids in release of energy from the three basic foodstuffs.	Found in meats, poultry, fish, peanuts, whole grain cereals and breads.	Deficiency can cause pellagra.	Excessive amounts can cause burning and tingling around face and hands.
B$_6$	Aids in absorption of protein and production of red blood cells.	Found in wheat germ, pork liver, dried beans, bananas, and potatoes.	Deficiency can cause kidney stones, muscle twitch, irritability.
B$_{12}$	Aids in red blood cell formation, nervous system development, and synthesis of genetic material.	Found in animal foods only, such as meat, fish, eggs, and cheese.	Deficiency can cause neurologic dysfunction.
Folacin	Aids in synthesizing genetic material and in formation of hemoglobin.	Found in whole wheat products, green vegetables, liver, and dried beans.	Deficiency can lead to anemia and diarrhea.
Pantothenic acid	Aids in metabolism of three foodstuffs and hormone synthesis.	Produced by intestinal bacteria and found in all plant and animal products.	Deficiency can produce fatigue and nausea.
Biotin	Aids in metabolism of amino acids and formation of fatty acids.	Found in vegetables, milk, liver, and egg yolks.	Deficiency can cause, fatigue, depression, and nausea.
C	Also known as ascorbic acid. It plays a role in tooth and bone formation and repair and wound healing and is necessary in production of collagen. It does *not* appear to provide any protection against the common cold.	Found in citrus fruits, strawberries, tomatoes, cabbage, potatoes, and raw vegetables.	Deficiency can cause scurvy.

TABLE 7-3 Minerals

Mineral	Function in Body	Source
Calcium	Calcium is necessary for acid-base equilibrium and balances potassium and sodium in maintaining muscle tone. It is also necessary for normal regulation of the heartbeat. Calcium absorbed from the food is readily transferred through the body; it has very little effect on the actual level of calcium in the blood because of the store of calcium in bones. The parathyroid gland controls the calcium level of the blood, and it is only with disease conditions that low calcium develops in the blood. Low blood calcium may cause hyperirritability of muscle and nerve which may result in tetany. Calcium is necessary for muscle contraction.	Dairy products, clams, oysters, dark green vegetables, peas, and beans.
Phosphorus	Phosphorus has been shown to be necessary in normal muscle metabolism, carbohydrate metabolism, fat metabolism, protein metabolism, brain and nerve metabolism in normal blood chemistry; skeletal growth, and tooth development. It is concerned with acid-base regulation and with vitamin and enzyme activity.	Fish, poultry, meat, dairy products, nuts, beans, and peas.
Sodium	About 0.2% of the body is composed of sodium, practically all of which is found in the extracellular fluids of the body. The importance of sodium as a regulator of neutrality in the body can be seen by the fact that sodium ions compose 93% of the basic ions in the blood. Sodium has also been shown to be associated with muscle contraction. In normal humans, 90% of sodium is excreted through the kidneys, usually in the form of sodium chloride or sodium phosphates. Under conditions of intense perspiration, the main excretory route can be in the form of perspiration; in persons who normally perspire profusely, it may be necessary to provide extra salt.	Salt and used in most foods as a preservative.
Potassium	Potassium is found mostly within the cells of the body. The formed elements of blood contain twenty times as much potassium as the plasma. The muscles are known to contain approximately six times as much potassium as sodium. Potassium is closely associated with the function of muscles and has been demonstrated to have a close balance	Mainly bananas, orange juice, and potatoes.

	with calcium in the maintenance of nerve irritability or excitability. Potassium is also closely associated with carbohydrate metabolism. Under normal conditions potassium deficiency is not to be expected, but it can occur in infants in conditions of extreme diarrhea or in cases of severe electrolyte depletion as in heat related problems.	
Iron	Iron is one of the most vital elements in body metabolism. It constitutes only 0.004% of the body but is vital as a part of the hemoglobin molecule and therefore is necessary for blood transport of oxygen and carbon dioxide. Iron is also closely associated with cellular oxidation. The iron level in the body is regulated by absorption of iron from food. Persons with a normal iron content absorb very little iron from the intestinal tract, whereas anemic persons or those with low iron stores absorb appreciable quantities. Injected iron is eliminated with some difficulty. The body does not appear to be able to control its iron reserves by selective excretion.	Kidney, liver, red meat, green vegetables, dried fruit, egg yolk, and whole grain products.
Copper	Copper is closely associated with iron because it is necessary for the formation of hemoglobin. Although copper is present in the blood, it does not constitute part of the hemoglobin molecule. Copper deficiency has been shown to result in an anemia, which is really an iron deficiency anemia. Under these circumstances, iron may be built up as a reserve in the liver and yet not form hemoglobin because of the deficiency of copper.	Liver, kidney, chocolate, nuts, and oysters.
Sulfur	Important in the formation of amino acids.	Beef, clams, peanuts, and wheat germ.
Magnesium	Involved in protein synthesis and transmission of nerve impulses to the muscle.	Green vegetables, nuts, whole grain products, peas, and beans.
Chlorine	Helps in the maintenance of water balance.	Salt.
Zinc	Zinc has vital functions within the body. It is associated with carbon dioxide metabolism. It appears to be essential for the normal functioning of the pancreas and in that way is tied in with carbohydrate metabolism.	Seafood, poultry, liver, eggs, meat, and whole grains.
Iodine	Forms the thyroid hormone and is essential in reproduction.	Shellfish and iodized salt.

sweating and subsequent losses of large amounts of water. Restriction of water during these times will result in dehydration. Dehydration's symptoms include fatigue, vomiting, nausea, exhaustion, fainting, and possibly death.

The United States Senate Select Committee on Nutrition and Human Needs published a report in 1977 entitled *Dietary Goals for the United States*. According to this respected committee, the guidelines in the box below are set forth for a nutritionally adequate diet.

U.S. Dietary Goals

To avoid being overweight, consume only as much energy (calories) as is expended; if overweight, decrease energy intake and increase energy expenditure. Increase the consumption of complex carbohydrates and "naturally occurring" sugars from about 28 percent of energy intake to about 48 percent of energy intake. Reduce the consumption of refined and processed sugars by about 45 percent to account for about 10 percent of total energy intake.

Reduce overall fat consumption from approximately 40 percent to about 30 percent of energy intake.

Reduce saturated fat consumption to account for about 10 percent of total energy intake; and balance that with polyunsaturated and monounsaturated fats, which should account for about 10 percent of energy intake each.

Reduce cholesterol consumption to about 300 mg. a day.

Limit the intake of sodium by reducing the intake of salt to about 5 grams a day.

The Goals Suggest the Following Changes in Food Selection and Preparation:

Increase consumption of fruits and vegetables and whole grains.

Decrease consumption of refined and other processed sugars and foods high in such sugars.

Decrease consumption of foods high in total fat and partially replace saturated fats, whether obtained from animal or vegetable sources, with polyunsaturated fats.

Decrease consumption of animal fat and choose meats, poultry, and fish that will reduce saturated fat intake.

Except for young children, substitute low-fat and non-fat milk for whole milk and low-fat dairy products for high-fat dairy products.

Decrease consumption of butterfat, eggs, and other cholesterol sources. Some consideration should be given to easing the cholesterol goal for premenopausal women, young children, and the elderly in order to obtain the nutritional benefits of eggs in the diet.

Decrease consumption of salt and foods high in salt content.

Reprinted from the Dietary Goals for the United States, Second Edition, December, 1977.

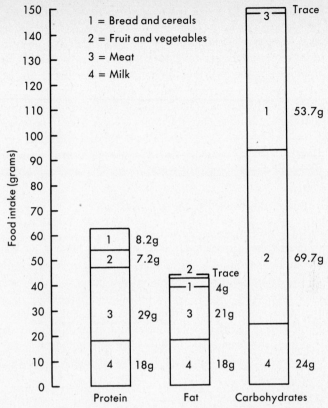

FIGURE 7-1

Recommendations for basic carbohydrate, fat, and protein intake as well as food sources for these nutrients.
From Howe, P. (1971). *Basic nutrition in health and disease*. Philadelphia: W.B. Saunders.

FIVE BASIC FOOD GROUPS

Foods are categorized in five basic groups on the basis of similarities in nutrient content. The five basic food groups are organized as follows:
   Cereals and grains: Flour, cereals, enriched breads and whole-grain products
   Meat and high proteins: Poultry, fish, meat, eggs, dried beans, peas, and nuts
   Milk and dairy products: Milk, cheese, ice cream, yogurt, and sour cream
   Vegetables and fruits: Yellow or dark green vegetables, tomatoes, and citrus
      fruits
   Fats and sugars: Candy, soft drinks
The key to achieving a well-balanced diet is to eat a variety of foods in each of the first four food groups. It is recommended that during a single 24-hour period

at least two servings from both the milk and dairy products group as well as the meat and high-protein group be consumed. It is also recommended that four servings from both the vegetables and fruits and the cereal and grains groups be eaten each day. The fats and sugars group contain relatively few nutrients and a high number of calories; thus daily intake from this group is not recommended.

As long as intake is balanced among the five food groups, there should be no problems in obtaining all necessary nutrients.[3] Thus vitamin supplementation is not necessary for persons who consume a well-balanced diet.

Fig. 7-1 indicates recommendations for intake from the various food groups in terms of the three basic foodstuffs—proteins, fats, and carbohydrates.

Vitamin Supplementation in Physical Activity

For many years improved performance has been associated with the increased intake of vitamin *supplements* by the physically active person. Recently, vitamin C and the B-complex vitamins have received a lot of attention and have been singled out as two vitamins that are depleted during physical activity. The fact is that the body generally cannot utilize additional quantities of any vitamin other than the amount required for normal function. As long as the diet provides the adequate nutrients, vitamin supplementation does nothing more than enhance the nutrient value of the urine. The typical college student in many cases does not have a well-balanced diet; for those persons, vitamin supplementation will definitely be helpful.

Nutritional Deficiencies and Physical Performance

A number of misconceptions exist regarding the value of dietary supplementation for the purpose of eliminating nutritional deficiencies that are thought to have a negative effect on physical performance.

It has been suggested that vitamins B_{12}, C, and E are deficient in the physically active person and require additional supplementation during physical activity.[3]

The B-complex vitamins, particularly B_{12}, have been recommended for the purpose of increasing strength and energy. It is true that the B-complex vitamins play a critical role in the metabolism of carbohydrates, fats, and proteins that supply energy for muscular work. However, vitamins have no caloric value whatsoever, and increased intake of B complex is not necessary for the athlete.

Megadoses of vitamin C have been recommended both for improving physical performance and as a preventive measure for the common cold. Although vitamin C does play a vital role in wound healing and the development of teeth and bones, there is no evidence to suggest that physical performance will be enhanced or that the chances of getting a cold will be reduced. Excessive intake of vitamin C may cause irritation of the gastrointestinal tract.

Vitamin E is said to increase resistance to fatigue, lower serum cholesterol, and increase sexual potency. Again, there is no evidence that ingestion of either vitamin E or large quantities of wheat germ oil has any of the suggested effects. The body requires only a small amount of vitamin E; ingestion of excessive amounts can be toxic.

Ingestion of Sweets before Physical Activity

It has been suggested that ingesting large quantities of glucose in the form of honey, candy bars, or pure sugar immediately before physical activity will significantly aid performance. The time for ingestion of large amounts of carbohydrates is during the week before an event, not immediately before. The problem with taking carbohydrates shortly before physical activity is that they raise blood insulin, which causes an inhibition of fat utilization during exercise. The muscles will rely on carbohydrates, using muscle glycogen more rapidly and driving down blood glucose.

Organic Foods and Physical Performance

Persons involved in some physical activity for the purpose of improving health sometimes consume foods that are said to be "natural," or organic, health foods.

Natural foods are those that contain no additives or preservatives, such as fruits, raw vegetables, and whole-grain products. Organic foods have been produced using no fertilizers or other chemical treatments. Stores that deal exclusively in these types of health foods have become extremely popular and advertise all types of benefits that may be derived from eating only organic or natural foods. Although some psychologic effects of eating only health foods may benefit performance, there is no evidence that physiologic performance is enhanced. Health food can be quite expensive, and thus consumption of this type of diet is not recommended.[5]

Effects of Caffeine on Performance

Caffeine is a stimulant of the central nervous system. Caffeine is contained in soft drinks, coffee, chocolate, and tea. Small amounts of caffeine are known to increase alertness and decrease fatigue; however, large amounts of caffeine tend to cause irritability, nervousness, and headaches.

Although small amounts of caffeine do not appear to be harmful to physical performance, there is little evidence that there are any real benefits to performance. There is evidence that caffeine enhances fat utilization during endurance exercise, thus postponing glycogen depletion.[6] This would help endurance performance.

Consumption of Alcohol

There are many negative effects of alcohol consumption on physical performance. There is no question that alcohol consumption will have a detrimental effect on both mental and physical performance in terms of decreased physical coordination, increased reaction time, and decreased mental alertness.

For a person exercising in a hot environment, alcohol consumption before activity can be dangerous because alcohol has a diuretic effect that leads to dehydration. Thus consumption of alcohol before or during physical activity is strongly discouraged.

Protein Supplementation

A common misconception among persons interested in developing muscle strength as well as muscle bulk is that additional amounts of protein will facilitate this growth. Consumption of large quantities of commercially manufactured protein powder, which is extremely expensive, is common practice among weight lifters and body builders. Protein supplementation is *not* needed to increase muscle mass in strength training, although protein consumption must be sufficient to supply muscle-building pathways that cause muscle hypertrophy.[1,4] Excess protein is not stored as protein but is instead converted to triglyceride and stored as fat.

Pre-event Meal

The importance and content of the pre-event meal is a topic that has been heatedly debated and discussed among coaches, trainers, and physical educators. The trend has been to ignore logical thinking about what should be eaten before competition in favor of upholding the tradition of "rewarding" the athlete for hard work by serving foods that may hamper his or her performance. For example, the traditional steak-and-eggs meal before football games is great for the coaches and trainers; however, the athlete gains nothing from this meal.

The important point is that too often people are concerned primarily with the pre-event meal and fail to realize that those nutrients consumed over several days before competition are much more important than what is eaten 3 hours before an event. The purpose of the pre-event meal should be to provide the competitor with sufficient nutrient energy and fluids for competition while taking into consideration the digestibility of certain foods and most importantly the eating preferences of the individual athlete. The box on p. 189 gives two examples of pre-event meals.

A physically active person should be encouraged to be conscious of his or her diet. There is no experimental evidence to indicate that performance may be enhanced by altering a diet that is basically sound. There are a number of ways that a balanced diet may be achieved, and the diet that is optimal for one person may not be the best for another. In many instances, the individual athlete will be the best judge of what he or she should or should not eat in the pre-event meal. It seems that the best guide for a person is to eat whatever he or she is most comfortable with, within the following basic guidelines:

1. Try to achieve the largest possible storage of carbohydrate in the form of

Sample Pre-Event Meals
(to be eaten 3 to 4 hours before event)

Meal 1

¾ c Orange juice	¾ c Orange juice
½ c Cereal with 1 tsp sugar	1-2 Pancakes with:
1 Slice whole wheat toast with:	1 tsp Margarine
1 tsp Margarine	2 tbsp Syrup
1 tsp Honey or jelly	8 oz Skim or lowfat milk
8 oz Skim or lowfat milk	Water
Water	(Approximately 450-500 kcal)
(Approximately 450-500 kcal)	

Meal 2

1 c Vegetable soup	1 c Spaghetti with tomato sauce and cheese
1 Turkey sandwich with:	½ c Sliced pears (canned) on ¼ c cottage
2 Slices bread	cheese
2 oz Turkey (white or dark)	1-2 Slices (Italian) bread with 1-2 tsp mar-
1 oz Cheese slice	garine (avoid garlic)
2 tsp Mayonnaise	½ c Sherbet
8 oz Skim or lowfat milk	1-2 Sugar cookies
Water	4 oz Skim or lowfat milk
(Approximately 550-600 kcal)	Water
	(Approximately 700 kcal)

From Anderson & others. (1982). *Teens, foods, fitness, sports*.

glycogen in both resting muscle and the liver. This is particularly important for endurance activities but may also be beneficial for intense, short-duration activities. Additionally, carbohydrates are broken down and digested more quickly than fats or protein.

2. The type of food eaten should allow for the quickest possible gastric emptying so that stomach volume will be as small as possible at the time of competition. Fats are the most difficult foodstuff to digest and may also prove to be extremely irritating to the gastrointestinal tract. Proteins, like fats, are not easily digested, and their breakdown results in production of fixed acids that may impede performance. A stomach that is not clear of food during contact sport is subject to acute injury.

3. Foods should not cause irritation or upset to the gastrointestinal tract. Foods high in cellulose, such as lettuce, cause increased need for defecation. Highly spiced foods or gas-forming foods (such as onions, baked beans, or peppers) must also be avoided because any type of disturbance in the gastrointestinal tract may be detrimental to performance.

4. Liquids consumed should be easily absorbed and low in fat content, and should not act as a laxative in the gastrointestinal tract. Fruit juices, whole

milk, coffee, and tea should be avoided. Water intake should be increased, particularly if the temperature is high.

5. The pre-event meal should be eaten approximately 3 to 4 hours before the event. This 3- to 4-hour period allows for adequate gastric emptying, but the athlete will not feel hungry during competition.

6. The athlete should not be required to eat any food that is not palatable. Most importantly, he or she must feel psychologically satisfied by the pre-event meal. If not, performance may very well be impaired more by psychologic factors than by physiologic factors.

Recently, liquid meals such as Nutrament and Sustagen have been recommended as extremely effective pre-event meals. These liquid meals have several advantages: (1) they are generally flavorful and palatable, (2) they contain large quantities of carbohydrate and limited quantities of protein and fat, (3) they generally have a high nutrient value, (4) they are liquid and aid in fluid replacement, and (5) they are easily absorbed, leaving little if any residue in the stomach by event time. Liquid meals provide a good but unfortunately expensive alternative to the traditional pre-event meal.

Specialized Diets

Many physically active persons are generally very conscious of good health and in most cases do everything they can to make their bodies as "healthy" as possible. They will generally try anything that they think may effectively improve their performance. As a result, specialized diets, such as the vegetarian diet, have gained popularity among many athletes.

The vegetarian diet and its many variations provide most of the nutrients needed. Unfortunately, the body needs fats in different forms for normal function, and many vegetarians are deficient in fat consumption. However, the main nutritional concern of vegetarians is receiving all the essential amino acids necessary for carrying on body functions.

GLYCOGEN LOADING

Glycogen supplies in muscle and liver can be increased by decreasing the training programs for about 48 hours before competition or by significantly increasing carbohydrate intake during the week before competition.

By reducing training 48 hours before an event, the body is able to eliminate metabolites that tend to inhibit performance and also to allow depleted glycogen stores to increase to more normal levels.

Increasing carbohydrate intake 3 to 4 days before an event and tapering the amount of exercise 5 to 6 days before an event has been commonly referred to as *glycogen loading*. The idea is that the quantity of glycogen stored in a muscle directly affects the endurance of that muscle. By depleting initial stores of glycogen, the body will overcompensate and replenish a greater quantity of glycogen than was originally present. Glycogen loading is accomplished over a 6-day period divided into three phases. In phase 1 (days 1-2), the athlete trains very hard and restricts dietary intake of carbohydrates. During phase 2 (days 3-5), training is cutback while the athlete loads up with carbohydrates. Studies have indicated that glycogen stores may be increased from 50% to 100%, theoretically enhancing endurance during a long-term event. Phase 3 (day 6) is the day of the event, during which a normal diet must be consumed. The effect of glycogen loading in improving performance during endurance activities has not as yet been clearly demonstrated. It has been recommended that glycogen loading not be done more than 2 to 3 times during a course of a year.[2] It must also be added that intake of large amounts of glucose up to 30 minutes before an event significantly increases blood insulin levels, which inhibits fat utilization during exercise. The muscles then rely on carbohydrates by using up muscle glycogen, thus decreasing blood glucose. The practice of giving sugar, dextrose tablets, candy, or honey to provide quick energy actually defeats the whole purpose and will likely hamper performance. It must be added that glycogen loading is only of value in events that could produce glycogen depletion such as a marathon.

ANEMIA IN PHYSICAL ACTIVITIES

An inadequate intake of iron from the diet may lead to what is clinically known as iron-deficiency *anemia*.[2] If the anemia is severe, the oxygen-carrying capacity of red blood cells becomes so reduced that muscle cells do not function properly. Other body tissues are similarly compromised. The net result is a reduction in functional performance. Obviously a person could not compete at peak level with a severe iron deficiency.

Women are more susceptible to low intakes of iron from the diet than men. This deficit occurs in women because they generally eat smaller amounts of food, especially the iron-containing foods, and also because of a loss of blood during menstration.

Whether sports activities such as long-distance running and training contribute in some way to iron-deficiency anemia is not clear. This type of anemia is referred to as "sports anemia." One common opinion is that it is simple dietary iron deficiency that contributes to the anemia associated with participation in endurance sports. However, trained athletes undergo an expansion of their blood volume. If the fluid portion of the blood (serum) increases while the amount of red blood cells remains constant, then the concentration of red blood cells (hematocrit) is reduced. Such persons may then appear to be anemic even though their blood still contains the same number of red blood cells.

In general, if a person is truly anemic and has reduced performance, it may be reasonable to assume that his or her dietary habits are not including sufficient iron-containing foods. Iron supplements and frequent blood checks are recommended by physicians when this is suspected.

ANOREXIA NERVOSA

Anorexia Nervosa is a disease in which a person for one reason or another develops a psychologic aversion to food of any variety. Over a period of weeks or months the person suffers a pathologic weight loss.

Anorexia has recently become a widespread problem seen most commonly in young women, but it has also been reported in men. For persons involved in sports, it seems to be found most frequently in those activities in which physical appearance is of great importance, such as gymnastics, dance, and to some degree tennis.

In many instances, anorexia begins as nothing more than a normal diet, an attempt to lose some body weight. Reasons for dieting vary, but most people seem to associate their body weight and appearance with their ability to perform successfully. The anorexic person becomes obsessed with dieting. He or she may begin skipping one meal a day but frequently will not eat anything for several days. It is not uncommon to find anorexic persons who will eat a good meal but then proceed to the restroom, where they force themselves to regurgitate the food that was just consumed. Obviously anorexia at this stage is a psychologic problem. Death from total starvation occurs occasionally with anorexia.

Because anorexia is a type of psychologic disorder, treatment of this problem is usually beyond the scope of a physical educator, trainer, or coach. The anorexic person is probably best treated by someone involved with health education or mental health (although the latter often carries some negative connotations). Unfortunately, simply referring an anorexic person to a health education clinic for help is not usually effective. The key to treatment of anorexia seems to be getting the patient to realize that some problem exists and that they could benefit from outside professional help. They must voluntarily accept this professional help if the treatment is to be successful.

Anorexia is a serious problem that can be extremely difficult to deal with. If handled improperly, anorexia nervosa can be a fatal disease. Early recognition of the problem seems to be the key to successful treatment.

BULIMIA

Bulimia is another type of eating disorder that involves recurrent episodes of binge-type eating. Usually this intake of high-calorie foods serves as a release from stress and typically is said to reduce depression and anger. People who go on these eating binges tend to do so when they are alone and generally end this binge by voluntary, self-induced vomiting. Binges usually produce heightened feelings of guilt, depression, and disgust, which tend to lead to vomiting, laxative or amphetamine abuse, and restricted dieting or fasting.

Persons with bulimia are most commonly preoccupied primarily with a fear of becoming fat. They become obsessed with food, dieting, and exercise, all of which contribute to being "fat." Bulimic persons also have low self-esteem and feelings of isolation, depression, and anxiety and seem to have problems with interpersonal relationships.

A typical binge involves the consumption of 1000 to as many as 50,000 calories during a 1- to 2-hour period as often as four times a day. The binge is always followed by purging with vomiting, laxatives, or fasting. It becomes very expensive to supply food and laxatives as this binge-purge problem becomes worse over time.

Bulimic persons tend to be women in their late teens or early twenties who are close to proper weight. These binge-purge episodes tend to go on for years until the person seeks professional help.

Perhaps the most vital treatment approach involves early detection and intervention by trained professionals. The treatment focus should be on small behavioral changes and successes, not failures, along with alternative methods for coping with stress. It is essential to be realistic about changing bulimic behavior; habits take time to change.

SUMMARY

- The three basic foodstuffs are fat, carbohydrates, and proteins. These three foodstuffs provide the energy required for muscular work during activity and also play a role in the function and maintenance of body tissues.
- Foodstuffs are metabolized to provide energy either aerobically or anaerobically, depending on the availability of oxygen.
- Vitamins are substances found in food that have no caloric value but produce specific physiologic effects. Vitamins may be either fat soluble (vitamins A, D, E, and K) or water soluble (vitamins B-complex, C, folacin, and biotin).
- The essential minerals: calcium, phosphorus, sodium, potassium, chlorine, magnesium, manganese, iodine, iron, copper, sulfur, zinc, cobalt, bromine, and fluorine are necessary in most physiologic functions of the body.
- Water is the most essential of all the nutrients and should be of great concern to anyone involved with physical activity.
- A well-balanced diet consists of eating a variety of foods from each of the basic food groups.
- If your diet resembles anything close to a well-balanced diet, vitamin supplementation is not necessary.
- The pre-event meal should be (1) higher in carbohydrates, (2) easily digested, (3) eaten 3 to 4 hours before an event, and (4) psychologically pleasing.
- Glycogen loading involves maximizing resting stores of glucose in the muscle, blood, and liver before a competitive event.
- It may be necessary to supplement the diet with extra iron to prevent anemia.
- Anorexia is a disease in which a person suffers a pathologic weight loss because of a psychologic aversion to food and eating.

GLOSSARY

amino acids The constituents of protein. Needed by the body to manufacture the proteins required for growth and repair of tissues

anemia Disorder in which the oxygen-carrying capacity of the blood is reduced because of inadequate intake of iron in the diet

anorexia nervosa Disease in which a person develops a psychologic aversion to food

caffeine Stimulant of the central nervous system

carbohydrates Primary food substance, mainly responsible for providing energy during high-intensity muscular activity

fats Primary food substance that can provide energy during long-term endurance activities

glucose End product of the breakdown of carbohydrates that is transported in the blood

glycogen loading Increasing carbohydrate intake in the days before competition for the purpose of enhancing endurance

glycolysis Process involving the breakdown of glucose stored in finite amounts in resting muscle

mineral Inorganic metal compounds found in small amounts in the body that, like vitamins, are essential for normal body function

natural foods Those foods that contain no additives or preservatives

proteins Primary food source that provides the basic building components for the cells and relatively small amounts of energy

vitamin Organic compounds that perform essential functions within the cell necessary for maintenance of good health

supplements Additional vitamins or minerals ingested in tablet or powder form

REFERENCES

1. American Alliance for Health, Physical Education and Recreation. (1971). *Nutrition for Athletes*. Washington, DC: Author.
2. Anderson, J., Burge, J., DeWalt, J., Earey, P., Hastedt, P., & Prentice, W. (1982). *Teens, Foods, Fitness and Sports*. Raleigh, NC: Department of Public Instruction.
3. Bogert, L., & others. (1973). *Nutrition and physical fitness*. Philadelphia: W.B. Saunders.
4. Felig, P., & Wahren, J. (1971). Amino acid metabolism in exercising man. *Journal of Clinical Investigation, 50*,2703.
5. Mayer, J. (1975). *A diet for living*. New York: David McKay.
6. McArdle, W., Katch, W., and Katch, V. (1981). *Exercise physiology, energy, nutrition, and human performance*. Philadelphia: Lea & Febiger.

SUGGESTED READINGS

Åstrand, P.O., and Rodahl, K. (1977). *Textbook of work physiology*. New York: McGraw-Hill.

Briggs, G.M., and Calloway, D.H. (1984). *Nutrition and Physical Fitness*. New York: CBS College Publishing.

Corbin, C., Linus, D., Lindsey, R., & Tolson, H. (1981). *Concepts in physical education with laboratories and experiments*. Dubuque, IA: William C. Brown.

deVries, H. (1980). *Physiology of exercise for physical education and athletics*. Dubuque, IA: William C. Brown.

Fox, E. (1984). *Sport physiology*. New York: CBS College Publishing.

Getchell, B. (1983). *Physical fitness: A way of life*. New York: John Wiley & Sons.

Hamilton, E., & Whitney, E. (1982). *Nutrition concepts and controversies*. St. Paul: West.

Howe, P. (1971). *Basic nutrition in health and disease*. Philadelphia: W.B. Saunders.

Jense, C., & Fisher, G. (1979). *Scientific basis of athletic conditioning*. Philadelphia: Lea & Febiger.

Miller, D., & Allen, E. (1982). *Fitness: A lifetime concept*. Minneapolis: Burgess.

Smith, V. (1976). *Food for sport*. Palo Alto, CA: Bull.

Stokes, R., & Farls, D. (1983). *Fitness everyone!* Winston-Salem, NC: Hunter Textbooks.

Williams, M. (1976). *Nutritional aspects of athletic performance*. Springfield, IL: Charles C Thomas.

COMMON FITNESS

INJURIES

After completing this chapter, you will be able to:

- Realize that participation in physical activity places a person in situations in which injury is likely to occur.
- Define and differentiate between muscle strain and muscle soreness.
- Discuss tendonitis in relation to the inflammatory process.
- Identify the causes of lower back pain and how it can best be avoided.
- Describe the most common overuse injuries that occur in the lower extremity.
- Describe the general principles of initial treatment of injuries.
- Describe the different types of heat-related problems.

Participation in any type of physical activity places you in situations in which injury can occur at any given moment. Although some of these injuries are serious, and a few life-threatening, most sport-related injuries are not serious and lend themselves to rapid rehabilitation.

The human body is composed of a system of bones that provide the primary structural support mechanism. The skeletal system serves as the point of attachment for the musculotendinous units. When contracted, the muscles produce angular movements of the skeletal bones that allow us to walk, run, throw, twist, and turn.

Unfortunately, the skeletal and muscular systems were not designed to meet all the demands that strenuous physical activity often places on them. Sooner or later the forces placed on these structures simply become too great for them to handle and injury occurs.

Although most sporting activities are not practiced with the idea of promoting health, there is certainly no reason to think of physical activities in terms of their capacity to impair it. Training programs such as those described in previous chapters will reduce the possibility of injury. The overload demands placed on the body during training enable it to handle added stresses and strains that occur during physical activity. Thus the first step in preventing injuries associated with physical activity involves designing a well-planned training program based on the basic principles discussed in Chapter 2; overload, gradual progression, consistency, individuality, and safety.

Perhaps the biggest mistake that people make when beginning a physical activity program is beginning at an inappropriate level and then trying to progress too quickly. Sedentary persons must begin at a much lower level and gradually increase their level of activity. Quite often, the persons most likely to be injured are those who at one time, usually during the college years, were very active physically but have been relatively inactive for some time since graduation. When they decide to return to activity and start exercising again, there is a tendency to try and begin where they left off. Unfortunately, it simply does not work that way.

No matter how much attention is directed toward these general principles, it is still very likely that some physical problems will occur that may be of either acute or chronic variety. In this chapter we will discuss some of the more generalized traumatic and overuse injuries that occur during physical activity. It is important to remember that caution must be exercised when trying to evaluate an injury. A considerable amount of experience and training is required to accurately determine not only what may have caused an injury but also exactly what the injury is. These evaluation skills are far beyond the capabilities of most college students. Injuries should be evaluated by persons experienced in dealing with these sport-related injuries. Physicians, athletic trainers, and physical therapists all have strong evaluation skills. However, the physician makes the injury diagnosis, whereas the athletic trainer or physical therapist assumes responsibility for injury rehabilitation.

In Chapter 2 it was mentioned that one of the basic essentials of any type of training is safety. If you are involved in some physical activity and you realize that a specific part of your body is causing you discomfort or pain that is affecting your performance during that activity, then it is strongly recommended that this problem be evaluated immediately. The sooner an injury is diagnosed and treatment begun, the less chance there is that continued activity will exacerbate the problem.

MUSCLE STRAINS

The musculotendinous unit was described and diagrammed in Chapter 4. Basically, the muscle is composed of separate fibers that are capable of simultaneous contraction when stimulated by the central nervous system. Each muscle is attached to bone at both proximal and distal ends by strong, relatively inelastic tendons that cross over joints.

If a muscle is overstretched or forced to contract against too much resistance,

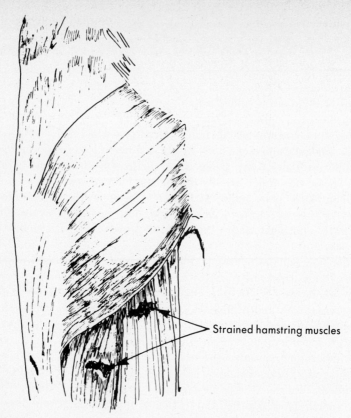

Strained hamstring muscles

FIGURE 8-1

A muscle strain results in tearing or separation of muscle fibers.

damage occurs to the muscle fibers. This separation or tearing of muscle fibers is referred to as a *strain* (Fig. 8-1). Muscle strains, like ligament sprains, are subject to various classification systems. The following is a simple system of classification of strains:

First-degree strain. Some muscle fibers have been stretched or actually torn. There is some tenderness and pain on active motion. Movement is painful but full range of motion is usually possible.

Second-degree strain. A number of muscle fibers have been torn, and active contraction of the muscle is extremely painful. There is usually a palpable depression or divot somewhere in the muscle belly at the spot at which the muscle fibers have been torn. Some swelling may occur because of capillary bleeding.

Third-degree strain. There is a complete rupture of a muscle either in the muscle belly, in the area where muscle becomes tendon, or at the tendinous attachment to the bone. There will be significant impairment to or perhaps

total loss of movement. Pain will be intense initially but will diminish
quickly because of complete separation of the nerve fibers.

Muscle strains can occur in any muscle and usually result from some uncoordinated activity between synergistic muscle groups. Third-degree strains are
most common in the biceps tendon of the upper arm or in the Achilles heel cord
in the back of the calf. When either of these tendons rupture, the muscle tends
to bunch toward its proximal attachment. Third-degree strains involving large
tendons that produce great amounts of force must be surgically repaired. Smaller
musculotendinous ruptures, such as those that occur in the fingers, may heal by
immobilization with a splint.

Regardless of the severity of the strain, there is no question that the time
required for rehabilitation is fairly lengthy. In many instances, rehabilitation
time for a muscle strain is longer than for a ligament sprain. These incapacitating
muscle strains occur most frequently in the large force-producing hamstring and
quadriceps muscles of the lower extremity. The treatment of hamstring strains
requires a healing period of 6 to 8 weeks and a considerable amount of patience.
Trying to return to activity too soon will frequently cause reinjury to the area of
the muscle that has been strained, and the healing process must begin again.

MUSCLE SORENESS

It is well known that overexertion in strenuous muscular exercise often results
in muscular pain. All of us at one time or another have experienced *muscle
soreness,* usually resulting from some physical activity to which we are unac-
customed. You will find that the older you get, the more easily muscle soreness
will seem to develop. Muscle soreness differs from a muscle strain in that soreness
generally does not involve damage to the muscle fibers.

There are two types of muscle soreness. The first type of muscle pain accom-
panies fatigue. It is transient, occurs during and immediately after exercise, and
can be attributed to the build-up of a product of anaerobic metabolism called
lactic acid. Lactic acid accumulates in the muscle because of insufficient oxygen
supply to the working muscle tissues, thus stimulating pain receptors in the
area.[1] In addition, fluid collects in the muscles during increased activity because
of an increase in hydrostatic pressure, resulting in swelling. The muscle becomes
shorter and thicker and thus more resistant to stretching. Therefore when a
muscle is stretched, there is a sensation of stiffness which may last for some
time and is a symptom of the second type of muscle pain.

The second type of soreness involves delayed muscle pain that appears approximately 12 hours after injury. It becomes most intense after 24 to 48 hours
and then gradually subsides so that the muscle becomes symptom-free after 4
to 6 days. This second type of pain may best be described as a syndrome of
delayed muscle pain that includes several components: muscle spasm, leading
to increased muscle tension, edema formation, increased stiffness, and resistance
to stretching.[2]

It has been hypothesized that delayed muscle pain is caused by tonic localized spasm of motor units varying in number with the severity of pain.[1] This theory, known as the spasm theory, can be explained on the basis that exercise causes varying degrees of ischemia in the working muscles. This ischemia causes pain, which results in reflex tonic muscle contraction that increases and prolongs the ischemia. Consequently a cycle of increasing severity is begun. To eliminate this muscle soreness, this cycle must be broken by allowing the muscle to rest over a period of days. Treatment of muscle soreness usually also involve static or PNF stretching activity.[2]

TENDONITIS

Of all the overuse problems associated with physical activity, tendonitis is probably the most common. Any term ending in the suffix *itis* means there is inflammation present; thus **tendonitis** means inflammation of a tendon. During muscle activity a tendon must move or slide on other structures around it whenever the muscle contracts. If a particular movement is performed repeatedly, the tendon becomes irritated and inflamed. This inflammation is manifested by pain on movement, swelling, possibly some warmth, and usually crepitus. Crepitus is a crackling sound similar to the sound produced by rolling your hair between your fingers by your ear. Crepitus is usually caused by the tendon adhering to surrounding structures as it slides back and forth. This adhesion is caused primarily by the chemical products of inflammation that accumulate on the irritated tendon.

At this point it is necessary to mention that the inflammatory process is an essential part of the healing process. Once a structure is damaged or irritated, inflammation must occur to initiate the healing process. Symptoms of inflammation include pain, swelling, warmth, and perhaps redness. During the inflammatory process, certain chemicals are released that facilitate the healing process. Inflammation is supposed to be an acute process that has an endpoint after its function in the healing process has been fulfilled. However, if the source of irritation (that is, the repetitive movements that cause stress to the tendon) is not removed, then the inflammatory process becomes chronic rather than acute. When this occurs, tendonitis may become a disabling problem.

The key to the treatment of tendonitis is rest. If the repetitive motion causing irritation to the tendon is eliminated, chances are the inflammatory process will allow the tendon to heal. Unfortunately, if you are seriously involved with some physical activity, you may find it difficult to totally stop what you have been doing and rest for 2 or more weeks while the tendonitis subsides. It is desirable to find some alternative activity that will allow you to maintain present fitness levels to a certain degree while allowing the tendon a chance to heal.

Tendonitis most commonly occurs in the Achilles tendon in the back of the lower leg in runners or in the muscle tendons of the shoulder joint in swimmers, although it can certainly flare up in any tendon in which overuse and repetitive movements occur.

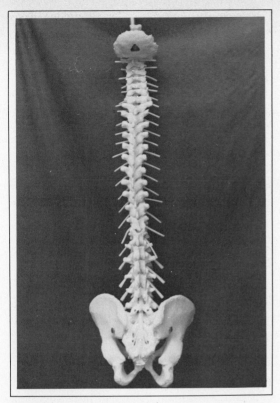

FIGURE 8-2

Spine and pelvis with nerve roots.

LOWER BACK PAIN

If you could come up with a foolproof method of eliminating lower back pain, you would probably become one of the richest and most respected people in America. There is no question that lower back pain is one of the most annoying and disabling ailments known. Many causes and cures for lower back pain have been proposed, but the problem is that there are so many different things that can cause pain in the area of the lower back that no single incriminating cause or absolute cure can be identified. In our discussion of lower back pain, we will concentrate on some of the most common causes.

One certainty is that generally the older you get, the more problems you tend to have in the lower back. Although lower back pain does not become a major problem for most people until their middle twenties, it is true that many people have minor congenital defects that are not realized until they become painful as a result of faulty body mechanics.

Herniated disc

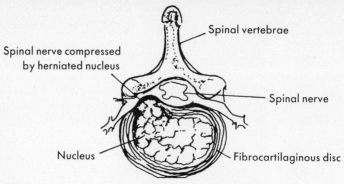

Spinal vertebrae

Spinal nerve compressed
by herniated nucleus

Spinal nerve

Nucleus

Fibrocartilaginous disc

FIGURE 8-3

A vertebral disc herniation.

The human spine is composed of 24 vertebral bodies, each separated from the others by a fibrocartilaginous disc. There are 7 cervical vertebrae in the neck region, 12 thoracic vertebrae in the thorax, and 5 lumbar vertebrae in the lower back. The sacrum is a large triangular bone that is also part of the spine that is located in the area below the small of the back in the pelvis (Fig. 8-2).

The function of the spine is twofold; to provide structural support for an upright posture and to protect the descending spinal cord and the spinal nerves as they exit from the spinal column to provide motor and sensory innervation.

The position of each vertebrae in the spinal column is maintained by a number of strong ligaments and muscles that attach to each vertebra. The vertebral discs that separate each segment serve a shock-absorptive function in the spinal column.

Herniated Disc

The traditional view of lower back pain maintains that although there may be many causes of lower back pain, disc degeneration and rupture is the most common cause. This hypothesis is somewhat questionable at this point; however, it is true that disc-related problems do produce many low back problems.

A vertebral disc is similar to the type of chewing gum that has a liquid center. A sudden twist or jerking movement can cause the liquid center, or nucleus, of the disc to protrude to one side, resulting in pressure on the spinal nerve at that segment. Pressure will usually cause pain to radiate down the leg. The most common areas for disc-related problems are in the discs between the fourth and fifth lumbar vertebrae and between the fifth lumbar vertebra and the sacrum. This condition is commonly referred to as a ***herniated disc.*** A disc herniation should definitely be treated by a qualified physician (Fig. 8-3).

Lumbosacral Sprains

Certainly not all lower back pain results from problems related to the vertebral disc. A more contemporary explanation of lower back pain involves a sprain of the intervertebral ligaments resulting from sudden rotation of the vertebrae. This type of injury is most common in the lower lumbar and sacral areas and is often referred to as a *lumbosacral sprain.*

Rotation of a vertebra can be caused by forces incurred from sudden twisting movements or bending over to pick up some object while the spine is twisted. The force from one of these motions can cause a vertebra to rotate out of its normal alignment.

A vertebra that is rotated tends to impinge on the spinal nerve in much the same manner as a herniated disc, causing pain. When pain is present because of a change in position of one vertebra, the muscles surrounding the area of pain in the vertebral column tend to go into spasm to protect the area and prevent additional injury. This muscle spasm only tends to pull the rotated vertebra further out of line, increasing the spinal nerve impingment and thus the pain. Any type of movement is very painful, and movement is at best restricted.

Sacroiliac Sprains

There are two strong ligaments on each side of the sacrum that connect this portion of the vertebral column to one of the bones of the pelvis, called the ilium. A sprain of either of these sacroiliac ligaments usually results from stepping off of a curb or into a hole, thus causing one sacroiliac joint to forcefully rotate either forward or backward with respect to the other and stretching at least one of the ligaments.

Stretching of the ligament produces pain, and once again the muscles in the surrounding area will go into spasm to protect the injured ligament, thus pulling one sacroiliac joint further out of line with respect to the other. Pain will be felt directly over the sacroiliac joint that has been sprained.

Many treatment and rehabilitation techniques involving mobilization and manipulation have been proposed for treatment of both lumbosacral and sacroiliac sprains. However, a discussion of these ideas and principles is far beyond the scope of this text. Again, treatment by qualified professionals who possess a sound understanding of these treatment techniques is highly recommended.

Prevention of Lower Back Pain

Some knowledge of the pathology of lower back pain is important, but it is more important to understand how lower back pain can be avoided.

To prevent lower back pain, the practice of avoiding unnecessary stresses and strains should be integrated into your daily life. The back is subjected to these stresses and strains when standing, lying, sitting, working, and exercising, and care should be taken to avoid postures and positions that can potentially cause injury.

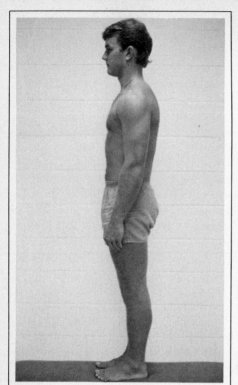

FIGURE 8-4

Ideal standing posture.

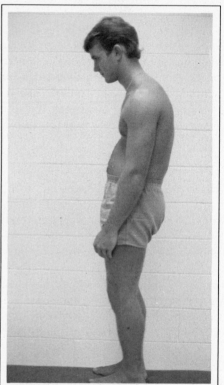

FIGURE 8-5

Poor standing posture can increase lower back pain.

Standing posture (Fig. 8-4). If standing posture is correct, it should be possible to draw a straight line from the ear, through the tip of the shoulder, over the middle of the hip bone, just behind the kneecap, and just in front of the ankle bone on the lateral side.

The biggest problems in standing posture are rounded shoulders and excessive curve in the lumbar area (Fig. 8-5). To get an idea of what good posture should feel like, back up against a wall. Press your shoulders and lower back flat, tighten all the muscles, and walk away from the wall in that position (Fig. 8-6). When standing for long periods of time, one foot should be elevated to eliminate the excessive curve in the lower back (Fig. 8-7). When bending over and leaning on some object, the knees should be flexed, not straight (Fig. 8-8).

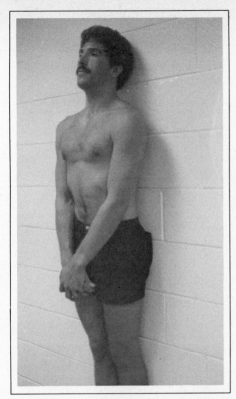

FIGURE 8-6

Standing with the lower back pressed firmly into the wall will give some indication of what correct posture should feel like.

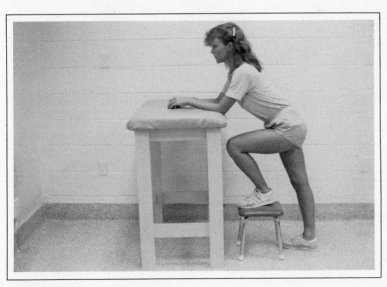

FIGURE 8-7

When standing for a long time, always have one leg flexed.

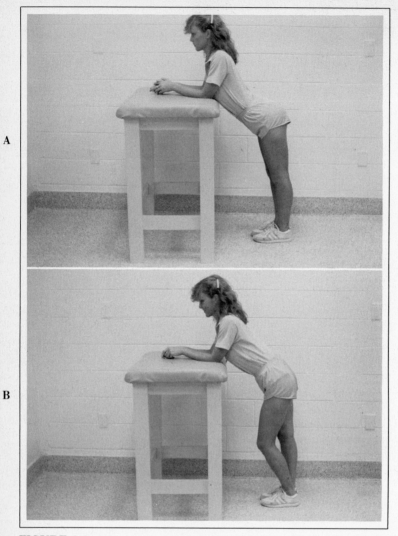

FIGURE 8-8

Always lean on an object with the knees bent. **A,** Incorrect; **B,** recommended.

Lying posture. The back is subjected to many stresses and strains while lying down. Most of us spend between 7 and 10 hours each day sleeping. Obviously, improper positions during sleep can cause chronic lower back pain. It is essential to have a good, firm mattress. Sleeping on a bed that is too soft can increase the tendency toward swayback.

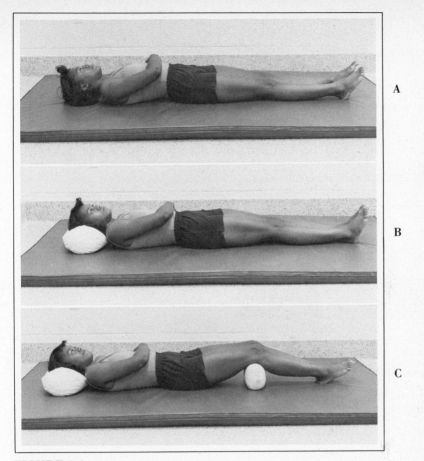

FIGURE 8-9

Sleeping on the back is safe only when both the knees and head are supported. **A,** Incorrect; **B,** incorrect; **C,** recommended.

Swayback can also result from sleeping flat on your back with no pillow. It is more correct when sleeping on the back to place a pillow under the knees or under the head so that the lower back will flatten (Fig. 8-9). This position is also recommended for resting or just lying around. It must be added that sleeping on your back using a pillow under the head may cause some additional problems with rounded shoulders.

Lying on the stomach face down also tends to enhance swayback (Fig. 8-10). Bending the knee and hip on one side does not take pressure off the lower back area (Fig. 8-11). The best position for sleeping is to sleep on your side with your knees flexed and your head on a pillow for support (Fig. 8-12). This flattens the lower back and almost totally eliminates stress.

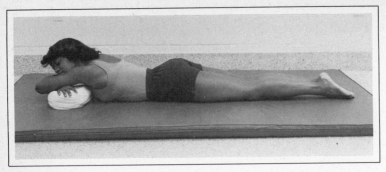

FIGURE 8-10

Sleeping on the stomach exaggerates swayback position.

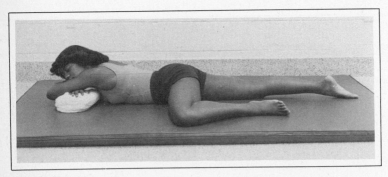

FIGURE 8-11

Lying on the stomach with one knee flexed does not eliminate pressure on the lower back.

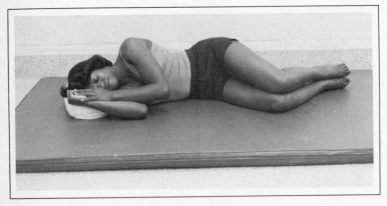

FIGURE 8-12

The sidelying sleeping position flattens the lower back. A pillow should support the head.

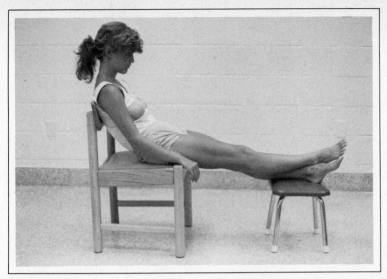

FIGURE 8-13

Slumping in a chair strains neck and shoulders.

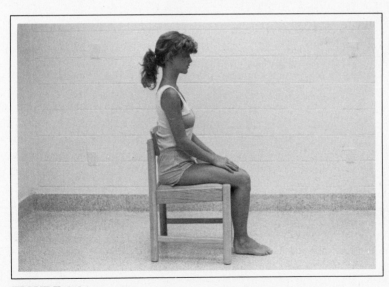

FIGURE 8-14

Ideal sitting position is with the lower back flat against support and the legs crossed or elevated.

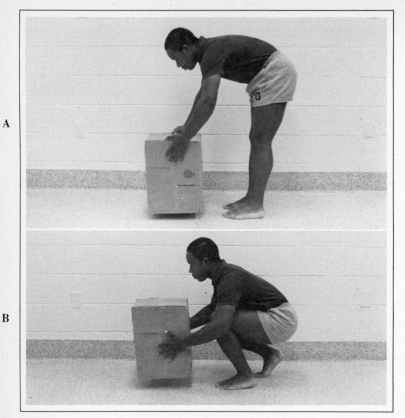

A

B

FIGURE 8-15

Always lift heavy objects with the legs and not the back. **A,** Incorrect; **B,** recommended.

Sitting posture. Of the postural positions discussed to this point, it is likely that the sitting posture causes the greatest stress and strain to the lower back. The slumping posture many of us use when watching television obviously produces significant stress to the shoulders and neck (Fig. 8-13).

When sitting, you should slide all the way up against the back of the chair so that the lower back has some support. The neck and back should be held erect in a straight line. The feet should be propped up or the legs crossed to further flatten out the lower back (Fig. 8-14). Any variation in the recommended correct sitting position will add stress to the lower back. When sitting in a car or driving for a long period of time, some type of support should be placed behind the lower back, and the position of the backrest should be changed periodically. Leaning forward away from the back support while driving is not recommended.

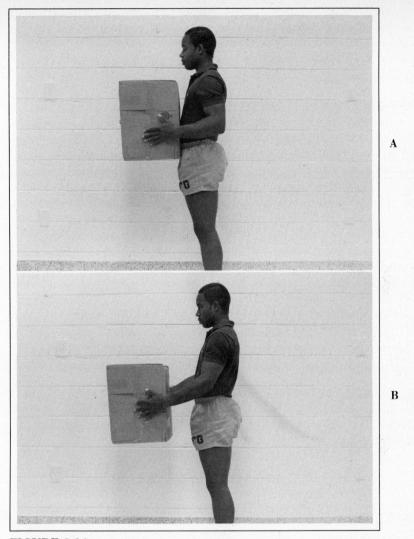

A

B

FIGURE 8-16

Heavy objects should be carried close to the body. **A,** Correct; **B,** incorrect.

Working posture. When lifting objects from the ground it is important to remember to use the legs to lift, not the back. Always turn and face the object you are going to lift. Bend at the knees and keep your lower back straight rather than trying to keep the legs straight and bend at the waist (Fig. 8-15). Don't try to lift the object higher than your waist. When carrying heavy objects, hold them close to you with the elbows locked at the sides (Fig. 8-16). It is best to remember that when you are working it pays to take a little extra time to position yourself properly for lifting and carrying heavy objects to avoid repetitive stress to the lower back.

Lower Back Exercises

For the normal person the biggest problem in the case of lower back pain is that the muscles in the lower back are too tight and the abdominal muscles are relatively weak. Preventive exercises should be directed toward improving flexibility of the lower back muscles while increasing the strength and tone of the abdominal muscles. Fig. 8-17 indicates an exercise for improving lower back flexibility.

Sit-ups are the best exercise for strengthening the abdominal muscles. Sit-ups must be done with the knees flexed to 90° to eliminate the curve in the lower back. The head should be lifted off the ground and the trunk should curl into the sit-up position. Alteration of this technique may cause additional strain to the lower back (Fig. 8-18).

The pelvic tilt exercise may also be used to strengthen abdominal muscles and loosen up lower back muscles to eliminate swayback. It is done by lying on the back on the floor and pressing the lower back flat against the floor (Fig. 8-19).

Additional Helpful Hints

1. Avoid wearing high-heeled shoes, which can increase the curvature in the lower back. You should buy shoes that have a consistent heel height.
2. When carrying heavy objects, try to balance the load and carry the weight as close to the body as possible.
3. Don't try to lift or move objects that are too heavy for you. Find someone else to help you.
4. Avoid sudden straining-type movements. This is a problem during athletic participation; however, if the lower back and abdominal muscles have been properly conditioned, the chances of injury are significantly reduced.
5. Avoid buying soft mattresses or chairs. Even though they may feel very comfortable initially, they can potentially cause significant low back pain over a period of time.
6. If lower back injury does occur, consult a qualified professional who is highly trained in the treatment of lower back pain. Many people who have lower back pain seem to be turning to chiropractors for treatment. There are good and bad chiropractors, just as there are good and bad physicians, athletic trainers, and physical therapists. It pays to talk to people about the skill of the person you choose to treat you. Remember that getting a second opinion is always a good idea.

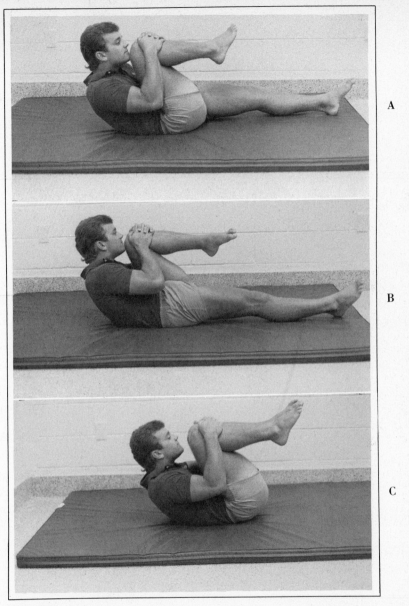

FIGURE 8-17

Exercise: Low back stretch.
Muscles stretched: Extensors of lumbar and sacral vertebrae.
Instructions: Lie flat on back. Bring right knee up and touch chin to knee (**A**); bring left knee up and touch chin to knee (**B**); bring both knees up and touch chin to knees (**C**). Repeat entire sequence 3 times, hold each position for 30 seconds.

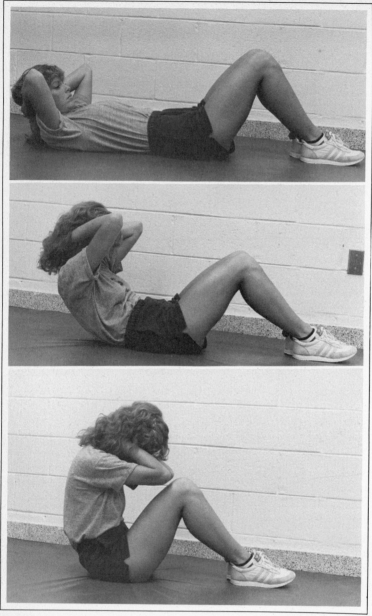

FIGURE 8-18

Sit-ups should be done with the knees flexed and the neck curled to avoid lower back strain.

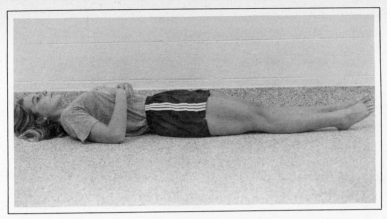

FIGURE 8-19

Pelvic tilt exercise is used to correct swayback by contracting the abdominal muscles to press the low back firmly against the ground.

INJURIES TO THE LOWER EXTREMITY

Chondromalacia Patella

There is little doubt that *chondromalacia patella* is the most common overuse type of injury to the lower extremity. Chondromalacia involves damage to the articular cartilage on the back of the patella, or kneecap. Through some kind of trauma, either falling directly on the knee or as a result of excessive stressful knee movements such as in running, this articular cartilage becomes damaged, and small cracks, splits, and tears develop. Normally the patella slides up and down very smoothly in its groove during knee flexion and extension. But when these cracks and splits form in the articular cartilage, the sliding movement is no longer smooth and it feels as if there is some grating, popping, or clicking around the joint.

Persons with chondromalacia patella commonly complain of pain when walking up or down stairs or when standing from a squatting position. They indicate a feeling that the knee is about to "go out from underneath them," although there is no instability whatsoever associated with chondromalacia patella. There are times when this condition is very painful and limiting and other times when there is absolutely no pain.

Chondromalacia is a form of osteoarthritis, which is known to involve some degeneration of the articular cartilage. Once the degeneration begins there is little that can be done to reverse the process; however, it may be possible to reduce the pain of chondromalacia to some extent by strength training of the quadriceps muscle group. We find that knee extension exercises (Fig. 8-20) that concentrate on strengthening through the last 20° of extension are helpful in

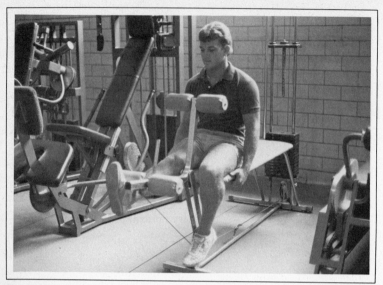

FIGURE 8-20

Strengthening of the quadriceps is essential in a knee rehabilitation program.

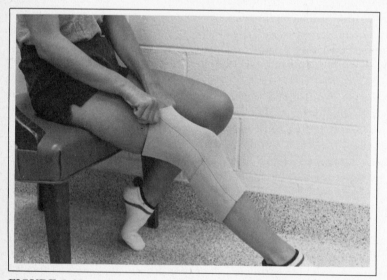

FIGURE 8-21

A Neoprene sleeve can be helpful for chondromalacia and jumper's knee.

reducing pain. It must be added, however, that doing knee extensions through a full range of motion during periods when chondromalacia is painful may only increase the pain. It may be necessary to instead perform isometric exercises by contracting the quadriceps muscle with the knee in full extension and trying to press the back of the knee into the ground.

When the knee is painful, it may be helpful to use a lot of cold therapy to take advantage of the analgesic effects of ice. Ice may well be of little therapeutic benefit but it will definitely help in pain reduction.

It may also be helpful to wear a neoprene sleeve around the knee joint during activity (Fig. 8-21). Neoprene is the material wet suits are made of. The knee sleeve provides pressure around the joint, which seems to provide a little support and also tends to keep the joint warm during activity. Wearing a knee sleeve is helpful to some persons but seems to have no effect in reducing pain for others.

Shin Splints

Shin splints is a catch-all term that refers to any pain that occurs in the anterior shin. Shin splints can result from several different conditions; pain may result from muscle strains at the point of attachment in the anterior compartment; inflammation of a broad ligamentous sheath that connects the tibia and fibula may also produce pain; and occasionally a stress fracture of either the tibia or fibula is classified as shin splints. Pain may occur anywhere in the anterior surface of the shin; however, shin splints seem to occur most often in the anterior medial surface of the lower half of the leg.

Once shin splints occur, they become a cause for concern because a stress fracture may be involved. Running should be stopped. Alternative conditioning activities such as swimming or cycling can be substituted. Ice massage is helpful for reducing pain. Therapeutic exercises for shin splints include stretching of the muscles that make up the Achilles heel cord complex (gastrocnemius and soleus) (see Fig. 5-24). A heel lift insert made of ¼-inch thick felt and inserted in the shoe may also be helpful.

Shin splints may be avoided by running as much as possible on soft surfaces, wearing well-padded, shock-absorbing shoes, and maintaining good flexibility of the Achilles heel cord through proper stretching.

Achilles Tendonitis

The gastrocnemius and soleus muscles come together to form the large Achilles tendon. The Achilles tendon, or heel cord, inserts into the calcaneus (heel bone) and when contracted produces plantar flexion. *Achilles tendonitis* occurs as a result of repetitive forceful plantar flexion of the foot in activities that involve a lot of running. Inflammation develops around the area of attachment to the

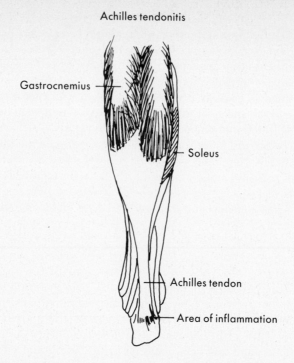

Achilles tendonitis

Gastrocnemius

Soleus

Achilles tendon

Area of inflammation

FIGURE 8-22

Achilles heel cord, showing most common area of inflammation.

calcaneus (Fig. 8-22). The area of inflammation becomes very painful, particularly during active movement. There may also be considerable swelling in the area of inflammation. Crepitus is easily detected in advanced stages.

Achilles tendonitis may become so painful that running must be stopped altogether, and walking will also be limited. Rest is essential to healing in Achilles tendonitis. Ice massage and anti-inflammatory medication (aspirin) will help reduce inflammation. During a rehabilitation program, the Achilles tendon must be stretched (see Fig. 5-24). Placing a heel lift made of ¼-inch felt in the heel of the shoe will take some stress off of the heel cord when walking.

ANKLE AND FOOT INJURIES

The ankle joint involves the articulation of three bones; the tibia and fibula of the lower leg, and the talus, which wedges up between the two long bones (Fig. 8-23).

The muscles that surround the ankle joint originate in the lower leg. Some of them produce movement only at the ankle joint, whereas others cause movement of the toes. The stability of the ankle joint is maintained primarily by strong

Ankle joint and ligaments

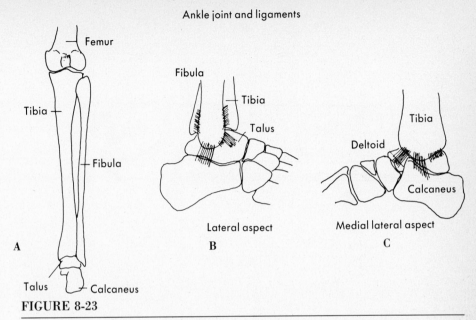

FIGURE 8-23

Ankle joint structure: **A,** bones; **B,** lateral ligaments; **C,** medial ligaments.

medial and lateral ligaments that prevent excessive inversion and eversion motion.

Ankle Sprains

Of all the problems discussed in this chapter, ankle sprains are probably the most common acute injury associated with physical activity.

Ankle sprains generally occur when the foot rolls underneath, causing a sprain of the ligaments on either the lateral or medial side of the joint. Sprains that involve the lateral ligaments are called inversion sprains because the sole of the foot turns inward. Sprains of the medial ligaments are referred to as eversion sprains because the sole of the foot turns outward (Fig. 8-24).

Inversion sprains are much more common than eversion sprains for two reasons. The malleolus (ankle bone) on the lateral side is much longer than the medial malleolus. When the talus tilts back and forth in the joint, the lateral malleolus prevents eversion. However, the medial malleolus does not stop inversion, and it is much more likely that the lateral ligaments will be injured. Also, the medial ligament is much thicker and stronger than the lateral ligaments and thus is less likely to be sprained.

If an ankle sprain does occur, it must be treated initially with ice, compression, and elevation. Long-term rehabilitation would be directed toward decreasing pain, improving range of motion through flexibility exercises, and strengthen-

Inversion/eversion movements causing sprains

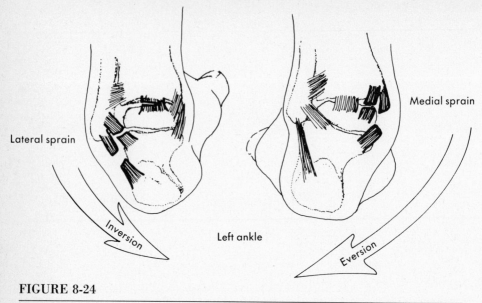

FIGURE 8-24

Ligament sprains caused by excessive inversion or eversion.

ing the muscles surrounding the ankle joint by doing resistive exercises with weights.

Plantar Fasciitis

The plantar fascia is a broad band of dense connective tissue that runs from its primary insertion on the inferior medial calcaneus, and fans out to insert at the base of the toes (Fig. 8-25). The plantar fascia supports the longitudinal arch in the foot and provides stability to the metatarsal bones.

The plantar fascia tends to be irritated during the early stages of activities involving a lot of repetitive jumping or running. It is placed under a great deal of stress when the toes are extended and the weight is on the ball of the foot or when the longitudinal arch is depressed. This occurs whenever there is plantar flexion and the toes forcefully push off the ground. *Plantar fasciitis* often results from changing from a rigid, inflexible street shoe to a soft, pliable running shoe.

Pain resulting from irritation of the plantar fascia is most often felt at the insertion on the inferior surface of the calcaneus. If inflammation of this area persists, a small calcium deposit or bone spur may appear, which becomes painful during weight bearing. Pain is increased whenever the toes, particularly the great toe, are extended.

Plantar fasciitis will respond to ice massage and stretching by passive extension of the great toe. A plastic heel cup that disperses forces around the heel may take some pressure off the irritated and painful site of origin (Fig. 8-26).

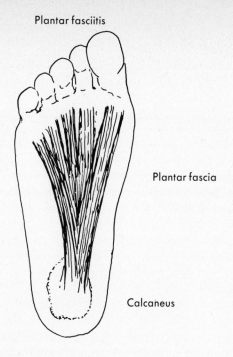

FIGURE 8-25

Plantar fascia attachments.

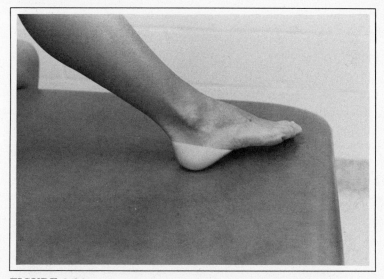

FIGURE 8-26

A plastic heel cup can take pressure off the tender point on the heel by dispersing forces over a larger surface area.

TREATMENT AND MANAGEMENT OF INJURIES

Initial first aid and management techniques for each of the above problems were not discussed individually because, fortunately, the methods of treatment for all are similar.

Regardless of which type of injury we are talking about, there is one problem they all have in common—swelling. Swelling may be caused by any number of factors, including bleeding, production of synovial fluid, an accumulation of inflammatory by-products, *edema*, which is nothing more than an accumulation of body fluid, or a combination of several factors. No matter which mechanism is involved, swelling produces an increased pressure in the injured area, and increased pressure causes pain. Swelling is most likely during the first 72 hours after an injury. Once swelling has occurred, the healing process is significantly retarded. The injured area cannot return to normal until all the swelling is gone.

Therefore everything that is done in terms of first-aid management of any of these conditions should be directed toward controlling the swelling. If the swelling can be controlled initially in the acute stage of injury, it is very likely that that time required for rehabilitation will be significantly reduced.

To control and severely limit the amount of swelling, the ICE principle can be applied. ICE stands for Ice, Compression, and Elevation. Each factor plays a critical role in limiting swelling, and all three should be used simultaneously.

Use of Ice Treatments

There is increasing agreement that in acute injury the use of cold is the initial treatment of choice for most conditions involving strains, sprains, and contusions.[2] It is most commonly used immediately after injury to decrease pain and promote local vasoconstriction, thus controlling hemorrhage and edema. It is also used in the acute phase of inflammatory conditions such as bursiitis, tenosynovitis, and tendonitis conditions in which heat may cause additional pain and swelling. Cold is also used to reduce the reflex muscle spasm and spastic conditions that accompany pain. Its analgesic effect is probably one of its greatest benefits. One explanation of the analgesic effect is that cold decreases the velocity of nerve conduction, although it does not entirely eliminate it. It is also possible that cold bombards central pain receptor areas with so many cold impulses that pain impulses are lost. With ice treatments, the patient usually reports an uncomfortable sensation of cold, followed by burning, then an aching sensation, and finally complete numbness.

Because of the low thermal conductivity of underlying subcutaneous fat tissues, applications of cold for short periods of time will be ineffective in cooling deeper tissues. For this reason longer treatments, 20 to 30 minutes in duration, are recommended. It is generally believed that cold treatments are more effective in reaching deep tissues than most forms of heat. Cold applied to the skin is capable of significantly lowering the temperature of tissues at a considerable depth. The extent of this lowered tissue temperature depends on the type of cold

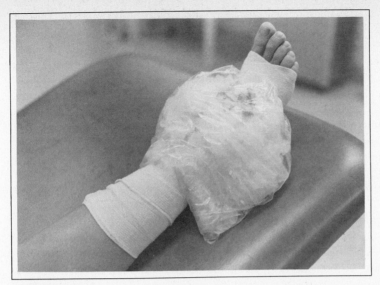

FIGURE 8-27

Ice-compression-elevation technique for treatment of a sprained ankle.

applied to the skin, the duration of its application, the thickness of the subcutaneous fat, and the region of the body to which it is applied.

Compression

Compression is equally as important as ice for controlling swelling. The purpose
of compression is to reduce the amount of space that is available for swelling
by applying pressure around an injured area. The best way of applying pressure
is to use an elastic wrap (such as an Ace bandage) to apply firm but even pressure
around the injury.

Because of the pressure buildup in the tissues, it may become painful to leave
a compression wrap in place for a long period of time. However, there is no
question that it is essential to leave the wrap in place even though there may
be significant pain because it is so important in the control of swelling. The
compression wrap should be left in place for at least 72 hours after an acute
injury. In many chronic overuse problems, such as tendonitis, tenosynovitis, and
particularly bursitis, the compression wrap should be worn until the swelling is
almost entirely gone.

Elevation

The third factor that assists in controlling swelling is elevation. The injured
part, particularly an extremity, should be elevated to eliminate the effects

of gravity on blood pooling in the extremities. Elevation assists venous drainage of blood and other fluids from the injured area back to the central circulatory system. The greater the degree of elevation, the more effective the reduction in swelling. For example, in an ankle sprain (Fig. 8-27), the leg should be placed in a position so that the ankle is virtually straight up in the air. The injured part should be elevated as much as possible during the first 72 hours.

The appropriate technique for initial management of acute injuries discussed in this chapter, regardless of where they occur, would be the following:

1. Apply a compression wrap directly over the injury. Wrapping should be from distal to proximal. Tension should be firm and consistent. It may be helpful to wet the elastic wrap to facilitate the passage of cold from ice packs.

2. Surround the injured area entirely with ice bags and secure them in place. Ice bags should be left on for 45 minutes initially and then 1 hour off and 30 minutes on as much as possible over the next 24 hours. During the following 48-hour period, ice should again be applied as often as possible.

3. The injured part should be elevated as much as possible during the initial 72-hour period after injury. It is particularly important to keep the injury elevated while sleeping.

Long-Term Rehabilitation

The initial management of an injury is extremely critical to the length of time required for rehabilitation. Although initial treatment will be virtually the same for everyone, long-term plans for rehabilitation are extremely variable and will be affected by many factors.

The goal of rehabilitation should be to return the person to physical activity as quickly and as safely as possible. Most persons involved in some physical activity, whether recreational or competitive, are interested in a speedy return to activity after injury. Thus the rehabilitation program philosophy should be extremely aggressive. Early movement involving both flexibility and strength training are important. The important thing to remember is that for a structure to heal properly it must perform the function for which it was designed. In the case of an injured muscle, it must be made to contract against resistance and produce movement. Strength training through a full range of motion is essential.

Long-term rehabilitation programs require the supervision of a trained professional if they are going to be safe and effective. Persons highly trained in the area of injury rehabilitation, such as athletic trainers or physical therapists, should be contacted to supervise rehabilitation programs. An injury that is not properly rehabilitated may continue to cause many problems with increasing age.

HEAT STRESS

Regardless of your level of physical conditioning, extreme caution must be taken when exericising in hot, humid weather. Prolonged exposure to extreme heat can result in heat cramps, heat exhaustion, or heatstroke. Heat stress is certainly preventable, but each year many people will suffer illness or perhaps death from some heat-related cause. People who exercise in the heat are particularly vulnerable to heat stress.

The physiologic processes in the body will only continue to function as long as body temperature is maintained within a normal range. Maintenance of normal temperature in a hot environment depends on the ability of the body to dissipate heat. Body temperature can be affected by four factors.

Metabolic heat production. Normal metabolic function in the body results in the production of heat. Consequently, metabolism will always cause a heat gain dependent on the intensity of the physical activity. The higher the metabolic rate, the more heat produced.

Convective heat exchange. Body heat can be either lost or gained, depending on the temperature of the circulating medium. A cool breeze will always tend to cool the body by removing heat from the body surface. Conversely, if the temperature of the circulating air is higher than the temperature of the skin, there will be a gain in body heat.

Radiant heat exchange. Radiant heat from sunshine will most definitely cause an increase in body temperature. However, on a cloudy day your body is also emitting radiant heat energy, and thus radiation may also result in either heat loss or heat gain.

Evaporative heat loss. Sweat glands in the skin allow water to be transported to the surface where it evaporates, taking large quantities of heat with it. When the temperature and radiant heat of the environment become higher than body temperature, loss of body heat becomes highly dependent on the process of sweat evaporation.

A normal person can sweat off about 1 quart of water per hour for about 2 hours. But the air must be relatively free of water for evaporation to occur. Heat loss through evaporation is severely impaired when the relative humidity reaches 65% and virtually stops when the humidity reaches 75%.

It should be obvious that heat-related problems have the greatest chance of occurrence on those days when the sun is bright and the temperature and relative humidity are very high. But it is certainly true that heat cramps, heat exhaustion, or heatstroke can occur whenever the body's ability to dissipate heat is impaired.

Heat Cramps

Heat cramps are extremely painful muscle spasms that occur most commonly in the calf and abdomen, although any muscle can be involved. The occurrence of heat cramps is related to some imbalance between water and several *electrolytes,* or ions (sodium, potassium, and calcium), which are each essential elements in muscle contraction.

Profuse sweating involves losses of large amounts of water and significant quantities of sodium and potassium, which destroys the balance in concentration of these elements in skeletal muscle and results in painful muscle contraction.

The person most likely to get heat cramps is one who is in fairly good condition but simply overexerts in the heat.

Heat cramps may be prevented by adequate placement of sodium, potassium, calcium, and water. Ingestion of salt tablets is not recommended. Simply salting food a bit more heavily can replace sodium; bananas are particularly high in potassium; and calcium can be gotten through milk and cheese products. The immediate treatment for heat cramps is ingestion of large quantities of water and mild stretching with ice massage of the muscle in spasm.

Heat Exhaustion

Heat exhaustion results from inadequate replacement of fluids lost through sweating. Clinically, the victim of heat exhaustion will collapse and manifest profuse sweating, flushed skin, mildly elevated temperature, dizziness, hyperventilation, and rapid pulse.

It is sometimes possible to spot a person who is having problems with heat exhaustion. They may begin to develop heat cramps. They become disoriented and light-headed, and their physical performance is not up to usual standards when fluid replacement has not been adequate. In general, persons in poor physical condition who attempt to exercise in the heat are most likely to get heat exhaustion.

Immediate treatment of heat exhaustion requires ingestion of large quantities of cool water. If possible, the person should be placed in a cool environment, although it is more essential to replace fluids.

Heatstroke

Unlike heat cramps and heat exhaustion, *heatstroke* is a serious, life-threatening emergency. The specific cause of heatstroke is unknown; however, it is clinically characterized by sudden collapse with loss of consciousness; pale, relatively dry skin; and most importantly, a core temperature of 106° or higher. Basically there is a breakdown of the sweating mechanism and the body loses the ability to sweat.

Heatstroke can occur suddenly and without warning. The victim will not usually experience signs of heat cramps or heat exhaustion. The possibility of death from heatstroke can be significantly reduced if body temperature is lowered to normal within 45 minutes.

Every first-aid effort should be directed to lowering body temperature. Strip *all* clothing off the victim and douse him or her with cool water and fan him or her with a towel. It is imperative that the victim be transported to a hospital as quickly as possible. Don't wait for an ambulance; transport the victim in whatever vehicle happens to be available. The replacement of fluid is not critical in initial first aid.

Prevention of Heat-Related Illness

Acclimatization. This is the process of gradually preparing the body to be able to work in heat by slowly exposing the system to the stresses of a hot, humid environment. Heat dramatically reduces performance capabilities, and abrupt exposure to these conditions can predispose a person to heat-related illness. Acclimatization to heat generally occurs rapidly, usually within 5 to 7 days of gradually increasing periods of exercise in the heat. It is enhanced by being in good physical condition and by adequate fluid replacement.

Fluid and electrolyte replacement. During hot weather it is essential to continually replace fluids lost through evaporation by drinking large quantities of water regardless of whether or not you are thirsty. To prevent heat cramps a balance must be maintained between water and the electrolytes. However, the time to be concerned about replacing electrolytes is not during physical activity. *Water should be the only fluid consumed during exercise.*

A number of commercial electrolyte drinks are available, including Gatorade, Pripps, Squencher, and Break Time. These electrolyte drinks are good for replenishing fluids and electrolytes before and after activity in the heat. However, ingestion of these drinks *during* activity may actually be harmful. In the stomach, hypertonic solutions such as these tend to draw fluids into the gastrointestinal tract, away from the working tissues. A cell needs water to be able to function normally and may be damaged if sufficient amounts of water are not available. Thus ingestion of electrolyte drinks during activity is not recommended.

Water breaks should be taken every 15 minutes during activity in a hot environment. There is no truth to the theory that drinking water during activity will produce stomach cramps.

Clothing. When exercising in the heat, wear as little clothing as possible to allow maximal evaporation. Light-colored cotton or nylon material allows maximal evaporation. A hat should never be worn because about 40% of all heat lost from the body is lost through the head.

Wearing a rubberized suit for the purpose of losing weight during hot weather is ineffective and dangerous. The only weight lost will be water weight, which must be replaced immediately after activity. Rubberized suits severely limit the body's ability to dissipate heat and may predispose you to heat exhaustion or possibly heatstroke.

Exercise your common sense when exercising. Avoid coming directly out of an air-conditioned environment and immediately beginning to exercise. Give yourself some time to adapt to the change in temperature.

If possible, do not exercise during the hottest part of the day between 11 AM and 4 PM. The temperature is usually highest at about 4 PM.

Try to avoid exercise on surfaces such as asphalt, concrete, or astroturf, which tend to absorb and hold heat.

If you experience any of the heat-related problems, stop activity immediately, get into a cool environment, and drink large quantities of cool water. Common sense is the best prevention for heat stress.

SUMMARY

- Injuries associated with a physical training program can be avoided by designing a well-planned program based on the principles of overload, progression, consistency, individuality, and safety.
- The best way to prevent injury is to begin at low levels of intensity and gradually progress at your own speed.
- Muscle strains involve a stretching or tearing of muscle fibers or their tendons, causing impairment to active movement.
- Muscle soreness results in spasms, which are caused by ischemia in working muscles.
- Tendonitis is an inflammation of a muscle tendon that usually occurs because of overuse, causing pain on movement.
- All injuries should be initially managed using ice, compression, and elevation for the purpose of controlling swelling and thus reducing the time required for rehabilitation.
- Lower back pain can result from many causes, but the three most common lower back problems are herinated discs, lumbosacral strains, and sacroiliac sprains.
- Lower back pain can be prevented by paying attention to standing, lying, sitting, and working postures to prevent the lower back from being placed in potentially injurious positions.
- Chondromalacia patella involves damage to the articular cartilage of the patella or femur, resulting in pain on flexion and extension movements.
- *Shin splints* is a term that applies to any kind of pain occurring in the anterior shin.
- Achilles tendonitis is an inflammation of the heel cord complex that usually occurs in running activities.
- Ankle sprains are most commonly inversion sprains that involve the lateral ligaments.

- Plantar fasciitis is an inflammation of the plantar fascia on the sole of the foot, usually occurring from excessive forceful extension of the toes.
- Particular caution must be used when exercising in a hot, humid, sunny environment. Failure to use some common sense in the heat may result in heat cramps, heat exhaustion, or heatstroke.
- Injuries that occur during physical activity should be diagnosed by a physician and rehabilitated by an athletic trainer or physical therapist.

GLOSSARY

achilles tendonitis Inflammation of the tendon on the lower portion of the back of the lower leg

chondromalacia patella Damage to the articular cartilage on the back of the kneecap and resulting from either direct trauma or overuse

edema Accumulation of body fluid in an area of injury

electrolytes Ions (sodium, potassium, calcium) that are essential elements for muscle contraction

heat cramps Painful muscle cramps that occur most commonly in the calf and abdomen and are related to some imbalance between water and electrolytes

heat exhaustion An illness associated with inadequate replacement of fluids lost through sweating

heatstroke A life-threatening emergency in which the sweating mechanism breaks down and the body is no longer able to dissipate heat

herniated disc Condition in which the nucleus of the vertebral disc is squeezed out of its normal position and presses on the spinal nerve, producing pain.

lumbosacral sprain Stretching or tearing of the ligaments between the vertebrae, resulting from twisting or sudden rotation

muscle soreness A syndrome of pain that includes muscle spasm and increased muscle tension that is usually observed after strenuous muscular exertion

plantar fasciitis Inflammation of the thick connective tissue running from the heel to the base of the toes that commonly occurs with running and jumping activities

sacroiliac sprain Stretching or tearing of the ligaments that connect the sacrum and the ilium in the lowest part of the back

shin splints A catch-all term that refers to any type of pain occurring in the anterior shin

stress fracture A fracture that results from overuse rather than acute trauma

strain The separation or tearing of muscle fibers

tendonitis Inflammation of a tendon that occurs as a result of trauma or overuse

REFERENCES

1. deVries, H. (1980). *Physiology of exercise for physical education and athletics*. Dubuque, IA: William C. Brown.
2. Prentice, W. (1982). An electromyographic analysis of the effectiveness of heat or cold and stretching for inducing muscular relaxation. *Journal of Orthopedics and Sports Physical Therapy*, 3, 133-140.

SUGGESTED READINGS

Albohm, M. *Health care for the female athlete*. North Palm Beach, FL: The Athletic Institute.

American Medical Association. (1966). *Standard nomenclature of athletic injuries*. Chicago: Author.

Arnheim, D. (1985). *Modern principles of athletic training*. St. Louis: Times Mirror/Mosby College Publishing.

Fox, E. (1984). *Sports physiology*. New York: CBS College Publishing.

Getchell, B. (1983). *Physical fitness: A way of life*. New York: John Wiley & Sons.

Morris, A. (1984). *Sports medicine: Prevention of athletic injuries*. Dubuque, IA: William C. Brown.

Muckle, D. (1982). *Injuries in sport: A guide for the accident department and general practice*. Boston: PSG Publishing.

O'Donoghue, D. (1984). *Treatment of injuries to athletes*. Philadelphia: W.B. Saunders.

Roy, S., & Irvin, R. (1983). *Sports medicine: Prevention evaluation management and rehabilitation*. Englewood Cliffs, NJ: Prentice-Hall.

Strauss, R. (1984). *Sports medicine*. Philadelphia: W.B. Saunders.

Vinger, P., & Hoerner, E. (1981). *Sports injuries—The unthwarted epidemic*. Boston: PSG Publishing.

THE MANAGEMENT

OF STRESS

After completing this chapter, you will be able to:

- Define the terms *stress*, *stressor*, *eustress*, and *distress*.
- Identify warning signs of stress.
- Describe various kinds of psychologic, physiologic, and sociologic stressors.
- Explain how stress can be both beneficial and harmful.
- Describe how the body responds to stress.
- Describe Seyle's general adaptation syndrome.
- Explain various acceptable ways of coping with stress as well as how defense mechanisms can be a questionable method.
- Describe the role of physical activity in coping with stress.
- Identify various relaxation techniques for coping with stress.
- List general guidelines for a college student for coping with stress.

The term *stress* comes from the Latin word *stringere*, meaning "to draw tight." The term refers to the responses that occur in the body as a result of what is called a *stressor*, or stimulus. Signs of stress may include insomnia, headaches, backaches, inability to cope, lack of concentration, anxiety, and irritability. Stress occurs when the homeostatic balance of the body is affected. Conditions that promote homeostatic imbalance can be either physiologic or psychologic.

Everyone experiences stress, and some stress is needed to perform the daily tasks of life. Stress can be beneficial, as when an athlete performs well after "psyching up" for an activity. However, too much stress, especially when it exists for a prolonged period of time and is unrelieved, can result in physical and mental illness. Stress is the body's way of reacting to any demand made on it.

Dr. Hans Seyle,[12] biologist and endocrinologist, defined stress as the "nonspecific response of the body to any demand made upon it." He further points out that stress is caused or triggered by stressors that may be physical, social, or psychologic and negative or positive in nature. Seyle called human reactions to positive stressors *eustress* and used the term *distress* to describe responses to negative stressors.

When a person is under stress, the brain activates two interrelated physiologic systems—the autonomic nervous system and the endocrine system. The result is an increased heart rate and blood pressure and elevated levels of oxygen and glucose in the blood. These responses prepare us for "fight" or "flight."

TYPES OF STRESSORS

There are many different types of stressors. Psychologic stressors arouse emotions such as fear, anxiety, anger, and love. There are biolecologic stressors such as noise, heat, and cold. Worrying about an examination is a stressor, as are vigorous exercise and strenuous sports activities. All illnesses are stressors. There are many environmental stressors, such as air pollution and overcrowding. Family or financial problems are examples of social stressors. Caffeine, sugar, white flour, and salt are physiologic stressors. Deprivational stress results from boredom and loneliness.

Each day in college life students encounter many stresses that are insignificant or great, pleasant or painful, physical or mental. Stressors in college may be tests, arguments with loved ones, money worries, or dislike for a subject, professor, or classmates. These stressors may cause headaches, muscle spasms, excessive sweating, constipation, rapid heart rate, stomachache, dermatitis, high blood pressure, nail biting, or heartburn.

Changes that occur during a person's lifetime are major stressors. Holmes and Rahe[6] have developed a life change scale to show how various life events can cause stress as they change a person's life-style. The scale was developed after hundreds of persons were surveyed and were asked how much stress they experienced in adapting to changes in their lives. Marriage was given a value of 50 points, and people were then requested to rate other events according to how much adjustment each event called for as compared to their marriage. For example, losing a spouse by death was rated 100 points, divorce received a rating of 73 points, personal injury or illness, 53 points, pregnancy, 40 points, sexual difficulties, 39 points, outstanding personal achievements, 28 points, beginning or ending school, 26 points, change in schools, 20 points, change in social activities, 18 points, change in eating habits, 15 points, and minor violations of the law, 11 points.

UNCONTROLLED STRESS

Uncontrolled stress can result in physical disorders that in turn result in a low level of fitness. To manage stress you must realize that you are responsible for

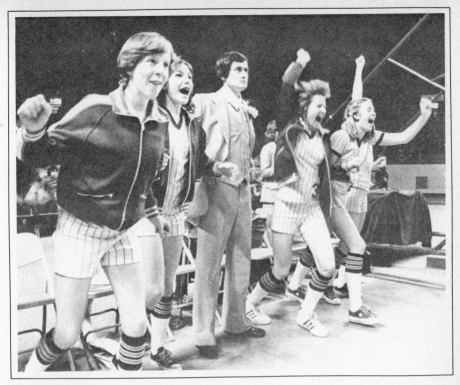

FIGURE 9-1

College students encounter many different types of stress each day, some
pleasant and others harmful.
From Coakley, J.J. (1978). *Sport in society*. St. Louis: C.V. Mosby.

your own emotional and physical well-being. Your perception of events, not the
events themselves, are under your control. You should not allow other people's
behavior to affect your ability to maintain a relatively stable condition (homeostatic balance). There are certain things that you can do to manage stress.

Although there are several methods and techniques to control stress, physical
activity is one of the most helpful.[4] It is believed that exercise burns up stress
hormones. Activity helps to release the tension that can accumulate when you
are under stress; inactivity inhibits natural expression. As a result, hormone-
induced tension is alleviated by activity. A stress-regulated and controlled life-
style is thought by some to provide a balance between work, play, rest, and
exercise.

WARNING SIGNS

Persons under stress tend to display certain warning signs and symptoms that vary from one person to the next. Seyle lists 31 signs of danger that anyone can easily detect (see box below). If you experience one or more of these symptoms, you are experiencing some degree of stress. You should also determine if your stress level is too high. If it is, try to reduce your stress level to avoid developing physical or emotional health problems.

Signs of Stress

Seyle lists stress symptoms that may represent danger signs. Check to see if you experience one or more of these symptoms:

	Yes	No
Irritability and depression	✓	
Heart palpitations	✓	
Dryness of throat and mouth	✓	
Impulsive behavior	✓	
Inability to concentrate	✓	
Feelings of weakness or dizziness	✓	
Crying		✓
Anxiety	✓	
Emotional tension	✓	
Nervous tics		✓
Vomiting		✓
Easily startled by small sounds		✓
Nervous laughter		✓
Trembling hands		✓
Stuttering or other speech problems		✓
Insomnia	✓	
Breathlessness		✓
Sweating		✓
Frequent urination		✓
Diarrhea and indigestion		✓
Migraine headaches		✓
Premenstrual tension or missed menstrual cycles	✓	
Pain in back		✓
Increased smoking		✓
Loss of appetite		✓
Nightmares	✓	
Fatigue	✓	

From Seyle, H. (1976). *The stress of life*. New York: McGraw-Hill.

You can see from Seyle's list that some physical and emotional signs of distress affect certain of the body's organic systems. Heart palpitations are cardiovascular in nature, vomiting is gastrointestinal in nature, and breathlessness is respiratory in nature. Some signs also reflect muscular tension, such as frequent headaches, fatigue, and trembling hands. Some signs also reflect conscious feelings, such as being fearful or apprehensive, crying, and mental disorientation and confusion.

Depression and anxiety are two common signs of stress. Depression can be characterized by sadness, lack of energy, and poor concentration with inability to perform routine activities. Anxiety can reflect a feeling of dread and apprehension, perhaps of some anticipated danger or lack of proper plans and strategy for coping with an anticipated danger. There may be worry about many things that can go wrong in accomplishing future plans.

Insomnia is a common sign of stress that drains a person's energy. The reason for insomnia may be that you are anxious or excited about future events. Although missing a night or two of sleep may be a normal thing for some people, for others it can be a symptom of stress.

There are many other signs of stress. Some people get pains in the back or neck when experiencing stress. This may be caused by a tensing of the muscles in these regions. Some people under stress let it affect their appetite. The result may be overeating or undereating. Others increase the number of cigarettes they smoke, feeling that relief comes with every puff on the cigarette. However, the chances are that the more you smoke, the more you are stressed because nicotine increases heart rate and acts on the body to temporarily raise blood pressure and levels of cholesterol and noradrenaline (which is closely associated with adrenalin).

An increase in the consumption of alcohol may also be a sign of stress. The danger here is that because drinking does permit a person to relax and forget some of the things that are causing stress, it may result in more and more drinking in order to experience additional psychic elation. However, such increased drinking can lead to further problems, including alcoholism.

There are some persons who also increase their caffeine intake when under stress. The average cup of coffee contains 100 to 150 mg of caffeine, and consumption of caffeine can cause or exacerbate insomnia, headaches, and nervousness.

Sexual dysfunction can also be a sign of stress. Furthermore, such a condition can lead to further stress if the condition continues to exist as a result of worry. Because sexual release is one method of alleviating stress, lack of this ability creates further problems.

THE BODY'S RESPONSE

Seyle described the body's response to stress as the *general adaptation syndrome* (GAS). His research showed that the response to stressors follows a three-stage pattern of alarm, resistance, and exhaustion.

Alarm. In the first stage, the body mechanisms are mobilized. Muscles tense, a queasy feeling appears in the stomach, the mouth is dry, and the pulse is rapid. Various hormones are secreted by the pituitary and adrenal glands, of which adrenalin is one of the best known. These hormones speed up the heartbeat, and the blood vessels become constricted. Respiration increases. Blood pressure goes up. These changes in the body are often referred to as the "fight or flight" syndrome. They are the body's normal reaction to danger and prepare a person to fight against a hostile stressor.

Resistance. At the resistance stage the body adjusts to stress and appears to return to its normal state of equilibrium. Heartbeat and respiration return to normal, and sweating disappears. Hormones known as ACTH and cortin, which are secreted by the pituitary gland and the adrenal cortex, have a calming effect and help the organism cope with the stressful situation. This is the stage of maximal ability of the body to withstand the stressor; it may continue for several days or longer, depending on the vitality of the person affected. However, sustained resistance can result in a strain on the body's resources.

Exhaustion. If stress continues and persists for a long time, exhaustion sets in. The hormones released by the pituitary gland to counter stress begin to weaken. Some of the symptoms that existed during the first (alarm) stage reappear, such as fatigue, headache, and muscle and joint pain. The person becomes progressively devitalized and loses the ability to resist stress. The various body functions are weakened. If this stage continues, it can result in death.

The body controls stress via the nervous system. The autonomic nervous system, which is usually beyond our control, goes into action when there is a stress response. The autonomic nervous system has two subsystems that also play a role in controlling stress, namely, the sympathetic and parasympathetic nervous systems. The sympathetic nervous system releases adrenalin into the bloodstream, producing the "fight or flight" response. This in turn, causes various changes to take place within the body, such as increased blood pressure and heart rate, that enable it to adapt to the stress response. The parasympathetic part of the autonomic nervous system, on the other hand, is responsible for lowering the heart rate and blood pressure. Techniques that reduce stress are utilized to increase the action of the parasympathetic system and decrease the action of the sympathetic nervous system.

As can be seen, stress can affect various body systems, particularly the digestive system. Most persons have at one time or other experienced nervous indigestion from emotional stress. This malady is the result of change of the rhythmic contractions of the muscle valves at the entrance and exit of the stomach. Under stress, muscle spasms can develop, resulting in the upper valve, the gateway to the stomach, becoming partially closed. The muscles of the esophagus then contract to force the food through the narrow valve, and this results in pain and indigestion. Furthermore, stress can affect the balance of the acid in the stomach, causing ulcers to develop, and contractions in the large intestine may result in diarrhea and constipation.

The cardiovascular system is also affected by stress. Heart rate and stroke volume increase, thus creating greater cardiac output, and blood vessels in the skin, kidneys, and internal organs become constricted, decreasing blood flow to these areas. Blood vessels in the skeletal muscles dilate, increasing the flow of blood to them; blood pressure and the volume of blood that is circulating are increased, which results in hypertension. Some authorities believe that emotional stress is one of the leading causes of cardiovascular disease. In identifying people at risk for cardiovascular disease, researchers commonly classify persons as "type A" or "type B" personalities. Drs. Meyer Friedman and Ray H. Rosenman[5] believe that the high-risk type A person, is a candidate for heart disease. This person is constantly on the go, never satisfied with what he or she has achieved, often seems tense, makes rapid body movements, suffers a sense of time urgency, and is impatient. In contrast, the "type B" person is more easygoing and relaxed, feels good about himself or herself, and is therefore thought to be less susceptible to heart disease.

The other systems of the body also are affected by prolonged stress. For example, the muscular system may respond to stress by the existence of uncontrolled spasms called *tics*. Furthermore, it has been suggested that more research should be conducted to see if there is any relationship between stress and problems affecting bones and joints (such as arthritis), the breakdown in the body's natural defense system (which can make a person more susceptible to illnesses such as cancer), and skin eruptions such as hives and acne.

COPING WITH STRESS

College life is filled with many challenges, some of which represent obstacles in the path of your career and life goals. When you face a challenge such as getting good grades in order to get into graduate school or have more free time, you may find that your body's homeostatic balance has been upset. This disruption may be short-lived as the challenge is met. On the other hand, there may be times when the disruption is long and difficult to control, and as a result, you find yourself under stress.

All students experience stress at times. Such stress may be helpful or harmful. It may motivate you to put forth greater effort and thus have positive growth effects, or, if it is exceptionally strong and recurring, it can contribute to several kinds of illness. Through proper procedures, however, you can improve mind-body harmony and thus reduce harmful stress and contribute to your health and fitness.

Coping skills to ward off stress are processes that allow people to deal with stress in a positive way. As people mature, they gain the competencies that keep their lives in equilibrium; however, these competencies are not always easily obtained. In most human endeavors there will be barriers to self-fulfillment, but as people manage stress in the form of pressures, conflicts, and frustrations, they strengthen their ability to select appropriate responses.

Of primary importance in life adjustment is the ability to face reality. This requires the courage to examine honestly and objectively the assumptions and values on which we base our judgments. Psychologists tell us that this self-examination or reality-testing implies maturity; however, for most of us it is difficult to test our basic assumptions against truth.

Learning to utilize reality-testing more effectively, we have to be aware that our behaviors are altered or controlled by the kinds of reinforcement we give ourselves or receive from others. In the end, each of us must manage our own emotions and make adjustments in order to control stress. People sometimes try to cope with stress by utilizing adjustment techniques called defense mechanisms.

Defense Mechanisms

In a very broad sense, every behavior or thought that satisfies some need is a defense mechanism. However, in psychology these mechanisms are usually cat-

Defense Mechanisms

Rationalization:	A mental mechanism that is used to avoid facing a loss of self-esteem or to prevent feeling guilty. For example, a student who flunks out of college remarks "Who needs it?"
Projection:	Attribution of unacceptable personal qualities to other people, as when the inability to make friends evokes the response, "The people are all unfriendly."
Compensation:	Substitution of an attainable goal for one that may be unattainable. For example, the physically inadequate student who wants to be a star athlete, but cannot, puts all his energies into journalism, at which he can excel.
Sublimation:	Change of direction of a basic drive toward a new goal when previous goal is impossible to obtain. For example, a student with a basic drive of aggression directs it to playing football rather than taking it out on classmates by picking fights with them.
Repression:	Removal from consciousness of memories that are painful and desires that produce strong guilt feelings. For example, a student fails to keep an appointment with a professor who failed him in another subject. This mechanism can be harmful when it creates stress and behavioral problems.
Fantasy:	Type of daydreaming involving substitution of imagination for reality. For example, a student imagines she is the top student in the class or the star athlete on the team.
Identification:	Identification with another person such as a professor, a coach, or a famous personality. This mental mechanism becomes harmful when it interferes with the development of a person's real self and identity.

egorized and defined by therapists as they interpret the meaning behind everyday behavior. Essentially, defense mechanisms protect the ego; they preserve harmony within a person and provide to some degree a sense of adequacy. They help a person cope with anxiety. We all use defense mechanisms, but if these mechanisms are allowed to become a habitual pattern of behavior, our behavior under any stress can become counterproductive.

The particular mechanism operating at a given moment depends on a particular situation and the past history of reinforcement. A person tends to use those forms of behavior that have worked most effectively in the past. A word of caution: these mechanisms are often deceptive devices; that is, they are not necessarily the most successful way to control stress. They may bolster the ego, but they also can circumvent real problems, in which case they are evasions (see box on opposite page).

Mental mechanisms are deceptive. They are often unconsciously originated, but the behaviors are observable. The better you understand your own behavior and motives, the better able you will be to cope with stress and develop into a productive human being. Inappropriate behavior can become habitual, particularly if you are encouraged (reinforced) by the behavior.

PHYSICAL ACTIVITY AND STRESS

Michael,[10] in *Stress Adaptation Through Exercise*, found that physical activity provides a low type of stress for the adrenal glands that strengthens them so that they can more effectively counter severe stress. Increased adrenal activity as a result of exercise appears to result in the creation and formation of reserves of steroids, which counteract stress.

deVries[4] found that activities such as jogging, bicycling, walking, and bench-stepping of durations from 5 to 30 minutes and with target heart rates of 30% to 60% of maximal rate resulted in significant relaxation for tense persons. Exercise appears to provide a mental diversion from problems and activities that could cause stress.

Seyle[13] suggests that the person who exercises regularly is able to resist stressors better, and that situations that are stressful do not represent as much harm to the trained person as to the sedentary person.

Matteson and Ivancevich,[8] in their book *Managing Job Stress and Health*, indicated that the general benefits of exercise include the following:
Greater strength and endurance, leading to more efficient utilization of energy
Improved cardiovascular function, including lowering of blood pressure and a lower heart rate
Less fatty tissue in the body
Better appearance and a more positive self-concept
Better muscle tone and posture
Better utilization of foods
Greater cardiac output

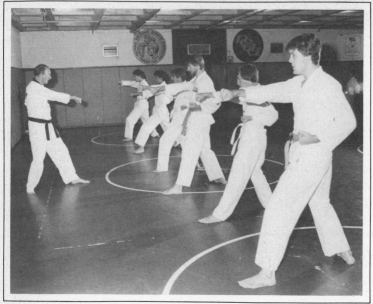

FIGURE 9-2

Physical activity is one of the most beneficial methods of stress reduction. These students are practicing karate.

Increased number of red blood cells, furthering oxygen delivery to cells
Better sleeping pattern
Less consumption of drugs, alcohol, tobacco, and sugar
Better control of body weight
Lower cholesterol levels in the blood

According to Anderson,[2] physical exercise provides three benefits for humans: (1) maintenance of good muscular tone, which makes it possible to engage in a variety of physical activities, (2) creation of a healthy cardiovascular system, and (3) a sense of well-being as a result of reduced stress. Yates[13] adds that a person is more relaxed after exercising.

Charlesworth and Nathan[3] point out that the human body and the image of that body that is held by some persons is a stressor, whether because of too much weight, poor muscular development, or poor posture. Exercise can improve your body development and in turn your self-image. They also point out that when problems confront you and appear difficult to solve, physical activity can provide a mental release and an opportunity to arrive at solutions in a more relaxed manner.

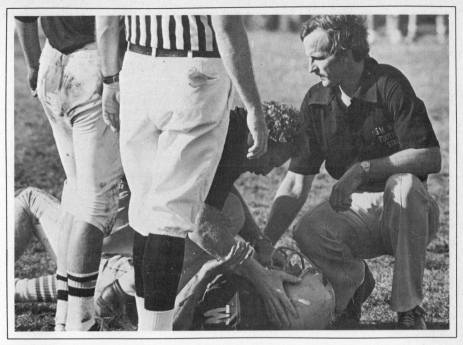

FIGURE 9-3

Athletic injuries can cause stress.
Courtesy Cramer Products, Inc., Gardner, Kan.

BENEFITS OF PHYSICAL ACTIVITY IN REDUCING STRESS

Improved Cardiovascular Function

Cardiovascular function is important in supplying the muscles with fuel and oxygen. The more efficient your cardiovascular function, the longer you will be able to sustain work. Cardiovascular efficiency represents the ability of the circulatory, respiratory, and other systems of the body to put forth an extended and persistent effort. Because of the benefits that are derived from improved cardiovascular function, such as the potential it has for preventing circulatory diseases, improving work capacity, providing greater resistance to fatigue, strengthening heart muscle, lowering resting heart rate, restricting the production of lactic acid, and enhancing endurance, this component, if properly developed, can render a major contribution to your ability to reduce stress.

Because the heart is a muscle, it must be exercised the same as any other muscle in the human body. Coronary heart disease appears to occur much more frequently in sedentary persons than in active persons. Also, diseases such as diabetes, duodenal ulcer, and lower back pain and certain emotional problems have been found to have a higher incidence among sedentary persons.

The cardiovascular system is improved by physical activity. A person who participates in regular and adequate amounts of exercise has a heart that usually beats more slowly than the heart of someone who does little exercise; furthermore, each beat of the heart moves a greater volume of blood. Exercise increases the blood-carrying capacity of the blood vessels, which permits the blood to circulate more efficiently throughout the body and at a lower pressure. The combination of a lower heart rate, lower blood pressure, and improved condition of the blood vessels helps in reducing circulatory disorders, which in turn reduces stress.

Less Body Fat

Body composition refers to the amount of fat in relation to the percentage of nonfat in the total body mass. It has been estimated that more than 50% of the adult population is overweight, a condition that can be extremely stressful to the body. Carrying around excess pounds has been related to such health problems as heart disease, arthritis, gallbladder disease, kidney disease, postural difficulties, and a shortened life span. Also, there is the problem of weakened endurance and capacity for work and study. On the other hand, proper body weight results in better appearance, less susceptibility to disease, greater efficiency, and less stress.

Obese persons have stores of fat that are utilized in response to needed calories. Studies of obese adults have shown that their weight gain began when their activity decreased but not their appetite. Eating is not stimulated by exercise, it is stimulated by habit.

Mental Health

The values of exercise are not limited to the physical; exercise also contributes to sound mental health. Those who exercise regularly never fail to mention that exercise makes them feel better. Psychiatrist William Menninger pointed out that physical activity provides an outlet for instinctive aggressive drives by enabling a person to "blow off steam," provides relaxation, and supplements daily work and study. He stressed the fact that "recreation, which is literally re-creating relaxation from regular activity, is a morale builder."

Flexibility

Poor joint flexibility can cause stress by resulting in health and fitness problems such as muscle strain caused by poor flexibility and backache caused by shortened lumbar and hip flexor muscles. (See chapter 5 for a further discussion of flexibility.)

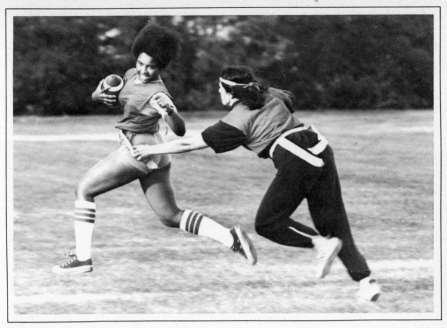

FIGURE 9-4

Taking part in games and sports is a good way to relieve stress. Flag football at The University of Mississippi.
Photo by Nelson D. Neal.

Strength and Endurance

Strength and endurance, capable of being developed through physical activity, provide major benefits in performing daily tasks and meeting emergencies with less fatigue. For example, they can help prevent lower back pain (see Chapter 8). Studies of 5000 patients at the Columbia Presbyterian Medical Center in New York and the Institute of Physical Medicine and Rehabilitation, New York University, indicated that approximately 80% of patients with lower back pain experienced this difficulty because of muscle weakness or stiffness. Follow-up studies showed that pain symptoms decreased as muscle strength and flexibility increased (see Chapter 4). If exercise was discontinued, the ailments returned.

How Physical Activity Reduces Stress

The human body responds to stress, as has been mentioned, by a response known as "fight or flight." As a result, a number of hormonal and physiologic changes take place as stress by-products are created for an overt physical response. By responding to the stressor by engaging in physical activity, the stress by-products are utilized. If not utilized by physical activity, the physiologic arousal that has been created continues to exist, and the body can be damaged.

Exactly how physical activity reduces stress is not completely understood at the present time. It has been generally established that the mind can influence the body, and it also is believed that the body influences the mind. The study of this subject is known as somatopsychics, and research in this area suggests

---

General Guidelines For Stress Reduction

Seyle set forth several suggestions for stress reduction, including:
Try not to be a perfectionist—instead, perform and work within your capabilities
Spend your time in ways other than trying to befriend those persons who don't
    want to experience your love and friendship
Enjoy the simple things of life
Strive and fight only for those things that are really worthwhile
Accent the positive and the pleasant side of life
On experiencing a defeat or setback, maintain your self-confidence by remembering
    past accomplishments and successes
Don't delay tackling the unpleasant tasks that must be done; instead, get at them
    immediately
Evaluate people's progress on the basis of their performance
Recognize that leaders, to be leaders, must have the respect of their followers
Adopt a motto that you will live in a way that will earn your neighbor's love
Try to live so that your existence will be useful to society
Clarify your values
Take constructive action to eliminate a source of stress

Other Suggestions
Maintain good physical and mental health
Accept what you cannot change
Serve other people and some worthy cause
Share worries with someone you can trust
Pay attention to your body
Balance work and recreation
Improve your qualifications for the realistic goals you aspire to
Avoid reliance on things such as drugs and alcohol
Don't be narcissistic
Manage your time effectively
Laugh at yourself
Get enough rest and sleep
Don't be too hard on yourself
Improve your self-esteem

*Seyle, H. (1976). *The stress of life*. New York: McGraw-Hill.
Seyle, H. (1974). *Stress without distress*. New York: Signet.

that physical activity can result in a positive psychologic response in a similar way to the fact that by changing a negative mental state, physical condition can be improved and the risk of psychosomatic and other disorders lessened.[1] Matteson and Ivancevich[8] outline some major explanations of this phenomenon:

- Changes that are psychologic in nature may be the result of physiologic and biochemical changes that come from exercise. More specifically, increased oxygen flow to the brain may increase glucose production, which in turn enhances mental functioning.
- Sweating as a result of physical activity reduces salt level in the brain, causing a better feeling of contentment and less tension.
- Neurotransmitter changes in the brain caused by exercise may be associated with mood changes.
- The awareness of physiologic changes taking place as a result of activity by the person exercising may lead to lower stress.
- Regular exercise may condition stress adaptation mechanisms in the body, causing an increased reserve of steroids to counter stress.
- The challenges offered by physical activity and meeting these challenges successfully may result in more positive responses to stress-provoking situations.

RELAXATION TECHNIQUES

Relaxation is essentially a mental phenomenon concerned with the reduction of tensions that could originate from muscular activity but are more likely to result from pressures of our hectic life-styles. The mounting pressures of modern society have resulted in an increase of certain mental and physical ailments.

The Jacobson Technique

Dr. Edmond Jacobson,[8] who made the first objective investigation of the relationship of exercise and relaxation, developed a technique of nervous re-education that has two basic steps.

1. *The person learns to recognize muscle tension in subtle as well as in gross forms.* Gross tension is easily identified. With fists tightly clenched, hold your arms outstretched to the side at shoulder height for 1 minute. Note the feeling of exertion and discomfort in the forearms and shoulders. Drop your arms to the side and relax the muscles of the arms and hands completely. Note the effortless relaxation, which Dr. Jacobson[8] calls the "negative of exertion."

Subtle tension, involving less muscle effort than that just illustrated, is sometimes difficult to detect. It takes concentration and practice to learn to recognize minor tension in the trunk, neck, face, throat, and other body parts.

2. *The person learns to relax completely.* First the large muscle groups in the arms, legs, trunk, and neck. Then the forehead, eyes, face, and even the throat have tension eased through a program of progressive relaxation.

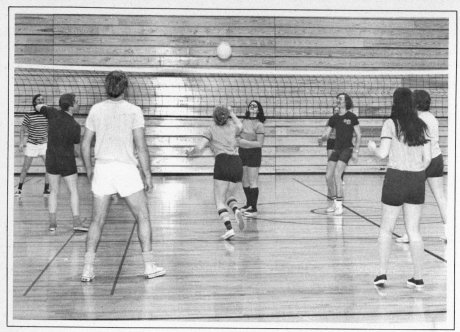

FIGURE 9-5

Exercise is conducive to relaxation.
Courtesy State University, College of Arts and Sciences, Potsdam, N.Y.

Carried out in the fashion outlined by Jacobson, the program teaches the person to relax his or her whole body to the point of negative exertion. The result is a release of tension, an antidote to fatigue, and also an inducement to sleep.

Exercises to Further Relaxation

The following exercises are designed to help remove tension. They are best practiced alone and in quiet surroundings.

1. Choose a particular time of day and make an effort to sit quietly for a few minutes each day at that time.
2. Sitting in a cross-legged position, rest your hands in your lap or on your knees. Gently close your eyes and concentrate on a single thing. Choose something pleasant to think about. Each time your mind is distracted, bring it back to your object of concentration.
3. Sitting quietly with your eyes closed, tighten your fists and mentally explore the feeling of tension in your hands. Slowly release the hands,

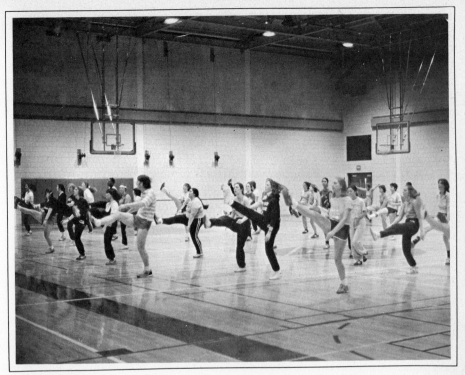

FIGURE 9-6

Physical activity may utilize the by-products of stress.
Courtesy Office of Public Relations, Smith College, Northampton, Mass.

studying the feeling of relaxation. Practice this several times until you are able to identify relaxation as it happens. Try this with different parts of your body.

4. Find a comfortable position lying on the floor. Try lying on your back, your head turned to one side, your arms away from your body, your feet and ankles loose. Turn your palms up and tighten your hands into a fist. Slowly let your hands relax. Concentrate on the feeling of relaxing your hands. Send the release up through your arms and relax the entire body.

5. Lying on the floor, roll to one side and curl up, bringing your knees to your chest. This is a position familiar to us as children. Turn your thoughts back to the day when you were a child and full of adventure and curiosity. As you return to the present, bring back with you that sense of wonder and open your eyes to the adventures that lie ahead.

6. Find a relaxing position. As you slowly close your eyes, let your thoughts wander and think of pleasant experiences that you have had.

7. Sitting quietly or lying down, empty your mind of unhappy thoughts—anger, irritation, resentment, disappointment—and adopt a positive outlook. Concentrate on being positive!

8. Think of yourself as a rag doll and collapse your body. Practice completely loosening every muscle you have.

9. Relax your mouth, lips, tongue, and throat.

10. Practice releasing the muscles in the different areas of your face—cheeks, temples, lips, chin. Your face should be blank of all expression.

Biofeedback

Biofeedback is a common form of stress management and relaxation therapy. Its main goals are to teach concentration, relaxation, and awareness. With the help of a machine it monitors various body functions and relays information to the subject in the form of either tones or lights. Some body functions, for example, those controlled by the autonomic nervous system, are often imperceptible to us. Biofeedback enables a person to actively control the responses and processes and take responsibility for his or her own well-being. For example, muscle biofeedback enables the subject, via the machine, to become aware of his or her muscle tension and learn how to control it as a result of becoming more aware of the feelings associated with relaxation. Biofeedback can also help in controlling body temperature by raising hand temperature by as much as 20° F—persons under stress may have cold hands. The patient does this by activating the parasympathetic nervous system, which is responsible for the stress response and the cold hands. Biofeedback helps people to become aware of tensions they had not previously perceived and learn to reduce them, eventually without relying on the machine.

Yoga

Yoga originated in India approximately 6000 years ago. Its basic philosophy is that most illness is related to poor mental attitudes, posture, and diet. Practitioners of yoga maintain that stress can be reduced by a mixture of mental and physical approaches. Through yoga it is possible to cope with such stress-induced maladies as obesity, hypertension, and smoking. Yoga's meditative aspects help, it is believed, in alleviating psychosomatic ailments. It aims to unite the body and mind to reduce stress; for example, Dr. Chandra Patel,[11] a yoga expert, has found that persons who practice yoga can reduce blood pressure indefinitely as long as they continue to practice yoga. Various body postures and breathing exercises are utilized in this activity.

Hatha-yoga utilizes a number of positions through which the practitioner may progress, beginning with the simplest and moving to the more complex. The purpose of the various positions is to increase mobility and suppleness of body.

Breathing Exercises

Some people use deep breathing as relief from stress. These persons maintain that as the body takes in more oxygen, you feel better and experience less stress. Also, by concentrating on the breathing, the source of stress is forgotten. A typical deep-breathing exercise for relaxation could involve getting in a sitting position, closing the eyes, inhaling slowly and deeply through the nose, and then exhaling slowly through the mouth. When inhaling, you could say "I am" and then during each exhalation, say the word "relaxed." This process should be repeated eight or ten times or as long as you wish and are comfortable. After this routine, you should breathe normally and rest quietly in a relaxed condition.

Benson's Techniques

Herbert Benson, a Harvard cardiologist, has also developed a system of relaxation through the use of breathing exercises. His technique calls for closing your eyes, relaxing all muscles beginning with the feet and then progressing to the face, and breathing through the nose and saying, "one in", and then exhaling and saying, "one out." This is continued for 10 to 20 minutes. The technique should be done once or twice daily but not within 2 hours after any meal because it may interfere with digestion.

Meditation

In most forms, meditation involves sitting quietly for a period of time, usually 15 to 20 minutes, and concentrating on a single word or image while breathing slowly and rhythmically. Utmost concentration is important in this process.

The response that underlies this transcendental awareness is sometimes called the relaxation response. Bringing about the relaxation response, meditation advocates say, helps the body to counteract the biochemical changes that cause stress. The goal of this technique is that the relaxation response is elicited whenever the practitioner confronts stressful situations. The relaxation response, it is believed, causes physiologic changes such as a decrease in respiratory rate, heart rate, blood pressure, and muscle tension.

Transcendental Meditation

Transcendental meditation (TM), the most widely used of the various forms of meditation, was popularized by Maharishi Mahesh Yogi, an Indian teacher. In this technique the meditator silently chants a mantra (a monosyllabic word or sound) for 20 minutes, twice a day, morning and evening. The word transcendental, meaning "going beyond," is used to illustrate that with this technique, one goes beyond a wakeful state to a state of restfulness characterized by a greater state of alertness. The mantra that a person uses is supposedly chosen

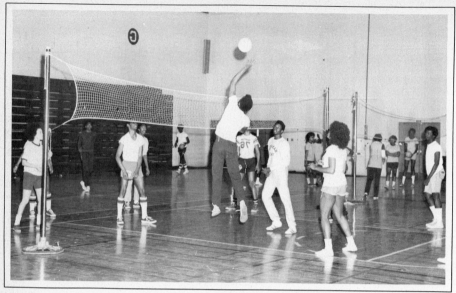

FIGURE 9-7

Maintaining good physical health is a good way to reduce stress.
Courtesy Hampton Institutes, Hampton, Va.

for that person alone and is kept secret in order to enhance attentiveness and quiet the conscious mind.

Imagery

Imagination can be used as a means of relaxation to cope stressful situations. The procedure is to sit relaxed, close your eyes, and concentrate on a pleasant, peaceful scene, such as a lake or a quiet place in the forest or mountains. Concentration is encouraged on all the details of the scene, such as the colors, smells, and sounds. The imagery can be continued as long as you wish. It is thought that by following this process you can relax your mind and body and thus relieve stress.

Massage

Massage can be a very relaxing and stress-reducing technique. Massage can be administered by yourself and applied to the neck, face, head, and shoulders; it also can be administered by another person.

Autogenic Training

This technique was developed by Johannes H. Schultz, a German psychiatrist, after observing that patients who were hypnotized had less fatigue and tension than those not under such a spell. Therefore he designed this technique to enable other persons to obtain the same benefits without having to go into hypnosis therapy. It involves a series of specific exercises and autohypnosis. It is designed to accomplish a deep mental and physical state of relaxation as the practitioner experiences two physical sensations during the progression through six different stages that are involved with this technique. First, the practitioner experiences a feeling of warmth as a psychologic perception of the dilation of the arteries is concentrated on. This perception results in a relaxed state. Second, the feeling of heaviness in the torso is concentrated on. This results in the actual relaxation of the muscles with which the practitioner is concerned.

SUMMARY

- Everyone experiences stress, and some stress is needed to perform the daily tasks of life.
- Two interrelated physiologic systems of the body are involved when a person encounters a stressor: the autonomic nervous system and the endocrine system.
- There are many different types of stressors, such as psychologic stressors and physiologic stressors.
- Each day in college life, students encounter many stresses of varying degree. Some are positive and some are negative. Stressors can be physical or mental stressors.
- Stress is not always harmful—it can also have a positive reaction.
- Uncontrolled stress can result in physical and mental disorders.
- Persons who are under stress tend to display certain danger signs and symptoms that indicate the body's malfunctioning.
- Seyle described the body's response to stress as the *general adaptation syndrome*.
- Stress can affect various body systems.
- Coping skills to ward off stress are those procedures that allow a person to deal with reality in a positive way.
- People sometimes try to cope with stress by using adjustment techniques called defense mechanisms.
- The better you understand your own behavior and motives, the better able you are to cope with stress and develop into a productive human being.
- Physical activity is one of the best ways to resist stressors and relax.
- Physical activity provides benefits such as a healthy cardiovascular system, a sense of well-being, mental release, and better self-concept.

- Regular and adequate amounts of exercise help to reduce stress by contributing to a lower heart rate, lower blood pressure, improved condition of the blood vessels, and fewer circulatory disorders.
- Physical activity can contribute to better body composition and thus prevent some forms of stress.
- Physical activity can help alleviate some cases of lower back pain, creating better flexibility, strength, and endurance.
- There are several relaxation techniques for coping with stress, including the Jacobson relaxation technique, biofeedback, yoga, breathing exercises, meditation, imagery, massage, and autogenic training.

GLOSSARY

autogenic training A series of exercises and autohypnosis designed to accomplish a deep mental and physical state of relaxation

Benson's relaxation techniques A system of relaxation accomplished through the use of breathing exercises

biofeedback A common form of stress management and relaxation therapy achieved with the help of a machine that monitors various body functions and is used to help a person control his or her own body responses

defense mechanism A psychologic device that is essentially designed to protect the ego, preserve inner harmony, and provide a sense of adequacy

distress A human reaction to negative stressors

eustress A human reaction to positive stressors

general adaptation syndrome (GAS) The body's response to stress as described by Seyle

hypokinetic disease Disease caused by insufficient exercise

imagery The use of imagination as a means of relaxation and to cope with stressful situations

Jacobson technique for relaxation A technique of nervous re-education designed to first recognize muscle tension and then learn to relax

meditation A technique for relieving stress that involves concentration on a single word or image

psychosomatic The development of physical symptoms as a result of emotional and mental disturbances

stress A term that comes from the Latin word *stringere*, meaning "to draw tight"—a response that occurs in the body, causing tension

stressor A stimulus that causes stress in the body

transcendental meditation (TM) A form of meditation in which the meditator silently chants a secret mantra and achieves a state of restfulness and a greater state of alertness

yoga A discipline that originated in India and maintains that stress can be reduced by a mixture of mental and physical approaches

REFERENCES

1. Allen, R.J., & Hyde, D.H. (1981). *Investigations in stress control*. Minneapolis: Burgess.
2. Anderson, R.A. (1978). *Stress power*. New York: Human Sciences.
3. Charlesworth, E.A., & Nathan, R.G. (1982). *Stress management: A comprehensive guide to wellness*. Houston: Behavioral Press.
4. deVries, H.A. (1975). Physical education, adult fitness programs: Does physical activity promote relaxation? *Journal of Physical Education and Recreation, 46*(7), 53-54.
5. Friedman, M., & Rosenman, R.H. (1974). *Type A behavior and your heart*. Greenwich, CN: Fawcett.
6. Holmes, T.H., & Rahe, T.E. (1967). The social readjustment rating scale. *Journal of Psychosomatic Research, 11*, 213-218.
7. Jacobson, E. (1938). *Progressive relaxation*. Chicago: University of Chicago Press.
8. Matteson, M.T., & Ivancevich, J.M. (1982). *Managing job stress and health*. New York: The Free Press.
9. Mayer J. (1960). Exercise and weight control. In W. Johnson (ed.), *Science and medicine of exercise and sport*. New York: Harper & Row.
10. Michael, E.D. (1957). Stress adaptation through exercise. *Research Quarterly, 28*,50-54.
11. Pelletier, K.R. (1977). *Mind as healer, mind as slayer*. New York: Delta.
12. Seyle. H. (1976). *The stress of life*. New York: McGraw-Hill.
13. Yates, J.E. (1979). *Managing stress*. New York: AMACOM.

SUGGESTED READINGS

Allen, J., (1983). *Human stress—its nature and control*. Minneapolis: Burgess.

Benson, H. (1975). *The relaxation response*. New York: Morrow.

Caplan, R. (1971). *Organizational stress and individual strain: A social-psychological study of risk factors*. Unpublished doctoral dissertation, University of Michigan, Ann Arbor.

Cooper, K. (1968). *Aerobics*. New York: Bantam Books.

Cooper, C.L., & Payne, R. eds. (1968). *Stress and work:* New York: John Wiley & Sons.

deVries, H.A. (1968). Immediate and long-term effects of exercise upon resting muscle action potential level. *Journal of Sports Medicine, 8*, 1-11.

Forbes, (1979). *Life stress*. Garden City, NJ: Doubleday.

Frew, D. (1977). *Management of stress: Using TM at work*. Chicago: Nelson-Hall.

Greenberg, J.S. (1985). *Comprehensive stress management*. Dubuque, IA: William C. Brown.

Ivanevich, J.M., & Matteson, M.T. (1980). *Stress and work: A managerial perspective*. Glenview, IL: Scott, Foresman.

Kory, R.B. (1976). *The TM program for business people*. New York: AMACOM.

Smith, L. (1975). Can you cope with stress? *Dun's Review, 106*, 89-91.

10

SELECTED LIFETIME

FITNESS ACTIVITIES

After completing this chapter, you will be able to:

- Describe how calisthenic exercises can improve muscle strength, cardiorespiratory endurance, flexibility, and body composition.

- Describe the advantages and disadvantages of a walking or running program.

- Describe the advantages and disadvantages of a swimming program.

- Describe the advantages of cycling as an activity for improving cardiorespiratory fitness.

- Describe the advantages of rope skipping as an aerobic activity.

- Describe the advantages of aerobic exercise as a means of improving cardiorespiratory endurance.

Until recently, the thought of doing calisthenic exercise probably conjured up the image of a hard-nosed Marine drill instructor leading a group of recruits through a boring, regimented exercise session. But add disco music and brightly colored exercise clothing and change the name to aerobic exercise, aerobic dance, or jazzercise, and you have a multimillion dollar industry that has swept a large segment of the American population into an exercise fanaticism. This new fascination with aerobic exercise has shown that calesthenic exercise can be enjoyable without being excessively regimented.

WHY DO CALISTHENIC EXERCISES?

We have already discussed weight training for the development of muscular strength and endurance, flexibility exercises, cardiorespiratory endurance, and maintenance of body composition. Calisthenic exercises, if done properly, can improve each of these four areas simultaneously. However, they are best suited as a supplemental activity to other previously discussed techniques

254

rather than as a substitute for weight training, walking, jogging, swimming, or cycling.

Muscle Strength

Calisthenics can help to increase muscular strength, tone, and endurance by using the weight of the body and its extremities as resistance. For example, chinning exercises (see Figure 10-3) use the weight of the body to resist the biceps muscles in elbow flexion. The primary advantage of calisthenics over training with weights is that you do not need any expensive equipment or machines to provide resistance for you. Most of these exercises can be accomplished without the use of any equipment whatsoever.

Flexibility

Calisthenic exercises can also help to improve flexibility as long as each exercise is done through a full range of motion. The weight of a body part can assist in passively stretching a muscle to its greatest length. However, caution must be used when doing calisthenic exercise to improve flexibility. The repetitive, bouncing nature of many of these exercises causes a muscle to be stretched ballistically, which can predispose a muscle to injury, particularly in an untrained person. Through calisthenic exercises the muscle should be progressively stretched during the set of exercises.

Cardiorespiratory Endurance

There is some question as to whether calisthenic exercises can increase resting heart rate significantly; but as stated in Chapter 3, if exercise is of sufficient intensity, frequency, and duration, cardiorespiratory endurance can be improved. Anyone who has gone through a 20 to 30 minute aerobic dance class will agree that heart rate is elevated to training levels. Calisthenic exercises should be done at a quick pace and without much rest between sets for optimal improvement of cardiorespiratory endurance.

Weight Control

Calisthenics can be important for increasing body firmness, but it must be re-emphasized that doing a specific calisthenic exercise to spot reduce, or get rid of fat in a particular area, is usually ineffective. Weight can only be lost when more calories are expended than are taken in. Thus these exercises can certainly help but cannot be expected to totally eliminate those "love handles" on the male abdomen or the "ledges" on the female buttocks; however, calisthenics can definitely help to improve muscle tone in these areas and thus firm up the muscles that lie underneath the fat layer. Maintenance of body weight requires a life-long commitment to consistent exercise and diet management. Calisthenic exercises can be an important component of any weight control program.

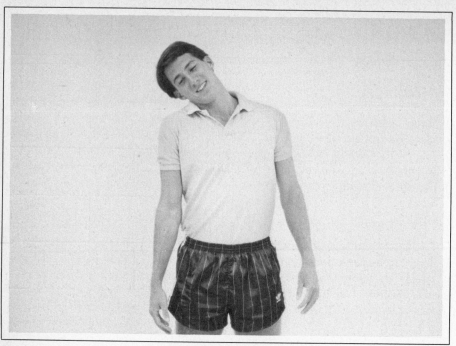

FIGURE 10-1

Head and neck rolls.
Purpose: Range of motion and strengthening.
Muscles: Flexors and extensors of neck.
Repetitions: Beginner   10 each direction
            Intermediate   15 each direction
            Advanced   20 each direction
Instructions: Circle head and neck in large circles in both directions.

Specific Exercises

The exercises illustrated in Figures 10-1 to 10-18 are recommended because they work on specific muscle groups and with a specific purpose. If all exercises are done, most of the major muscle groups in the body will be both stretched and contracted against resistance with the objective of improving strength, flexibility, and endurance. Each exercise can be done at your own pace, although the greater the pace, the greater the stress placed on the cardiorespiratory system. Thus it is recommended that you work quickly and move from one exercise to the next without delay.

These exercises can be done to music if you so desire. Most people find it easier to exercise to fast-paced music with a hard, rhythmic beat such as disco music. However, you should select the type of music most enjoyable to you.

Text continued on p. 277.

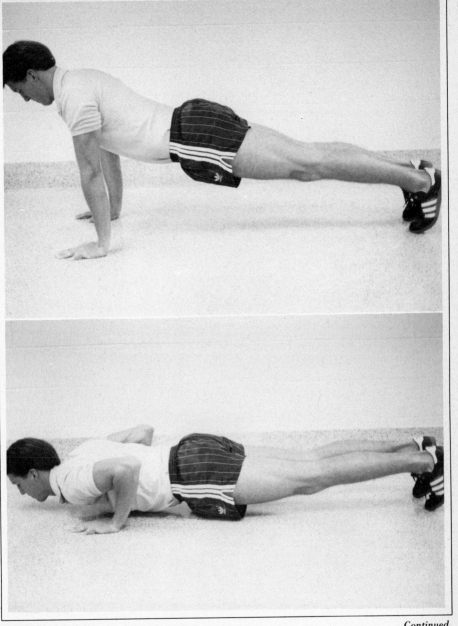

A

FIGURE 10-2

A, Push-ups; **B,** modified push-ups.
Purpose: Strengthening.
Muscles: Triceps and pectoralis major.
Repetitions: Beginner   10
           Intermediate 20
           Advanced   30
Instructions: Keep the upper trunk and legs extended in a straight line. Touch
floor with chest.

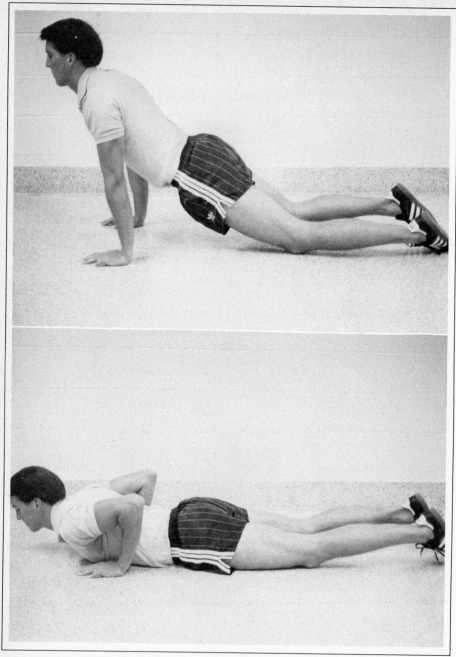

B

FIGURE 10-2, cont'd

For legend see p. 257.

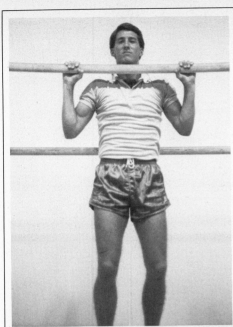

A

FIGURE 10-3

A, Chin-ups; **B,** modified chin-ups.
Purpose: Strengthening and stretch
of shoulder joint.
Muscles: Biceps and latissimus ⋅
dorsi.
Repetitions: Beginner   7
               Intermediate 10
               Advanced   15
Instructions: Pull up until chin
touches top of bar.

B

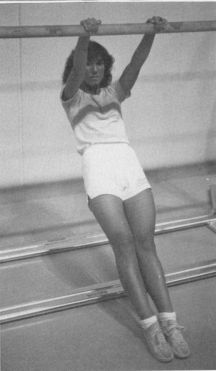 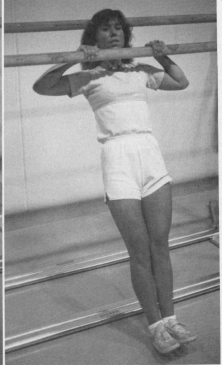

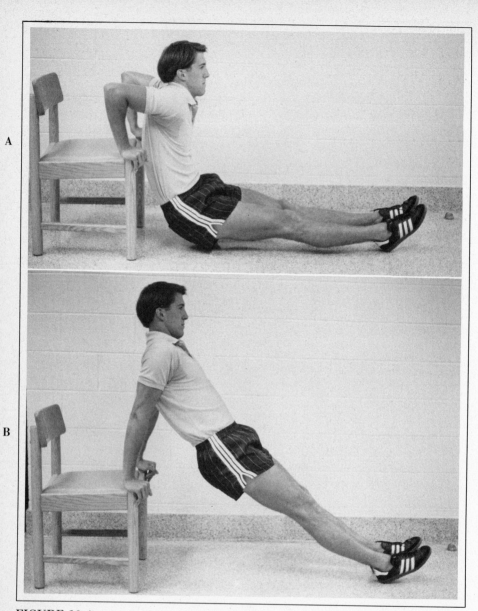

A

B

FIGURE 10-4

Tricep extensions.
Purpose: Strengthening and range of motion at shoulder joint.
Muscles: Triceps and trapezius.
Repetitions: Beginner   7
              Intermediate 12
              Advanced   18
Instructions: Begin with arms extended and body straight. Lower buttocks until they touch the ground and then press back up.

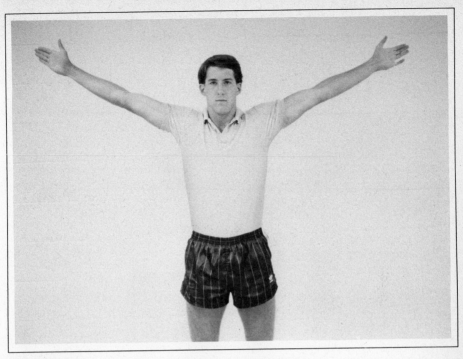

FIGURE 10-5

Arm circles.
Purpose: Range of motion at shoulder joints.
Muscles: All muscles surrounding shoulder joint.
Repetitions: Beginner   10 each direction
             Intermediate   15 each direction
             Advanced   20 each direction
Instructions: Arms should be circled in both directions.

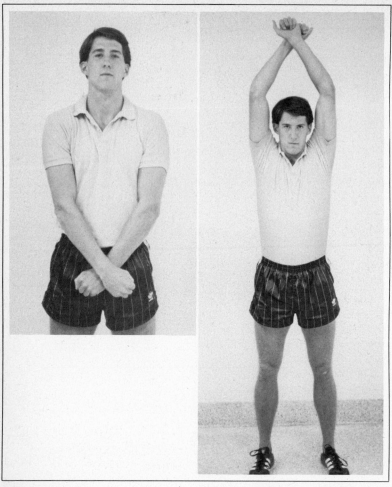

FIGURE 10-6

Arm wind-ups.

Purpose: Strengthening and range of motion at shoulder.

Muscles: Deltoid, trapezius, and shoulder rotators.

Repetitions: Beginner   10
            Intermediate   15
            Advanced   20

Instructions: Begin with arms crossed below waist and finish with them crossed above head.

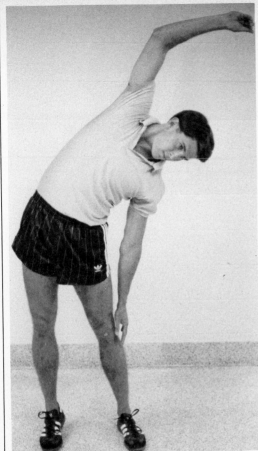

FIGURE 10-7

Side bends. **A,** Standing; **B,** sitting.
Purpose: Strengthening and range of motion.
Muscles: Lateral trunk flexors.
Repetitions:
Beginner   10 each side
Intermediate   20 each side
Advanced   30 each side
Instructions: Side bend as far as possible in both directions in either standing or sitting position.

A

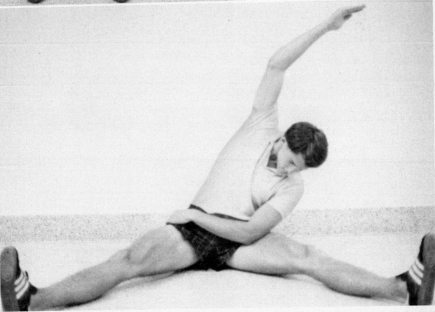

B

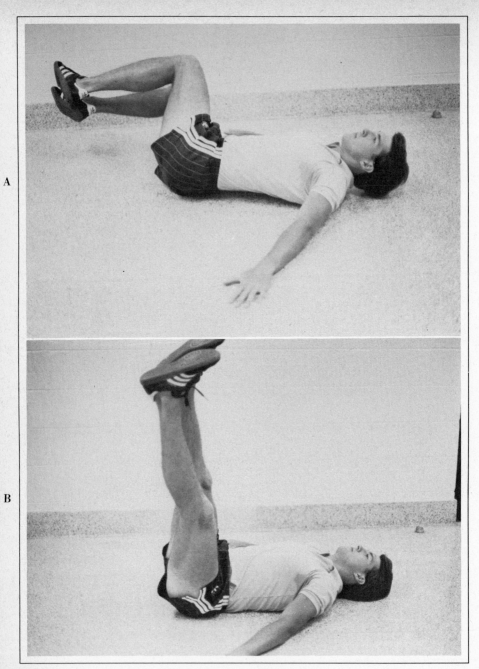

FIGURE 10-8

Trunk rotation. A, Beginner; B, advanced.
Purpose: Strengthen and stretch low back.
Muscles: Internal and external obliques.
Repetitions: Beginner   10 each direction
              Intermediate 15 each direction
              Advanced   20 each direction
Instructions: Rotate trunk from side to side until knees touch the ground.

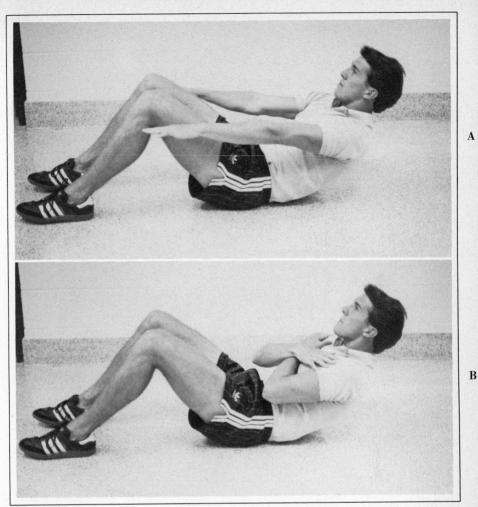

FIGURE 10-9   *Continued.*

Sit-ups. **A,** Beginner; **B,** intermediate; **C,** advanced.
Purpose: Strengthen abdominals and stretch lower back.
Muscles: Rectus abdominus and erector muscles in lower back.
Repetitions: Beginner   10-15
             Intermediate   16-30
             Advanced   31-50
Instructions: Knees should be flexed to 90°. Begin sit-up by curling neck, then
upper back before you come up.

C

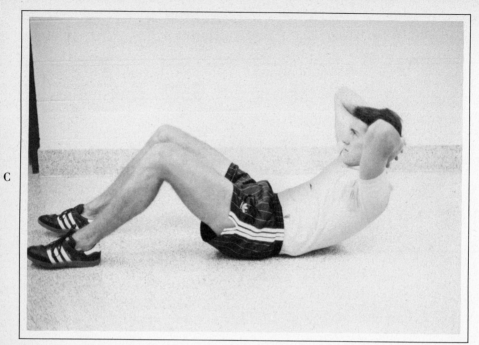

FIGURE 10-9, cont'd

For legend see p. 265.

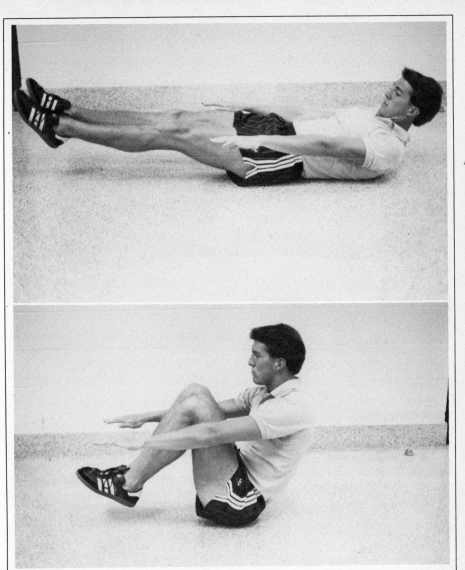

FIGURE 10-10

Sitting tucks.
Purpose: Strengthen abdominals and stretch lower back.
Muscles: Rectus abdominus and erector muscle in lower back.
Repetitions: Beginner   10
             Intermediate 20
             Advanced   30
Instructions: Keep legs and upper back off the ground and pull knees to chest.

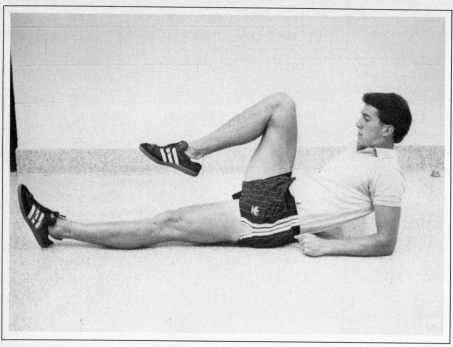

FIGURE 10-11

Bicycle.
Purpose: Strength hip flexors and stretch lower back.
Muscles: Iliopsoas.
Repetitions: Beginner   10 each side
            Intermediate   20 each side
            Advanced   30 each side
Instructions: Alternately flex and extend legs as if you were pedaling a bicycle.

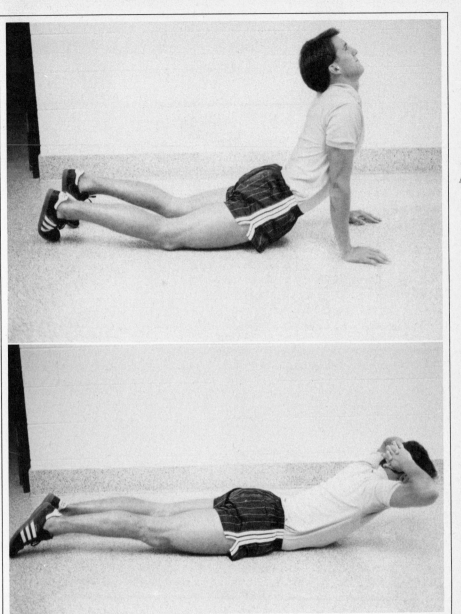

A

B

FIGURE 10-12

Back extensions. **A,** Beginner; **B,** intermediate and advanced.
Purpose: Strengthen lower back and stretch abdominals.
Muscles: Paravertebral erectors and rectus abdominus.
Repetitions: Beginner   10
              Intermediate   12
              Advanced   15
Instructions: Extend trunk as high off the floor as possible.

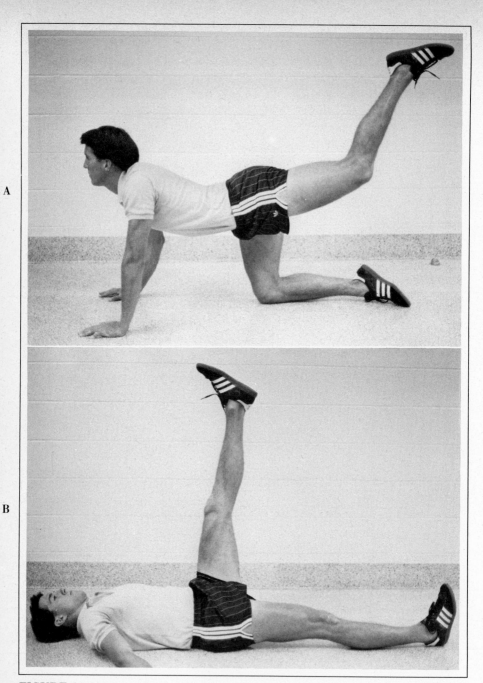

FIGURE 10-13

Leg lifts. **A,** Front; **B,** back; **C,** side (leg up); **D,** side (leg down).
Purpose: Strengthen **A,** hip flexors; **B,** hip extensors; **C,** hip abductors; and **D,** hip adductors.
Muscles: **A,** Iliopsoas; **B,** gluteus maximus; **C,** gluteus medius; and **D,** adductor group.
Repetitions: Beginner   10 each leg
                Intermediate   15 each leg
                Advanced   20 each leg
Instructions: Raise the exercising leg up as far as possible in each position.

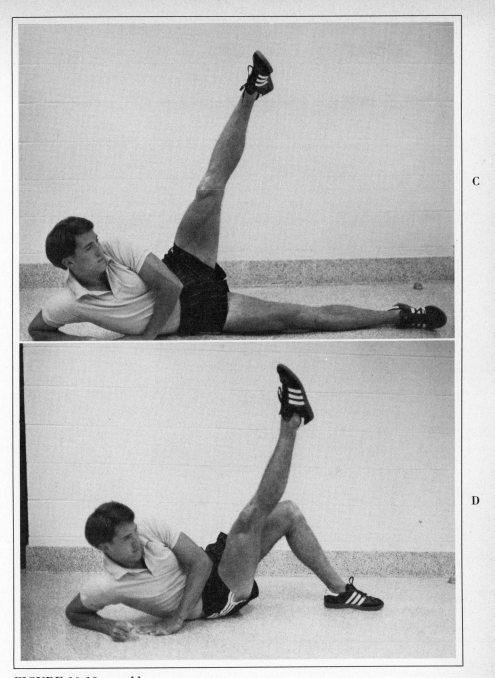

C

D

FIGURE 10-13, cont'd

For legend see opposite page.

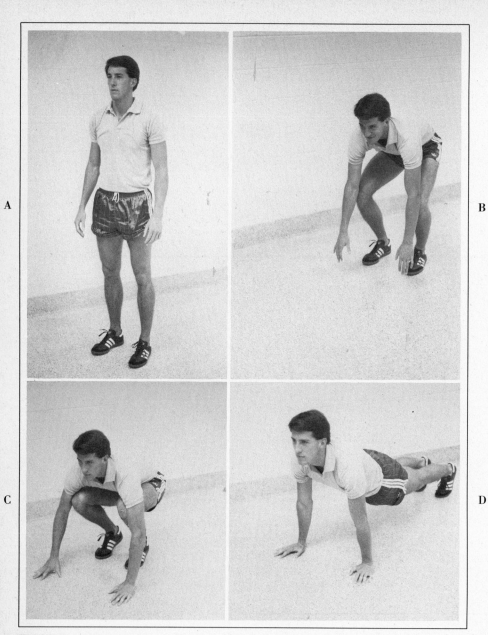

FIGURE 10-14

Squat thrusters.
Purpose: Strengthen hip flexors and extensors.
Muscles: Gluteus maximus and iliopsoas.
Repetitions: Beginner   10
              Intermediate 12
              Advanced   15
Instructions: Keep the lower back flat and only bend at the hips and knees.

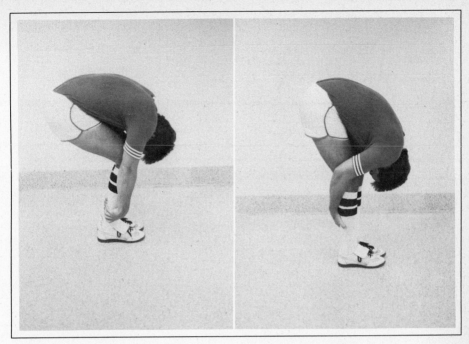

A   B

FIGURE 10-15

Hamstring stretches.
Purpose: Stretch hamstrings.
Muscles: Hamstrings.
Repetitions: Beginner   10
              Intermediate   15
              Advanced   20
Instructions: Grasp the lower leg as low as possible and straighten out the knees.

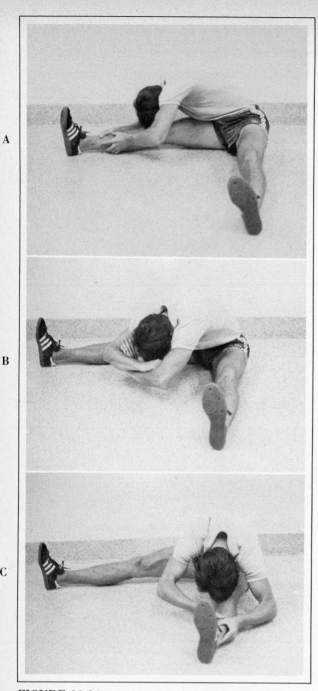

FIGURE 10-16

Chest to floor.
Purpose: Stretch of hip adductors and hamstrings.
Muscles: Adductors and hamstrings.

Repetitions: Beginner   10 each direction
            Intermediate   12 each direction
            Advanced   15 each direction

Instructions: With the legs straight and flat out on the floor, lean forward as far as possible in each direction.

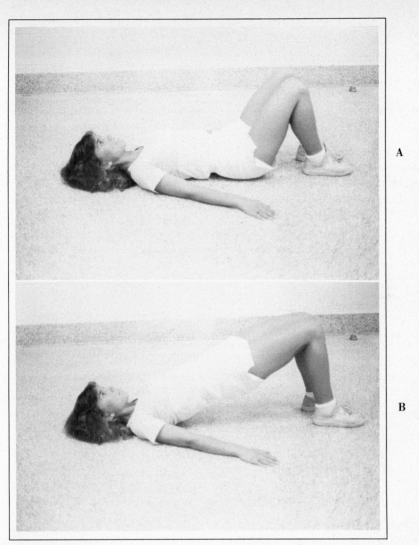

A

B

FIGURE 10-17

Buttock tucks.
Purpose: Strengthen muscles of buttocks.
Muscles: Gluteus maximus and hamstrings.
Repetitions: Beginner   10
             Intermediate   15
             Advanced   20
Instructions: Lying flat on back with knees bent, arch back and thrust the pelvis upward.

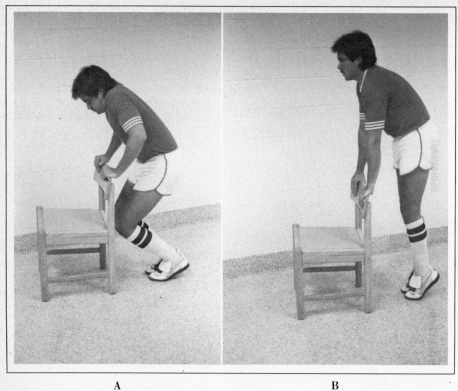

A   B

FIGURE 10-18

Calf and ankle exercise.
Purpose: Stretch and strengthen calf muscles.
Muscles: Gastrocnemius and soleus.
Repetitions: Beginner   10
                     Intermediate   20
                     Advanced   30
Instructions: Begin with feet flat on the floor, knees bent, then extend until you
are on your toes.

RUNNING

Perhaps no other physical fitness activity has become as much a part of our American way of life as walking or running. Running has long been accepted as an essential training component for the competitive athlete in almost every sport. But within the last 10 years, millions of people have taken to the streets and now run on a regular basis. Some 17,000 men and women began the 1983 New York Marathon, and it was estimated that more than 88% of these people completed the 26-plus mile run.

The running phenomenon doesn't seem to be restricted to any one segment of the population. Young children, college students, office personnel, laborers, elderly persons, people of all backgrounds and both sexes regularly put on their running shoes and go for a run.

Why has running attracted such widespread attention? Different people offer different reasons, but it seems that most people run for two major reasons; either for the effects that a regular running program can have on physical appearance or for some important health-related reason.

Running is an aerobic exercise that involves whole-body large muscle activities performed repetitively. This muscular activity requires energy, so calories are expended during the activity. Thus many people run as a means of controlling weight and burning off additional calories.

The number of calories expended during running depends on the intensity and the duration of the activity. Regardless of whether you walk, jog, or run 1 mile, it is estimated that an average-sized adult will burn off approximately 100 calories. It doesn't seem to matter whether you run 1 mile at a 6-minute pace or walk 1 mile at a 12-minute pace, the caloric expenditure is about the same. Of course, the person who runs for 30 minutes at a 6-minute per mile pace will burn off considerably more calories than another who walks for the same 30-minute period but at a 12-minute pace.

The 100-calorie-per-mile figure is a bit misleading. Assuming that 1 pound of fat contains approximately 3500 calories, persons who run a 26-mile marathon would only burn off 2600 calories, far less than 1 pound of body fat. However, the fact that the metabolic rate is increased during activity and remains elevated while slowly returning to normal during a several-hour period after the activity accounts for the expenditure of a large amount of additional calories (see Chapter 6).

Although many people run to control their weight and attain a healthful physical appearance, other people run for other physiologic benefits a running program offers. The effects of a sedentary life-style on the cardiovascular system have been previously discussed. Physically active persons seem to be less prone to cardiovascular heart disease than are those who are sedentary. Running seems to increase the efficiency of the cardiovascular system and also alters the build up of cholesterol on the arterial walls.

Many people report that running (or jogging) is relaxing and alleviates stress,

tension, and depression. They express feelings of greater self-worth and enthusiasm toward life after a run. The euphoric feeling has been called a "runner's
high," and although most people agree that this is a psychologic phenomenon,
it has been shown that there is a physiologic explanation for this "high."[2] The
brain releases opiate-like substances, called *endorphins*, that are endogenous
to the nervous system and are thought to be responsible for this calming, psychologically stimulating effect. Regardless of the underlying mechanisms, running does seem to be able to produce an escape from normal daily pressures.

Perhaps the biggest advantage that running has is that, unlike swimming and
cycling, the only equipment required is a pair of running shoes and some shorts.
Many people choose to invest large sums of money on expensive running outfits
and warm-up suits; however, these are not necessary to get started on a jogging
program.

There are some disadvantages to running. Because the feet and legs are
subjected to repetitive pounding on the running surface, overuse injuries are
very likely. Most of these injuries involve the muscles, tendons, ligaments, and
occasionally bones of the lower extremity. Proper running and training techniques
and properly fitted running shoes can reduce the number of injuries associated
with running.

Proper Running Technique

Running is a skill that most of us learn at an early age. Because no two persons
are anatomically exactly the same, each person will have a slightly different
running style or form. However, there are certain things that all runners should
pay attention to in terms of running style and proper form to help make running
more efficient and reduce the possibility of injury: (1) foot strike and stride
length, (2) proper body position, (3) arm movement, and (4) breathing pattern.

Foot strike and stride length. Foot strike and stride length vary according to
running speed. The faster the running speed, the longer the stride length. Regardless of how fast you are running, the foot should always strike the ground
directly under the knee at its farthest point of advance. The knee should always
be slightly flexed to absorb the impact of the foot strike. These two factors can
significantly reduce the forces being transferred through the ankle, knee, and
hip joints, reducing the possibility of injuries resulting from overuse (Figure
10-19).

The point of impact on the sole of the foot depends on the running speed
(Figure 10-20). During sprinting, the ball of the foot should contact the ground
first with the heel never coming in contact. When running at a moderate speed,
the contact is almost flat-footed, with most of the pressure in the metatarsal area.
In long-distance running, the heel should strike first, followed by the lateral
border of the foot and the push-off from the ball of the great toe. The biggest
mistake made by a runner is taking too much impact on the toes and not enough
on the heels.

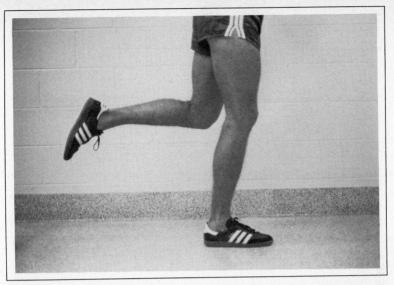

FIGURE 10-19

The foot should strike the ground directly under the knee, which should be flexed to absorb impact.

Proper body position. By far the most comfortable posture for the trunk is erect, with the spinal vertebrae supporting most of the weight. To facilitate this erect posture the shoulders should be slightly back and the pelvis rotated slightly forward. The head and face should be upright, looking far forward. The most critical factor is to be relaxed. If you are tense while running, you tend to be stiff, and this results in fatigue.

Arm movement. The faster you run, the more the arms tend to move. Some arm movement is necessary to maintain balance. But in slow, long-distance running, arm swing should be kept at a minimum. The arms should be held slightly away from the trunk, with the forearms parallel to the ground. The fists should not be clenched, and the fingers and thumb should be slightly flexed. Again, the arms and hands should be relaxed and swing rhythmically with foot strike. Excessive arm motion results in trunk rotation, which over an extended period of time causes fatigue and an unnecessary expenditure of energy. Occasionally, the arms should be totally relaxed and dropped to the side momentarily.

Breathing. Adequate breathing while running is essential; if sufficient oxygen is not supplied to the working muscles, activity cannot be continued for very long. In short sprint races such as the 60- or 100-yard dash, many sprinters do

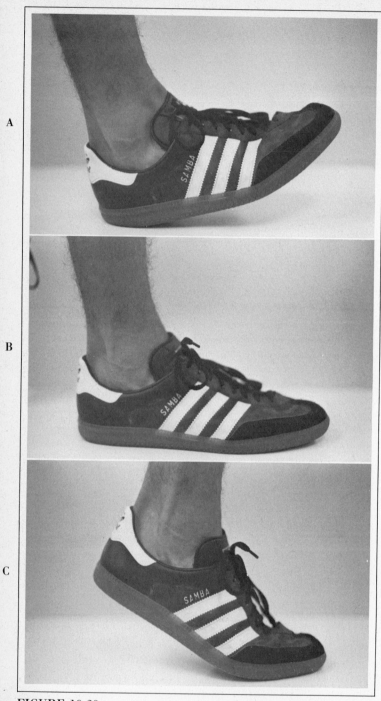

A

B

C

FIGURE 10-20

Foot contact in running. **A,** Heel; **B,** foot flat; **C,** toe.

not breathe at all and rely on anaerobic metabolism to provide sufficient oxygen. However, in long-distance running, which is aerobic, oxygen must be supplied continuously to working muscle. Breathing is best accomplished using the abdominal rather than diaphragmatic (chest) muscles.

Abdominal breathing may prevent a so-called *stitch in the side* that is more likely to occur with diaphragmatic breathing. The cause of the stitch in the side is unknown but is most often associated with some inability of the diaphragm muscle to utilize oxygen.

Breathing should be rhythmic and closely related to stride. Most runners breathe after every 2 to 4 strides. Concentrating on breathing often allows you to "lose yourself" and become more attuned to your body functions during a period of strenuous exercise.

Running shoes. We stated earlier that all the equipment you really need to become involved in a running program is a pair of training shoes. This makes the process of buying an appropriate running shoe sound very simple when in fact the purchase of running shoes may be a confusing experience. It is not uncommon for a shopper to enter a sporting goods store and be confronted by an entire wall filled with different types of running shoes. The logical question in this situation is, Where do you begin?

The running shoe manufacturing industry has become extremely sophisticated and offers a number of options on running shoes. Terms like *forefoot varus support* or *rear foot valgus wedge* are confusing to a person who simply wants to buy a pair of good running shoes. Most people are interested in finding a long-lasting shoe that will provide good support and comfort. *Runner's World* magazine publishes a yearly study that critically analyzes all current brands and models of running shoes. For the more serious runner it is recommended that this source be consulted for detailed information because the more you run, the more critical it is that a running shoe be built precisely for your foot.

For the less serious runner, the following points should be considered when buying running shoes (Figure 10-21).

Toe box. There should be plenty of room for the toes in your running shoe. Most experts recommend a $^{1}/_{2}$- to $^{3}/_{4}$-inch distance between your toes and the front of the shoe. Few running shoes are made in varying widths. If you have a very wide or narrow foot, most shoe salespersons can recommend a specific shoe for your foot. The best way to make sure there is adequate room in the toe box is to have your foot measured and then try on the running shoe.

Sole. The sole should possess two qualities. First, it must provide a shock absorptive function; second, it must be durable. Most shoes have three layers on the sole: a thick spongy layer, which absorbs the force of foot strike under the heel, a midsole, which cushions the midfoot and toes, and a hard rubber layer, which comes in contact with the ground. The average runner's feet strike the ground between 1500 and 1700 times per mile. Thus it is essential that the force of the heel strike be absorbed by

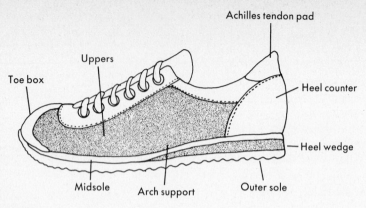

FIGURE 10-21

Parts of a well-designed running shoe.

the spongy layer to prevent overuse-type injuries from occurring in the ankles and knees. The sole must provide good traction and must be made of a tough material that is resistant to wear. Most of the better-known brands of running shoes tend to have well-designed, long-lasting soles.

Heel counters. The heel counter is the portion of the shoe that prevents the foot from rolling from side to side at heel strike. The counter should be firm but well-fitted to minimize movement of the heel up and down or side to side. A good heel counter may prevent ankle sprains as well as painful blisters.

Shoe uppers. The upper part of the shoe is made of some combination of nylon and leather. The uppers should be lightweight, capable of quick drying, and well-ventilated. The uppers should have some type of extra support in the saddle area, and there should also be some extra padding in the area of the Achilles tendon just above the heel counter.

Arch support. The arch support should be made of some durable yet soft supportive material and should smoothly join with the insole. The support should not have any rough seams or ridges inside the shoe, which may tend to cause blisters.

Price. Unfortunately, for many people price is the primary consideration in buying running shoes. Running shoes range between $20 and $100 per pair. One thing that should be remembered when buying running shoes is that they are the only piece of equipment that you really need; thus it certainly would be to your advantage to buy a quality pair of shoes. A little extra investment is worthwhile in terms of preventing injury.

Guidelines

In Chapter 3 we indicated that you should begin at your own level and progress at your own rate by gradually increasing the amount of training time and training

TABLE 10-1   Recommended Training Sessions for College-age Runners

Level	Activity	Time for 1 Mile (min:sec)	Speed (mph)	Approximate HR intensity	Approximate Distance Covered (20 min)
Beginner	Slow jog	12:00	5 mph	60%	1.66 miles
	Intermediate jog	10:00	6 mph	65%	2.00 miles
Intermediate	Brisk jog	8:34	7 mph	70%	2.33 miles
	Slow run	7:34	8 mph	75%	2.66 miles
Advanced	Intermediate run	6:40	9 mph	80%	3.00 miles
	Fast run	6:00	10 mph	85%	3.33 miles

intensity (as indicated by monitoring heart rate changes). Table 10-1 indicates recommended training sessions for beginning, intermediate, and advanced college-age runners.

SWIMMING

Like running, swimming is an excellent method of developing cardiorespiratory fitness. Swimming, like running, has broad appeal, and we find all types of people engaging in swimming fitness programs.

The physiologic benefits of swimming are similar to those of running; however, there are several differences that should be addressed.

The first difference is that in swimming not only must the arms and legs be used to propel the body through the water but also some energy must be expended to keep the body afloat. The drag of the water provides an excellent resistance for improving muscle strength and endurance. For these reasons it has been estimated that the amount of energy required to swim a given distance is approximately four times as great as running an equal distance.

Swimming also eliminates a lot of stresses and strains on the weight-bearing joints that are commonly found in runners. Although it is true that the shoulder joint receives a significant amount of overuse-type stress, the ankle and knee joints are spared the trauma of the foot repeatedly banging into a hard surface. It is common for trainers and therapists to recommend swimming as a substitute for a runner who has sustained some injury to the lower extremity. A runner who continues to train via running may well exacerbate the injury, whereas swimming used in the injury rehabilitation process maintains cardiorespiratory conditioning until the injured person can return to the track.

A swimsuit and perhaps a pair of goggles for persons whose eyes are irritated by chlorine are the only equipment necessary to get started with a swimming program. Perhaps the biggest drawback of a swimming program as a means of

TABLE 10-2   Guidelines for a Swimming Program

Level	Swimming Distance	Time Required	Approximate HR Intensity
Beginner	700-800 yards 28-30 lengths*	20 minutes	60%-70%
Intermediate	1200-1300 yards 48-52 lengths	30 minutes	70%-80%
Advanced	1900-2000 yards 76-80 lengths	40 minutes	80%-90%

*1 Length = 25 yards.

cardiorespiratory conditioning, is the unavailability of a swimming pool or a free lane to swim in. There are usually a number of outdoor pools available during the summer months; however, when the weather turns cold it becomes difficult to find an indoor pool that allows free swimming. Indoor pools are typically available at a YMCA, on most college campuses, at some high schools, and at many private health clubs or spas.

Although it is true that almost everyone can go out and run with little or no training, not everyone can jump into a pool and begin to swim. Simply being able to propel yourself through the water is a skill that must be learned, and swimming efficiency may only be considered once the basic skills have been mastered. Thus a detailed discussion of specific techniques of the crawl, backstroke, sidestroke, breaststroke, and butterfly techniques is well beyond the scope of this text. Several other books on swimming are recommended at the end of this chapter. Table 10-2 indicates recommended training sessions for beginning, intermediate, and advanced college-age swimmers.

CYCLING

Cycling is another of the aerobic activities and is excellent for improving cardiorespiratory endurance. Cycling is another activity that is enjoyed by all ages, primarily because of the ease with which anyone can learn to ride without formal training.

As with running and swimming, cycling produces some very desirable physiologic responses in terms of strength, endurance, and weight control. There is very little data to suggest that cycling produces any overuse-type injuries; therefore cycling is frequently used by trainers and therapists as an alternative training method for an injured athlete.

Bicycles come in thousands of different makes and models with countless numbers of available accessories and options. Prices range anywhere from about $60 for a standard 3-speed bike all the way up to several thousand dollars for professional touring or racing bikes. For the average person the cost of getting

TABLE 10-3   Guidelines for a Cycling Program

Level	Cycling Distance	Time Required	Approximate HR Intensity
Beginner	4 miles	20 min	60%-70%
Intermediate	6 miles	30 min	70%-80%
Advanced	9-10 miles	40 min	80%-90%

involved in some type of cycling activity is not much more than a pair of good running shoes.

Perhaps the biggest problem with cycling is locating a safe place to ride. No matter how safety-conscious you are on the bicycle, there is always a potential problem with traffic. For this reason, stationary exercise bikes, or ergometers, have become popular. Prices for these stationary bikes range from about $70 to about $900. The stationary bike allows you to gain all the cardiovascular benefits of cycling without having to worry about dealing with traffic safety. Additionally, it allows you to exercise regardless of outdoor conditions; it affords privacy and allows you to watch television or listen to music while working out.

However, to many, sitting in one place and pedaling is extremely boring because much of the thrill of riding a bicycle and looking at the scenery is lost.

Regardless of which cycling method you choose, the same principles of continuous training apply as indicated in Chapter 3. The intensity must be great enough to elevate the heart rate to between 60% and 90% of maximal rate, and this activity should be sustained for at least 20 minutes. This training level will assure improvement of cardiorespiratory endurance over a period of time.

There are numerous considerations for cycling, including selection of a bicycle, adjusting it to fit your body, maintaining it in good condition, and safety while cycling. Before getting started, we recommend that you consult some of the texts listed in the references at the end of the chapter.

ROPE SKIPPING

Rope skipping has many advantages for someone looking for an inexpensive and convenient form of exercise. It contributes to all the components of physical fitness, particularly in the area of cardiorespiratory endurance.

Rope skipping can be done alone or in pairs. The ends of the rope are held loosely in the fingers. Elbows should be close to the sides and the arms pointed away from the body. The arms and shoulders move in a circular motion; as the rope follows a circular motion, further momentum can be provided by rotating the wrists. Jump by pushing off from the toes just high enough to allow the rope to pass under your feet.

Some physical educators believe that rope skipping expends as much energy as running. Another advantage is the relatively short time it takes to perform the activity. Some people rope skip for 10 minutes and feel that this is similar to jogging for 30 minutes, at least in terms of energy expenditure. An added advantage of rope skipping as an activity for many students is that they do not have to skip on hard surfaces. Some students find jogging difficult because of the need to run on hard surfaces. Rope skipping, on the other hand, may be performed indoors or outdoors on a hard or soft surface. Rope skipping can be done almost anywhere at anytime, providing there is space enough for the rope to make a complete revolution.

Rope skipping raises the heart rate, and as you continue to use this activity in your fitness program it not only improves cardiorespiratory endurance but also muscular endurance. These qualities enable the muscular system to perform the activity for prolonged periods of time with less strain and fatigue. Because rope skipping requires a degree of coordination, speed, and agility it can also have a beneficial effect in these areas.

The equipment needed for rope skipping is inexpensive. The cost of a jump rope ranges from $3.50 to $20, depending on type. There are various types of jump ropes: sash, cord, plastic, and plain rope. Handles may be wooden or plastic. Weighted handles are available, or the participant may choose not to use handles but instead tie a knot at the ends of the rope. To be sure the rope is of a proper length, bring the handles up to the side of the body. The handles should be at armpit height. It is helpful to wear proper clothing. The ideal outfit would include a pair of proper-fitting shoes with gym socks, a pair of comfortable shorts, and a T-shirt or blouse. Variations in clothing may be used as long as they do not interfere with the rope-skipping activity.

Guidelines and Precautions

If you have been sedentary or have had health problems, you should see a physician and get a physical evaluation before beginning rope skipping as a fitness activity. It is also wise to do some warm-up exercises to increase blood flow, heart rate, flexibility, and respiration rate. Begin jumping for a short period of time, then gradually increase the time you are able to jump. Alternating jumping with walking is a good way to develop cardiovascular fitness. Jumpers should be cautioned that rope jumping is extremely vigorous and should be started gradually. In the beginning you should jump for just a few seconds, walk to catch your breath, then jump again. Ultimately you should be able to jump for 15 to 20 minutes.

As always, there should be a cool-down period after a vigorous workout. The cool-down prevents blood pooling and returns the body to a pre-activity level of respiration and heart rate. See Chapter 2 for specific cool-down techniques.

Program Suggestions

Rope-skipping routines should be designed to help you progress from a short series of workouts to extended workouts. Your program development plan should be flexible and should take into consideration your own goals and level of fitness; otherwise the activity could become boring or too physically difficult. An example of a beginning rope-jumping program is as follows:

Jumping on the balls of both feet, turning rope forward

Jumping on the right foot

Jumping on the left foot

Alternating jumping on the right and left feet

Jumping sideways

Turning the rope backward and following the above routine

AEROBIC DANCE

To understand aerobic dance, you need to have an understanding of aerobic exercise. Aerobic exercise is any physical activity that requires your heart rate to reach at least 60% of your maximal heart rate for an extended period of time. It is activity that can be sustained for an extended period of time without developing an oxygen debt (see pp. 56-57). An aerobic dance program contributes to physical fitness by providing aerobic exercise and improving cardiorespiratory endurance, strength, flexibility, and muscular endurance. Aerobic dance is a combination of choreographed fitness dance routines set to music. In other words, it is movement to music for fitness.

Most anyone can do aerobic dance; your physical condition will determine at what pace you should work. We recommend that the target heart rate (see pp. 56-57) be maintained for at least 20 minutes during the aerobic dance portion of the workout.

Aerobic dance utilizes various stretching, strength, and other exercises to achieve the target heart rate and produce a vigorous workout. The dance routines can be broken down to several different exercises, such as the following:

Bicycling. Sit on the floor and lean back, resting your weight on bent arms. With legs extended overhead, rotate legs in a circular motion similar to that of riding a bicycle.

Jumping jacks. Stand with legs together and arms at side. Jump to straddle position as arms move upward and hands touch overhead. Jump back to starting position with arms returning to sides. Repeat.

Circle jogging. Jog while turning in a circle. The circle can be as large as or as small as desired.

Jumping. Keep feet together and stand erect. Jump high, with both feet leaving the floor together and returning together. Repeat.

Hopping. Hop on one foot, hop on the other foot, hop on both feet. Repeat.

Floor touch. Stand erect and in a straddle position. Bend from the waist and touch first the left and then the right foot with both hands. Repeat.

Knee lifts. Stand erect with hands on hips. Lift right knee to chest and then return to starting position. Lift left knee to chest and return to starting position. Repeat.

Trunk circle. Stand erect in a straddle position, arms overhead. Bend from waist and swing trunk first clockwise and then counterclockwise. Repeat.

Aerobic dance is a vigorous physical activity that can provide an inexpensive and practical workout for most people. It increases the working capacity of the cardiovascular and pulmonary systems. If done on a regular basis, it should result in increased energy and stamina and better ability to handle life's stresses and tensions. It contributes to weight control and can be a means of relaxation.

Very little equipment is needed for aerobic dance. Comfortable clothing could include items such as leotard, shorts, t-shirt, and sneakers (or you can go barefoot). If you are not a member of an organized class or group, a record player, cassette player, or other equipment will be needed to play music. Aerobic dance can be performed almost anywhere, as very little space is needed to perform the range of motion involved with the exercises that are utilized. Some television stations feature aerobic fitness classes, so viewers can exercise in the privacy of their own living rooms.

Guidelines and Precautions

If you have not been active physically or have had health problems, see a physician before beginning an aerobic dance program. Persons who are overweight or have a family history of heart disease should have a physician's approval or a stress test before beginning an aerobic fitness program.

Periodically during an aerobic fitness class, you should stop and check your heart rate to be certain that it is within the recommended limits for safe exercise.

A warm-up program of stretching exercises is recommended. Warm-up could include exercises such as trunk stretching, trunk circles, half-knee bends, twists, and reaches. Follow a developmental sequence by going from simple tasks at the beginning of the program to more complex tasks later on. At the end of each workout, take time for cool-down period. Cool-down exercises should be done at your own speed and strength and in a relaxed manner.

Program development should be flexible to allow you to engage in activities appropriate for your interest and level of ability. Programs will vary according to each person's needs, interests, and physical condition. The object in most cases is to structure the aerobic dance program so that the intensity and length of the activity are gradually increased.

SUMMARY

- If done properly, calisthenic exercise can improve muscular strength and endurance, cardiorespiratory endurance, flexibility, and body composition.
- Calisthenic exercises should work on specific muscle groups with a specific purpose in mind.
- Running has become the most popular form of exercise in American society.

- Many people run to control their weight and attain a healthful appearance, whereas others run for the many physiologic benefits.
- Running also produces a psychologically stimulating effect.
- Proper running technique requires that you pay attention to the way your foot strikes the ground, your body position, your arm movement, and your breathing pattern.
- There are many considerations involved with buying a pair of running shoes, and some understanding of critical features is essential.
- Swimming offers physiologic benefits similar to running; however the physical stresses and strains to the lower extremity that occur with running are eliminated.
- Swimming requires approximately four times more energy to cover a given distance than does running.
- Swimming requires some specialized training in one or all five of the basic strokes before you can begin a program.
- Both swimming and cycling are used as substitute activities for an injured person who is incapable of running.
- Cycling is an aerobic activity that offers physiologic benefits similar to swimming and running.
- Rope skipping has many advantages for a person looking for an inexpensive and convenient form of exercise and offers an opportunity to improve personal fitness.
- Some physical educators feel that rope skipping is equivalent to jogging in terms of energy expenditure.
- Rope skipping raises the heart rate, and as students continue to actively use this activity in their fitness program, it improves not only cardiorespiratory endurance but also muscular endurance.
- If you are interested in rope skipping as a fitness activity, you should see a physician and get a physical evaluation if you have been largely sedentary or have had health problems.
- Rope skipping routines should be designed to help you progress from a short series of workouts to more extended workouts.
- Aerobic dance is movement to music for fitness.
- Aerobic dance contributes to physical fitness by providing aerobic exercise and involving such elements as cardiorespiratory endurance, balance, strength, flexibility, and muscular endurance.
- Aerobic dance utilizes various stretching, strength, and other exercises to achieve the target heart rate and produce a vigorous workout.
- An aerobic dance program should follow a developmental sequence by going from simple, easy tasks at the beginning of the program to more complex tasks later on.
- Periodically during an aerobic fitness class, you should stop and check your heart rate to be certain that it is within the recommended limits for safe exercise.

GLOSSARY

calisthenics Exercises done to improve strength, endurance, flexibility, and body composition

endorphins Chemicals that are endogenous to the nervous system and thought to be primarily responsible for the so-called "runners high"

abdominal breathing A type of breathing using the abdominal muscles that is recommended during strenous activity

stitch in the side Pain in the side often associated with some weakness or cramping of muscles in the abdomen or the diaphragm

REFERENCES

1. deVries, H. (1980). *Physiology of exercise for physical education and athletics*. Dubuque, IA: William C. Brown.
2. Fixx, J. (1980). *Jim Fixx's second book of running*. New York: Random House.
3. McArdle, W., Catch, F., Katch, V. (1981). *Exercise physiology, nutrition and human performance*. Philadelphia: Lea & Febiger.

SUGGESTED READINGS

American National Red Cross. (1981). *Adapted aquatics*. Washington, DC: Author.
Bailey, C. (1978). *Fit or fat?* Boston: Houghton Mifflin.
Coles, C., & Glenn, H. (1973). *Glenn's complete bicycle manual*. New York: Crown.
Cooper, K. (1977). *The aerobics way*. New York:M. Evans.
Cooper, K. (1980). *Aerobics for women*. Boston:Bantam Books.
Cooper, K. (1981). *The new aerobics*. Boston:Bantam Books.
DeLong, F. (1974). *DeLong's guide to bicycles and bicycling*. Radnon, PA:Chilton.
Douglas, P. (1983). *Handbook on tennis*. New York: Alfred A. Knopf.
Editors of *Runner's World*. (1981). Sixth annual *Runner's World* special shoe survey. *Runner's World 10*,36-65.
Fisher, G., & Allsen, P. (1980). *Jogging*. Dubuque, IA: William C. Brown.
Fonda, J. (1975). *Jane Fonda's workout book*. New York: Simon & Schuster.
Gabrielson, M., Spears, B., & Gabrielson, B. (1968). *Aquatics handbook*. Englewood Cliffs, NJ: Prentice-Hall.
Geline, R. (1978). *The practical runner*. New York:Collier.
Getchell, B. (1983). *Physical fitness: A way of life*. New York: John Wiley & Sons.
Henderson, J. (1977). *Jog, run, race*. Mountain View, CA:World Publications.
Hockey, R. (1985). *Physical fitness: The pathway to healthful living*. St. Louis:Times Mirror/ Mosby.
Hoyt, C., & Hoyt, J. (1978). *Cycling*. Dubuque, IA:William C. Brown.
Midtlyng, J. *Swimming*. (1982). Philadelphia:Saunders.
Miller, D., & Allen, E. (1982). *Fitness: A lifetime concept*. Minneapolis: Burgess.
President's Council of Physical Fitness and Sports. (1977). *Aqua dynamics*. Washington, DC: U. S. Government Printing Office.
Reeves, S. (1979). *Power walking*. New York: Merrill.
Sloane, E. (1970). *The complete book of cycling*. New York: Trident Press.
Sorenson, J. (1982). *Aerobic dancing*. New York:Rawson, Wade.
Stokes, R., & Farls, D. (1983). *Fitness everyone!* Winston-Salem, NC: Hunter Textbooks.
Torney, J., & Clayton, R. (1981). *Teaching aquatics*. Minneapolis: Burgess.
Williams, C., & Moore, C. (1983). *Jogging everyone*. Winston-Salem, NC: Hunter Textbooks.
Yankee, G.D. (1982). *Exercise walking*. Chicago:Contemporary Books.

APPENDIXES

APPENDIX A   NUTRITIVE VALUE OF THE EDIBLE PARTS OF FOODS

Foods, Approximate Measures, Units, and Weight (Edible Part Unless Footnotes Indicate Otherwise)	(Grams)	Water (Percent)	Food Energy (Calories)	Protein (Grams)	Fat (Grams)	Carbohydrate (Grams)	Calcium (Milligrams)	Iron (Milligrams)	Vitamin A Value (International Units)	Thiamin (Milligrams)	Riboflavin (Milligrams)	Ascorbic Acid (Milligrams)
Dairy Products (Cheese, Cream, Imitation Cream, Milk; Related Products)												
Cheese:												
Natural												
Blue	1 oz	28	100	6	8	1	150	0.1	200	0.01	0.11	0
Cheddar:												
Cut pieces	1 oz	28	115	7	9	Trace	204	.2	300	.01	.11	0
Shredded	1 cup	113	455	28	37	1	815	.8	1,200	.03	.42	0
Creamed (cottage cheese, 4% fat):												
Large curd	1 cup	225	235	28	10	6	135	.3	370	.05	.37	Trace
Small curd	1 cup	210	220	26	9	6	126	.3	340	.04	.34	Trace
Uncreamed (cottage cheese dry curd, less than ½% fat)	1 cup	145	125	25	1	3	46	.3	40	.04	.21	0
Cream	1 oz	28	100	2	10	1	23	.3	400	Trace	.06	0
Mozzarella, made with:												
Whole milk	1 oz	28	90	6	7	1	163	.1	260	Trace	.08	0
Part skim milk	1 oz	28	80	8	5	1	207	.1	180	.01	.10	0
Parmesan, grated:												
Tablespoon	1 tbsp	5	25	2	2	Trace	69	Trace	40	Trace	.02	0
Provolone	1 oz	28	100	7	8	1	214	.1	230	Trace	.09	0
Ricotta, made with												
Romano	1 oz	28	110	9	8	1	302	—	160	—	.11	0
Swiss	1 oz	28	105	8	8	1	272	Trace	240	.01	.10	0
Pasteurized process cheese:												
American	1 oz	28	105	6	9	Trace	174	.1	340	.01	.10	0
Swiss	1 oz	28	95	7	7	1	219	.2	230	Trace	.08	0
Cream, sweet:												
Half-and-half (cream and milk)	1 cup	242	315	7	28	10	254	.2	260	.08	.36	2
	1 tbsp	15	20	Trace	2		16	Trace	20	.01	.02	Trace

Food	Measure	Grams	Water (%)	Food energy (cal)	Protein (g)	Fat (g)	Saturated fatty acids (g)	Oleic (g)	Linoleic (g)	Carbohydrate (g)	Calcium (mg)	Iron (mg)	Vitamin A (IU)	Thiamin (mg)	Riboflavin (mg)	Niacin (mg)	Ascorbic acid (mg)
Light, coffee, or table	1 cup	240	74	470	6	46	28.8	11.7	1.0	9	231	.1	1,730	.08	.36	.1	2
	1 tbsp	15	74	30	Trace	3	1.8	.7	.1	1	14	Trace	110	Trace	.02	Trace	Trace
Whipping																	
Light	1 tbsp	15	64	45	Trace	5	2.9	1.5	.1	Trace	10	Trace	170	Trace	.02	Trace	Trace
Heavy	1 cup	238	58	820	5	88	54.8	22.3	2.0	7	154	.1	3,500	.05	.26	.1	1
	1 tbsp	15	58	80	Trace	6	3.5	1.4	.1	Trace	10	Trace	220	Trace	.02	Trace	Trace
Whipped topping, (pressurized)	1 cup	60	61	155	2	13	8.3	3.4	.3	6	61	Trace	550	.02	.04	Trace	0
	1 tbsp	3	61	10	Trace	1	.4	.2	Trace	Trace	3	Trace	30	Trace	Trace	Trace	0
Cream, sour	1 tbsp	12	71	25	Trace	3	1.6	.6	.1	1	14	Trace	90	Trace	.02	Trace	Trace
Cream products, imitation																	
Powdered	1 cup	94	2	515	5	33	30.6	.9	Trace	52	21	.1	190	0	.16	0	0
	1 tsp	2	2	10	Trace	1	.7	Trace	Trace	1	Trace	Trace	Trace	0	Trace	0	0
Whipped topping:																	
Frozen	1 cup	75	50	240	1	19	16.3	1.0	.2	17	5	.1	650	0	0	0	0
	1 tbsp	4	50	15	Trace	1	.9	.1	Trace	1	Trace	Trace	30	0	0	0	0
Powdered, made with whole milk	1 cup	80	67	150	3	10	8.5	.6	.1	13	72	Trace	290	.02	.09	Trace	1
	1 tbsp	4	67	10	Trace	1	.4	Trace	Trace	1	4	Trace	10	Trace	Trace	Trace	Trace
Ice cream. See Milk desserts, frozen																	
Ice milk. See Milk desserts, frozen																	
Milk:																	
Fluid:																	
Whole (3.3% fat)	1 cup	244	88	150	8	8	5.1	2.1	.2	11	291	.1	310	.09	.40	.2	2
Lowfat (2%)	1 cup	244	89	120	8	5	2.9	1.2	.1	12	297	.1	500	.10	.40	.2	2
Nonfat (skim)	1 cup	245	91	85	8	Trace	.3	.1	Trace	12	302	.1	500	.09	.34	.2	2
Buttermilk	1 cup	245	90	100	8	2	1.3	.5	Trace	12	285	.1	80	.08	.38	.1	2
Canned:																	
Evaporated, unsweetened — Whole milk	1 cup	252	74	340	17	19	11.6	5.3	.4	25	657	.5	610	.12	.80	.5	5
Skim milk	1 cup	255	79	200	19	1	.3	.1	Trace	29	738	.7	1,000	.11	.79	.4	3
Sweetened, condensed	1 cup	306	27	980	24	27	16.8	6.7	.7	166	868	.6	1,000	.28	1.27	.6	8
Dried	1 cup	68	4	245	24	Trace	.3	.1	Trace	35	837	.2	1,610	.28	1.19	.6	4
Milk beverages:																	
Chocolate milk (commercial) — Regular	1 cup	250	82	210	8	8	5.3	2.2	.2	26	280	.6	300	.09	.41	.3	2
Lowfat	1 cup	250	84	180	8	5	3.1	1.3	.1	26	284	.6	500	.10	.42	.3	2
Eggnog (commercial)	1 cup	254	74	340	10	19	11.3	5.0	.6	34	330	.5	890	.09	.48	.3	4
Malted milk	1 cup of milk plus ¾ oz of powder	265	81	235	9	9	5.5	2.3	.2	29	304	.5	330	.14	.43	.7	2

Adapted from United States Department of Agriculture, Home and Garden Bulletin No. 72 (Revised April 1981). Washington, DC: Superintendent of Documents, U.S. Government Printing Office.

Continued.

APPENDIX A NUTRITIVE VALUE OF THE EDIBLE PARTS OF FOODS—cont'd

Foods, Approximate Measures, Units, and Weight (Edible Part Unless Footnotes Indicate Otherwise)		(Grams)	Water (Percent)	Food Energy (Calories)	Protein (Grams)	Fat (Grams)	Carbohydrate (Grams)	Calcium (Milligrams)	Iron (Milligrams)	Vitamin A Value (International Units)	Thiamin (Milligrams)	Riboflavin (Milligrams)	Ascorbic Acid (Milligrams)
Dairy Products (Cheese, Cream, Imitation Cream, Milk; Related Products)—cont'd													
Milk beverages—cont'd													
Shakes, thick:													
Chocolate, container, net wt, 10.6 oz	1 container	300	72	355	9	8	63	396	.9	260	.14	.67	0
Vanilla, container, net wt. 11 oz	1 container	313	74	350	12	9	56	457	.3	360	.09	.61	0
Milk desserts, frozen:													
Ice cream:													
Regular:													
Hardened	1 cup	133	61	270	5	14	32	176	.1	540	.05	.33	1
	3 fl oz container	50	61	100	2	5	12	66	Trace	200	.02	.12	Trace
Soft serve (frozen custard)	1 cup	173	60	375	7	23	38	236	.4	790	.08	.45	1
Ice milk:													
Hardened	1 cup	131	69	185	5	6	29	176	.1	210	.08	.35	1
Soft serve	1 cup	175	70	225	8	5	38	274	0.3	180	0.12	0.54	1
Sherbet	1 cup	193	66	270	2	4	59	103	.3	190	.03	.09	4
Milk desserts, other:													
Custard, baked	1 cup	265	77	305	14	15	29	297	1.1	930	.11	.50	1
Puddings:													
Tapioca cream	1 cup	165	72	220	8	8	28	173	.7	480	.07	.30	2
From mix (chocolate) and milk:													
Regular (cooked)	1 cup	260	70	320	9	8	59	265	.8	340	.05	.39	2
Instant	1 cup	260	69	325	8	7	63	374	1.3	340	.08	.39	2
Yogurt:													
Made with lowfat milk:													
Fruit-flavored	1 container, net wt, 8 oz	227	75	230	10	3	42	343	.2	120	.08	.40	1
Plain	1 container, net wt, 8 oz	227	85	145	12	4	16	415	.2	150	.10	.49	2

Nutrients in Indicated Quantity

Made with nonfat milk	1 container, net wt, 8 oz	227	85	125	13	Trace	17	452	.2	20	.11	.53	2
Eggs													
Eggs, large (24 oz per dozen):													
Raw:													
Whole, without shell	1 egg	50	75	80	6	6	1	28	1.0	260	.04	.15	0
White	1 white	33	88	15	3	Trace	Trace	4	Trace	0	Trace	.09	0
Yolk	1 yolk	17	49	65	3	6	Trace	26	.9	310	.04	.07	0
Cooked:													
Fried in butter	1 egg	46	72	85	5	6	1	26	.9	290	.03	.13	0
Hard-cooked, shell removed	1 egg	50	75	80	6	6	1	28	1.0	260	.04	.14	0
Poached	1 egg	50	74	80	6	6	1	28	1.0	260	.04	.13	0
Scrambled (milk added)	1 egg	64	76	95	6	7	1	47	.9	310	.04	.16	0
Fats, Oils; Related Products													
Butter:													
Stick (½ cup)	1 stick	113	16	815	1	92	Trace	27	.2	3,470	.01	.04	0
Tablespoon (about ⅛ stick)	1 tbsp	14	16	100	Trace	12	Trace	3	Trace	430	Trace	Trace	0
Pat	1 pat	5	16	35	Trace	4	Trace	1	Trace	150	Trace	Trace	0
Fats, cooking (vegetable shortenings)	1 cup	200	0	1,770	0	200	0	0	0	—	0	0	0
	1 tbsp	13	0	110	0	13	0	0	0	—	0	0	0
Lard	1 cup	205	0	1,850	0	205	0	0	0	0	0	0	0
	1 tbsp	13	0	115	0	13	0	0	0	0	0	0	0
Margarine:													
Regular (1 brick or 4 sticks per lb):													
Stick (½ cup)	1 stick	113	16	815	1	92	Trace	27	.2	3,750	.01	.04	0
Tablespoon (about ⅛ stick)	1 tbsp	14	16	100	Trace	12	Trace	3	Trace	470	Trace	Trace	0
Pat	1 pat	5	16	35	Trace	4	Trace	1	Trace	170	Trace	Trace	0
Soft, two 8 oz containers per lb	1 container	227	16	1,635	1	184	Trace	53	.4	7,500	.01	.08	0
	1 tbsp	14	16	100	Trace	12	Trace	3	Trace	470	Trace	Trace	0
Whipped (6 sticks per lb)	1 stick	76	16	545	Trace	61	Trace	18	.1	2,500	Trace	.03	0
Tablespoon	1 tbsp	9	16	70	Trace	8	Trace	2	Trace	310	Trace	Trace	0
Oils, salad or cooking:													
Corn	1 cup	218	0	1,925	0	218	0	0	0	—	0	0	0
	1 tbsp	14	0	120	0	14	0	0	0	—	0	0	0
Olive	1 cup	216	0	1,910	0	216	0	0	0	—	0	0	0
	1 tbsp	14	0	120	0	14	0	0	0	—	0	0	0

Continued.

APPENDIX A NUTRITIVE VALUE OF THE EDIBLE PARTS OF FOODS—cont'd

Foods, Approximate Measures, Units, and Weight (Edible Part Unless Footnotes Indicate Otherwise)		(Grams)	Nutrients in Indicated Quantity										
			Water (Percent)	Food Energy (Calories)	Protein (Grams)	Fat (Grams)	Carbohydrate (Grams)	Calcium (Milligrams)	Iron (Milligrams)	Vitamin A Value (International Units)	Thiamin (Milligrams)	Riboflavin (Milligrams)	Ascorbic Acid (Milligrams)
Fats, Oils; Related Products—cont'd													
Salad dressings:													
Commercial:													
Blue cheese:													
Regular	1 tbsp	15	32	75	1	8	1	12	Trace	30	Trace	.02	Trace
Low calorie (5 cal per tsp)	1 tbsp	16	84	10	Trace	1	1	10	Trace	30	Trace	.01	Trace
French:													
Regular	1 tbsp	16	39	65	Trace	6	3	2	.1	—	—	—	—
Low calorie (5 cal per tsp)	1 tbsp	16	77	15	Trace	1	2	2	.1	—	—	—	—
Italian:													
Regular	1 tbsp	15	28	85	Trace	9	1	2	Trace	Trace	Trace	Trace	—
Low calorie 2 cal per tsp)	1 tbsp	15	90	10	Trace	1	Trace	Trace	Trace	Trace	Trace	Trace	—
Mayonnaise	1 tbsp	14	15	100	Trace	11	Trace	3	.1	40	Trace	.01	—
Mayonnaise type:													
Regular	1 tbsp	15	41	65	Trace	6	2	2	Trace	30	Trace	Trace	—
Low calorie (8 cal per tsp)	1 tbsp	16	81	20	Trace	2	2	3	Trace	40	Trace	Trace	—
Tartar sauce, regular	1 tbsp	14	34	75	Trace	8	1	3	.1	30	Trace	Trace	Trace
Thousand Island:													
Regular	1 tbsp	16	32	80	Trace	8	2	2	.1	50	Trace	Trace	Trace
Low calorie (10 cal per tsp)	1 tbsp	15	68	25	Trace	2	2	2	.1	50	Trace	Trace	Trace
Fish, Shellfish, Meat, Poultry; Related Products													
Fish and shellfish:													
Bluefish, baked with butter or margarine	3 oz	85	68	135	22	4	0	25	0.6	40	0.09	0.08	—
Clams:													
Canned, solids and liquid	3 oz	85	86	45	7	1	2	47	3.5	—	.01	.09	—
Crabmeat, canned	1 cup	135	77	135	24	3	1	61	1.1	—	.11	.11	—
Fish sticks, breaded, cooked	1 fish stick or 1 oz	28	66	80	5	3	2	3	.1	0	.01	.02	—
Haddock, breaded, fried	3 oz	85	66	140	17	5	5	34	1.0	—	.03	.06	2

Ocean perch, breaded, fried	1 fillet	85	59	195	16	11	6	28	1.1	—	.10	.10	—
Oysters, raw, meat only	1 cup	240	85	160	20	4	8	226	13.2	740	.34	.43	—
Salmon, pink, canned, solids and liquid	3 oz	85	71	120	17	5	0	167	.7	60	.01	.16	—
Scallops, frozen, breaded, fried, reheated	6 scallops	90	60	175	16	8	9	—	—	—	—	—	—
Shrimp:													
Canned meat	3 oz	85	70	100	21	1	1	98	2.6	50	.01	.03	—
French fried	3 oz	85	57	190	17	9	9	61	1.7	—	.03	.07	—
Tuna, canned in oil, drained solids	3 oz	85	61	170	24	7	0	7	1.6	70	.04	.10	—
Tuna salad	1 cup	205	70	350	30	22	7	41	2.7	590	.08	.23	2
Meat and meat products:													
Bacon, broiled or fried	2 slices	15	8	85	4	8	Trace	2	.5	0	.08	.05	—
Beef, cooked:													
Cuts braised, simmered or pot roasted:													
Lean and fat	3 oz	85	53	245	23	16	0	10	2.9	30	.04	.18	—
Lean only	2.5 oz	72	62	140	22	5	0	10	2.7	10	.04	.17	—
Ground beef, broiled:													
Lean with 10% fat	3 oz or patty	85	60	185	23	10	0	10	3.0	20	.08	.20	—
Roast, oven cooked, no liquid added:													
Lean and fat	3 oz	85	40	375	17	33	0	8	2.2	70	.05	.13	—
Lean only	1.8 oz	51	57	125	14	7	0	6	1.8	10	.04	.11	—
Steak:													
Lean and fat	3 oz	85	44	330	20	27	0	9	2.5	50	.05	.15	—
Lean only	2.0 oz	56	59	115	18	4	0	7	2.2	10	.05	.14	—
Beef, canned:													
Corned beef	3 oz	85	59	185	22	10	0	17	3.7	—	.01	.20	—
Corned beef hash	1 cup	220	67	400	19	25	24	29	4.4	—	.02	.20	0
Beef, dried, chipped	2½ oz jar	71	48	145	24	4	0	14	3.6	—	.05	.23	—
Beef and vegetable stew	1 cup	245	82	220	16	11	15	29	2.9	2,400	.15	.17	17
Beef potpie	1 piece	210	55	515	21	30	39	29	3.8	1,720	.30	.30	6
Chili con carne with beans, canned	1 cup	255	72	340	19	16	31	82	4.3	150	.08	.18	—
Chop suey with beef and pork (home recipe)	1 cup	250	75	300	26	17	13	60	4.8	600	.28	.38	33
Lamb, cooked:													
Chop, rib, (broiled													
Lean and fat	3.1 oz	89	43	360	18	32	0	8	1.0	—	.11	.19	—
Lean only	2 oz	57	60	120	16	6	0	6	1.1	—	.09	.15	—

APPENDIX A NUTRITIVE VALUE OF THE EDIBLE PARTS OF FOODS—cont'd

Foods, Approximate Measures, Units, and Weight (Edible Part Unless Footnotes Indicate Otherwise)	(Grams)	Water (Percent)	Food Energy (Calories)	Protein (Grams)	Fat (Grams)	Carbohydrate (Grams)	Calcium (Milligrams)	Iron (Milligrams)	Vitamin A Value (International Units)	Thiamin (Milligrams)	Riboflavin (Milligrams)	Ascorbic Acid (Milligrams)
Fish, Shellfish, Meat, Poultry; Related Products—cont'd												
Liver, beef, fried	3 oz	85	56	195	22	9	5	9	7.5	45,390	.22	3.56	23
Pork, cured, cooked:												
Ham, light cure, lean and fat, roasted	3 oz	85	54	245	18	19	0	8	2.2	0	.40	.15	—
Luncheon meat:												
Boiled ham, slice	1 oz	28	59	65	5	5	0	3	.8	0	.12	.04	—
Canned	1 slice	60	55	175	9	15	1	5	1.3	0	.19	.13	—
Pork, fresh, cooked:												
Chop, loin, broiled:												
Lean and fat	2.7 oz	78	42	305	19	25	0	9	2.7	0	0.75	0.22	—
Lean only	2 oz	56	53	150	17	9	0	7	2.2	0	.63	.18	—
Roast, oven cooked, no liquid added:												
Lean and fat	3 oz	85	46	310	21	24	0	9	2.7	0	.78	.22	—
Lean only	2.4 oz	68	55	175	20	10	0	9	2.6	0	.73	.21	—
Sausages (see also Luncheon meat)												
Bologna	1 slice	28	56	85	3	8	Trace	2	.5	—	.05	.06	—
Braunschweiger	1 slice	28	53	90	4	8	1	3	1.7	1,850	.05	.41	—
Brown and serve	1 link	17	40	70	3	6	Trace	—	.3	—	—	.01	—
Deviled ham, canned	1 tbsp	13	51	45	2	4	0	1	.3	0	.02	.01	—
Frankfurter	1 frankfurter	56	57	170	7	15	1	3	.8	—	.08	.11	—
Meat, potted (beef, chicken, turkey), canned	1 tbsp	13	61	30	2	2	0	—	—	—	Trace	.03	—
Pork link	1 link	13	35	60	2	6	Trace	1	.3	0	.10	.04	—
Salami:												
Dry type, slice	1 slice	10	30	45	2	4	Trace	1	.4	—	.04	.03	—
Cooked type	1 slice	28	51	90	5	7	Trace	3	.7	—	.07	.07	—
Vienna sausage	1 sausage	16	63	40	2	3	Trace	1	.3	—	.01	.02	—
Veal, medium fat, cooked, bone removed:												

Food	Measure	Weight (g)	Water (%)	Food energy (cal)	Protein (g)	Fat (g)	Carbohydrate (g)	Calcium (mg)	Iron (mg)	Vitamin A (I.U.)	Thiamin (mg)	Riboflavin (mg)	Ascorbic acid (mg)
Cutlet (4⅛ by 2¼ by ½)	3 oz	85	60	185	23	9	0	9	2.7	—	.06	.21	—
Poultry and poultry products:													
Chicken, cooked:													
Breast, fried, bones removed ½ breast	2.8 oz	79	58	160	26	5	1	9	1.3	70	.04	.17	—
Drumstick, fried, bones removed	1.3 oz	38	55	90	12	4	Trace	6	.9	50	.03	.15	—
Half broiler, broiled, bones removed	6.2 oz	176	71	240	42	7	0	16	3.0	160	.09	.34	—
Chicken, canned, boneless	3 oz	85	65	170	18	10	0	18	1.3	200	.03	.11	3
Chicken a la king, cooked	1 cup	245	68	470	27	34	12	127	2.5	1,130	.10	.42	12
Chicken and noodles	1 cup	240	71	365	22	18	26	26	2.2	430	.05	.17	Trace
Chicken chow mein:													
Canned	1 cup	250	89	95	7	Trace	18	45	1.3	150	.05	0.10	13
Chicken potpie	1 piece	232	57	545	23	31	42	70	3.0	3,090	.4	.31	5
Turkey, roasted,													
Dark meat	4 pieces	85	61	175	26	7	0	—	2.0	—	.03	.20	—
Light meat	2 pieces	85	62	150	28	3	0	—	1.0	—	.04	.12	—
Fruits and Fruit Products													
Apples, raw, unpeeled	1 apple	212	84	125	Trace	1	31	15	.6	190	.06	.04	8
Apple juice, bottled or canned	1 cup	248	88	120	Trace	Trace	30	15	1.5	—	.02	.05	2
Applesauce, canned:													
Sweetened	1 cup	255	76	230	1	Trace	61	10	1.3	100	.05	.03	3
Unsweetened	1 cup	244	89	100	Trace	Trace	26	10	1.2	100	.05	.02	2
Apricots:													
Raw	3 apricots	107	85	55	1	Trace	14	18	.5	2,890	.03	.04	11
Canned in heavy syrup	1 cup	258	77	220	2	Trace	57	28	.8	4,490	.05	.05	10
Dried	1 cup	130	25	340	7	1	86	87	7.2	14,170	.01	.21	16
Apricot nectar, canned	1 cup	251	85	145	1	Trace	37	23	.5	2,380	.03	.03	36
Avocados	1 avocado	216	74	370	5	37	13	22	1.3	630	.24	.43	30
Banana	1 banana	119	76	100	1	Trace	26	10	.8	230	.06	.07	12
Blackberries, raw	1 cup	144	85	85	2	1	19	46	1.3	290	.04	.06	30
Blueberries, raw	1 cup	145	83	90	1	1	22	22	1.5	150	.04	.09	20
Cantaloupe. See Muskmelons													
Cherries:													
Sour (tart), red, pitted, canned water pack	1 cup	244	88	105	2	Trace	26	37	.7	1,660	.07	.05	12
Sweet, raw, without pits and stems	10 cherries	68	80	45	1	Trace	12	15	.3	70	.03	.04	7
Cranberry juice cocktail	1 cup	253	83	165	Trace	Trace	42	13	.8	Trace	.03	.03	81
Cranberry sauce	1 cup	277	62	405	Trace	1	104	17	.6	60	.03	.03	6

Continued.

APPENDIX A   NUTRITIVE VALUE OF THE EDIBLE PARTS OF FOODS—cont'd

Foods, Approximate Measures, Units, and Weight (Edible Part Unless Footnotes Indicate Otherwise)		(Grams)	Water (Percent)	Food Energy (Calories)	Protein (Grams)	Fat (Grams)	Carbohydrate (Grams)	Calcium (Milligrams)	Iron (Milligrams)	Vitamin A Value (International Units)	Thiamin (Milligrams)	Riboflavin (Milligrams)	Ascorbic Acid (Milligrams)
Fruits and Fruit Products—cont'd													
Dates:													
Whole, without pits	10 dates	80	23	220	2	Trace	58	47	2.4	40	.07	.08	0
Chopped	1 cup	178	23	490	4	1	130	105	5.3	90	.16	.18	0
Fruit cocktail, canned, in heavy syrup	1 cup	255	80	195	1	Trace	50	23	1.0	360	.05	.03	5
Grapefruit:													
Raw	½ grapefruit with peel	241	89	50	1	Trace	13	20	.5	540	.05	.02	44
Canned	1 cup	254	81	180	2	Trace	45	33	.8	30	.08	.05	76
Grapefruit juice:													
Raw, pink, red, or white	1 cup	246	90	95	1	Trace	23	22	.5	—	.10	.05	93
Canned, white:													
Unsweetened	1 cup	247	89	100	1	Trace	24	20	1.0	20	.07	.05	84
Sweetened	1 cup	250	86	135	1	Trace	32	20	1.0	30	.08	.05	78
Frozen, concentrate, unsweetened	1 cup	247	89	100	1	Trace	24	25	.2	20	.10	.04	96
Grapes	10 grapes	50	81	35	Trace	Trace	9	6	.2	50	.03	.02	2
Grape drink, canned	1 cup	250	86	135	Trace	Trace	35	8	.3	—	.03	.03	—
Grape juice:													
Canned or bottled	1 cup	253	83	165	1	Trace	42	28	.8	—	.10	.05	Trace
Frozen concentrate, sweetened (diluted) by volume	1 cup	250	86	135	1	Trace	33	8	.3	10	.05	.08	10
Lemonade concentrate, frozen (diluted)	1 cup	248	89	105	Trace	Trace	28	2	.1	10	.01	02	17
Limeade concentrate, frozen (diluted)	1 cup	247	89	100	Trace	Trace	27	3	Trace	Trace	Trace	Trace	6
Muskmelons, raw:													
Cantaloupe	½ melon with rind	477	91	80	2	Trace	20	38	1.1	9,240	.11	.08	90
Honeydew	1/10 melon with rind	226	91	50	1	Trace	11	21	.6	60	.06	.04	34

Nutrients in Indicated Quantity

Food	Measure	Grams	Water %	Cal.	Protein	Fat	Carb.	Calcium	Iron	Vit. A	Thiamin	Riboflavin	Vit. C
Oranges, all commercial varieties, raw: Whole	1 orange	131	86	65	1	Trace	16	54	.5	260	.13	.05	66
Orange juice: Raw, all varieties	1 cup	248	88	110	2	Trace	26	27	.5	500	.22	.07	124
Canned, unsweetened	1 cup	249	87	120	2	Trace	28	25	1.0	500	.17	.05	100
Frozen concentrate (diluted)	1 cup	249	87	120	2	Trace	29	25	.2	540	.23	.03	120
Papayas, raw, ½-in cubes	1 cup	140	89	55	1	Trace	14	28	.4	2,450	.06	.06	78
Peaches: Raw: Whole	1 peach	100	89	40	1	Trace	10	9	.5	1,330	.02	.05	7
Sliced	1 cup	170	89	65	1	Trace	16	15	.9	2,260	.03	.09	12
Canned: Syrup pack	1 cup	256	79	200	1	Trace	51	10	.8	1,100	.03	.05	8
Water pack	1 cup	244	91	75	1	Trace	20	10	.7	1,100	.02	.07	7
Frozen, sliced, sweetened: 10-oz container	1 container	284	77	250	1	Trace	64	11	1.4	1,850	0.03	0.11	116
Cup	1 cup	250	77	220	1	Trace	57	10	1.3	1,630	.03	.10	103
Pears: Raw, with skin Bartlett	1 pear	164	83	100	1	1	25	13	.5	30	.03	.07	7
Canned	1 cup	255	80	195	1	1	50	13	.5	10	.03	.05	3
Pineapple: Raw, diced	1 cup	155	85	80	1	Trace	21	26	.8	110	.14	.05	26
Canned: Crushed, chunks, tidbits	1 cup	255	80	190	1	Trace	49	28	.8	130	.20	.05	18
Slices and liquid:	1 slice; 1¼ tbsp liquid	58	80	45	Trace	Trace	11	6	.2	30	.05	.01	4
Pineapple juice, unsweetened, canned	1 cup	250	86	140	1	Trace	34	38	.8	130	.13	.05	80
Plums: Raw, without pits: Japanese and hybrid	1 plum	66	87	30	Trace	Trace	8	8	.3	160	.02	.02	4
Prune-type	1 plum	28	79	20	Trace	Trace	6	3	.1	80	.01	.01	1
Prunes, dried, "softenized," with pits: Uncooked	4 extra large or 5 large prunes	49	28	110	1	Trace	29	22	1.7	690	.04	.07	1
Cooked, unsweetened	1 cup	250	66	255	2	1	67	51	3.8	1,590	.07	.15	2
Prune juice, canned or bottled	1 cup	256	80	195	1	Trace	49	36	1.8	—	.03	.03	5

Continued.

APPENDIX A NUTRITIVE VALUE OF THE EDIBLE PARTS OF FOODS—cont'd

Foods, Approximate Measures, Units, and Weight (Edible Part Unless Footnotes Indicate Otherwise)		(Grams)	Water (Percent)	Food Energy (Calories)	Protein (Grams)	Fat (Grams)	Carbohydrate (Grams)	Calcium (Milligrams)	Iron (Milligrams)	Vitamin A Value (International Units)	Thiamin (Milligrams)	Riboflavin (Milligrams)	Ascorbic Acid (Milligrams)
Fruits and Fruit Products—cont'd													
Raisins, seedless:													
Cup, not pressed down	1 cup	145	18	420	4	Trace	112	90	5.1	30	.16	.12	1
Packet, ½ oz (1½ tbsp)	1 packet	14	18	40	Trace	Trace	11	9	.5	Trace	.02	.01	Trace
Raspberries, red:													
Raw, capped, whole	1 cup	123	84	70	1	1	17	27	1.1	160	.04	.11	31
Frozen, sweetened, 10-oz container	1 container	284	74	280	2	1	70	37	1.7	200	.06	.17	60
Rhubarb, cooked, added sugar (frozen)	1 cup	270	63	385	1	1	98	211	1.9	190	.05	.11	16
Strawberries:													
Raw, whole berries, capped	1 cup	149	90	55	1	1	13	31	1.5	90	0.04	0.10	88
Frozen, sweetened:													
Sliced, 10-oz container	1 container	284	71	310	1	1	79	40	2.0	90	.06	.17	151
Whole, 1-lb container	1 container	454	76	415	2	1	107	59	2.7	140	.09	.27	249
Tangerine	1 tangerine	86	87	40	1	Trace	10	34	.3	360	.05	.02	27
Watermelon, raw, 4 by 8 in wedge with rind and seeds	1 wedge	926	93	110	2	1	27	30	2.1	2,510	.13	.13	30
Grain Products													
Bagel (egg) 3-in diam.:	1 bagel	55	32	165	6	2	28	9	1.2	30	.14	.10	0
Biscuits	1 biscuit	28	29	90	2	3	15	19	.6	Trace	.08	.08	Trace
Breadcrumbs	1 cup	100	7	390	13	5	73	122	3.6	Trace	.35	.35	Trace
Breads:													
Boston brown bread	1 slice	45	45	95	2	1	21	41	.9	0	.06	.04	0
Cracked-wheat bread	1 slice	25	35	65	2	1	13	22	.5	Trace	.08	.06	Trace
French or vienna bread, enriched													
French	1 slice	35	31	100	3	1	19	15	.8	Trace	.14	.08	Trace
Vienna	1 slice	25	31	75	2	1	14	11	.6	Trace	.10	.06	Trace
Italian bread, enriched	1 slice	30	32	85	3	Trace	17	5	.7	0	.12	.07	0

Nutrients in Indicated Quantity

Food	Measure	Grams	Water (%)	Food energy (cal.)	Protein (g)	Fat (g)	Carbohydrate (g)	Calcium (mg)	Iron (mg)	Vitamin A (I.U.)	Thiamin (mg)	Riboflavin (mg)	Ascorbic acid (mg)
Raisin bread, enriched	1 slice	25	35	65	2	1	13	18	.6	Trace	.09	.06	Trace
Rye bread:													
American, light	1 slice	25	36	60	2	Trace	13	19	.5	0	.07	.05	0
Pumpernickel	1 slice	32	34	80	3	Trace	17	27	.8	0	.09	.07	0
White bread, enriched:													
Loaf, 1 lb	1 loaf	454	36	1,225	39	15	229	381	11.3	Trace	1.80	1.10	Trace
Slice (18 per loaf)	1 slice	25	36	70	2	1	13	21	.6	Trace	.10	.06	Trace
Slice, toasted	1 slice	22	25	70	2	1	13	21	.6	Trace	.08	.06	Trace
Whole-wheat bread:													
Loaf, 1 lb	1 loaf	454	36	1,095	41	12	224	381	13.6	Trace	1.37	.45	Trace
Slice (16 per loaf)	1 slice	28	36	65	3	1	14	24	.8	Trace	.09	.03	Trace
Slice, toasted	1 slice	24	24	65	3	1	14	24	.8	Trace	.07	.03	Trace
Breakfast cereals:													
Hot type, cooked:													
Corn (hominy) grits, degermed enriched	1 cup	245	87	125	3	Trace	27	2	.7	Trace	.10	.07	0
Farina, enriched	1 cup	245	89	105	3	Trace	22	147	—	0	.12	.07	0
Oatmeal or rolled oats	1 cup	240	87	130	5	2	23	22	1.4	0	.19	.05	0
Wheat, rolled	1 cup	240	80	180	5	1	41	19	1.7	0	.17	.07	0
Wheat, whole-meal	1 cup	245	88	110	4	1	23	17	1.2	0	.15	.05	0
Ready-to-eat:													
Bran flakes (40% bran)	1 cup	35	3	105	4	1	28	19	5.6	1,540	.46	.52	0
Corn flakes:													
Plain	1 cup	25	4	95	2	Trace	21	—	—	—	—	—	13
Sugar-coated	1 cup	40	2	155	2	Trace	37	1	—	1,760	.53	.60	21
Corn, oat flour, puffed	1 cup	20	4	80	2	1	16	4	5.7	880	.26	.30	11
Corn, shredded	1 cup	25	3	95	2	Trace	22	1	.6	0	.33	.05	13
Oats, puffed	1 cup	25	3	100	3	1	19	44	4.0	1,100	.33	.38	13
Rice, puffed:													
Plain	1 cup	15	4	60	1	Trace	13	3	.3	0	.07	.01	0
Presweetened	1 cup	28	3	115	1	0	26	3	—	1,240	—	—	15
Wheat flakes	1 cup	30	4	105	3	Trace	24	12	4.8	1,320	.40	.45	16
Wheat, puffed:													
Plain	1 cup	15	3	55	2	Trace	12	4	.6	0	.08	.03	0
Presweetened	1 cup	38	3	140	3	Trace	33	7	—	1,680	.50	.57	20
Wheat, shredded, plain	1 oblong biscuit or ½ cup spoon-size biscuits	25	7	90	2	1	20	11	.9	0	.06	.03	0
Wheat germ	1 tbsp	6	4	25	2	1	3	3	.5	10	.11	.05	1

Continued.

APPENDIX A NUTRITIVE VALUE OF THE EDIBLE PARTS OF FOODS—cont'd

Foods, Approximate Measures, Units, and Weight (Edible Part Unless Footnotes Indicate Otherwise)		(Grams)	Nutrients in Indicated Quantity										
			Water (Per-cent)	Food Energy (Cal-ories)	Protein (Grams)	Fat (Grams)	Carbo-hydrate (Grams)	Cal-cium (Milli-grams)	Iron (Milli-grams)	Vitamin A Value (Inter-national Units)	Thia-min (Milli-grams)	Ribo-flavin (Milli-grams)	Ascorbic Acid (Milli-grams)
Grain Products—cont'd													
Cakes made from cake mixes with enriched flour:													
Angelfood	1 piece 1/12 of cake	53	34	135	3	Trace	32	50	.2	0	.03	.08	0
Coffeecake	1 piece (1/16 of cake)	72	30	230	5	7	38	44	1.2	120	.14	.15	Trace
Cupcakes													
Without icing	1 cupcake	25	26	90	1	3	14	40	.3	40	.05	.05	Trace
With chocolate icing	1 cupcake	36	22	130	2	5	21	47	.4	60	.05	.06	Trace
Devil's food with chocolate icing	1 piece (1/16 of cake)	69	24	235	3	8	40	41	1.0	100	.07	.10	Trace
Cupcake	1 cupcake	35	24	120	2	4	20	21	.5	50	.03	.05	Trace
Gingerbread:	1 piece (1/9 of cake)	63	37	175	2	4	32	57	.9	Trace	.09	.11	Trace
White, 2 layer with chocolate icing	1 piece (1/16 of cake)	71	21	250	3	8	45	70	.7	40	.09	.11	Trace
Yellow, 2 layer with chocolate icing	1 piece (1/16 of cake)	69	26	235	3	8	40	63	.8	100	.08	.10	Trace
Cakes made from home recipes using enriched flour:													
Boston cream pie with custard filling:	1 piece (1/12 of cake)	69	35	210	3	6	34	46	.7	140	.09	.11	Trace
Fruitcake, dark	1 slice	15	18	55	1	2	9	11	.4	20	.02	.02	Trace
Plain, sheet cake:													
Without icing	1 piece (1/9 of cake)	86	25	315	4	12	48	55	.9	150	.13	.15	Trace
With uncooked white icing	1 piece (1/9 of cake)	121	21	445	4	14	77	61	.8	240	.14	16	Trace
Pound	1 slice	33	16	160	2	10	16	6	.5	80	.05	.06	0

Spongecake	1 piece (1/12 of cake)	66	32	195	5	4	36	20	1.1	300	.09	.14	Trace
Cookies made with enriched flour:													
Brownies with nuts:													
From home recipe	1 brownie	20	10	95	1	6	10	8	.4	40	.04	.03	Trace
Frozen, with chocolate icing	1 brownie	25	13	105	1	5	15	10	.4	50	.03	.03	Trace
Chocolate chip (commercial)	4 cookies	42	3	200	2	9	29	16	1.0	50	.10	.17	Trace
Fig bars, square	4 cookies	56	14	200	2	3	42	44	1.0	60	.04	.14	Trace
Gingersnaps	4 cookies	28	3	90	2	2	22	20	.7	20	.08	.06	0
Macaroons	2 cookies	38	4	180	2	9	25	10	.3	0	.02	.06	0
Oatmeal with raisins	4 cookies	52	3	235	3	8	38	11	1.4	30	.15	.10	Trace
Plain	4 cookies	48	5	240	2	12	31	17	.6	30	0.10	0.08	0
Sandwich type (chocolate or vanilla)	4 cookies	40	2	200	2	9	28	10	.7	0	.06	.10	0
Vanilla wafers	10 cookies	40	3	185	2	6	30	16	.6	50	.10	.09	0
Crackers:													
Graham, plain	2 crackers	14	6	55	1	1	10	6	.5	0	.02	.08	0
Rye wafers, whole-grain	2 wafers	13	6	45	2	Trace	10	7	.5	0	.04	.03	0
Saltines, made with enriched flour	4 crackers or 1 packet	11	4	50	1	1	8	2	.5	0	.05	.05	0
Danish pastry (enriched flour), plain without fruit or nuts:													
Round piece, about 4¼-in diam. by 1 in	1 pastry	65	22	275	5	15	30	33	1.2	200	.18	.19	Trace
Ounce	1 oz	28	22	120	2	7	13	14	.5	90	.08	.08	Trace
Doughnuts, made with enriched flour:													
Cake type, plain	1 doughnut	25	24	100	1	5	13	10	.4	20	.05	.05	Trace
Yeast-leavened, glazed	1 doughnut	50	26	205	3	11	22	16	.6	25	.10	.10	0
Macaroni, enriched, cooked (cut lengths, elbows, shells)	1 cup	130	64	190	7	1	39	14	1.4	0	.23	.13	0
Macaroni (enriched) and cheese:													
Canned	1 cup	240	80	230	9	10	26	199	1.0	260	.12	.24	Trace
From home recipe (served hot)	1 cup	200	58	430	17	22	40	362	1.8	860	.20	.40	Trace
Muffins made with enriched flour:													
From home recipe:													
Blueberry	1 muffin	40	39	110	3	4	17	34	.6	90	.09	.10	Trace
Bran	1 muffin	40	35	105	3	4	17	57	1.5	90	.07	.10	Trace
Corn (enriched degermed cornmeal and flour)	1 muffin	40	33	125	3	4	19	42	.7	120	.10	.10	Trace
Plain, 3-in diameter	1 muffin	40	38	120	3	4	17	42	0.6	40	0.09	0.12	Trace

Continued.

APPENDIX A   NUTRITIVE VALUE OF THE EDIBLE PARTS OF FOODS—cont'd

Foods, Approximate Measures, Units, and Weight (Edible Part Unless Footnotes Indicate Otherwise)	(Grams)	Water (Per-cent)	Food Energy (Cal-ories)	Protein (Grams)	Fat (Grams)	Carbo-hydrate (Grams)	Cal-cium (Milli-grams)	Iron (Milli-grams)	Vitamin A Value (Inter-national Units)	Thia-min (Milli-grams)	Ribo-flavin (Milli-grams)	Ascorbic Acid (Milli-grams)
Grain Products—cont'd												
Muffins made with enriched flour—cont'd												
From mix, egg, milk	1 muffin	40	30	130	3	4	20	96	.6	100	.08	.09	Trace
Noodles (egg noodles), enriched, cooked	1 cup	160	71	200	7	2	37	16	1.4	110	.22	.13	0
Noodles, chow mein, canned	1 cup	45	1	220	6	11	26	—	—	—	—	—	—
Pancakes, (4-in diam.):												
Made from home recipe using en-riched flour	1 cake	27	50	60	2	2	9	27	.4	30	.06	.07	Trace
Made from mix with enriched flour, egg and milk added	1 cake	27	51	60	2	2	9	58	.3	70	.04	.06	Trace
Pies, piecrust made with enriched flour, vegetable shortening (9-in diam.):												
Apple	1 sector (⅐ of pie)	135	48	345	3	15	51	11	.9	40	.15	.11	2
Banana creme	1 sector (⅐ of pie)	130	54	285	6	12	40	86	1.0	330	.11	.22	1
Blueberry	1 sector (⅐ of pie)	135	51	325	3	15	47	15	1.4	40	.15	.11	4
Cherry	1 sector (⅐ of pie)	135	47	350	4	15	52	19	.9	590	.16	.12	Trace
Custard	1 sector (⅐ of pie)	130	58	285	8	14	30	125	1.2	300	.11	.27	0
Lemon meringue	1 sector (⅐ of pie)	120	47	305	4	12	45	17	1.0	200	.09	.12	4
Mince	1 sector (⅐ of pie)	135	43	365	3	16	56	38	1.9	Trace	.14	.12	1
Peach	1 sector (⅐ of pie)	135	48	345	3	14	52	14	1.2	990	.15	.14	4
Pecan	1 sector (⅐ of pie)	118	20	495	6	27	61	55	3.7	190	.26	.14	Trace
Pumpkin	1 sector (⅐ of pie)	130	59	275	5	15	32	66	1.0	3,210	.11	.18	Trace
Pizza (cheese) baked ⅛ of 12-in diam. pie	1 sector	60	45	145	6	4	22	86	1.1	230	0.16	0.18	4
Popcorn, popped:												
Plain, large kernel	1 cup	6	4	25	1	Trace	5	1	.2	—	—	.01	0
With oil (coconut) and salt added, large kernel	1 cup	9	3	40	1	2	5	1	.2	—	—	.01	0

Food	Measure	Grams	Water (%)	Food energy	Protein (g)	Fat (g)	Carbohydrate (g)	Calcium (mg)	Iron (mg)	Vitamin A	Thiamin (mg)	Riboflavin (mg)	Ascorbic acid (mg)
Pretzels, made with enriched flour:													
Dutch, twisted	1 pretzel	16	5	60	2	1	12	4	.2	0	.05	.04	0
Thin, twisted	10 pretzels	60	5	235	6	3	46	13	.9	0	.20	.15	0
Stick, 2¼ in long	10 pretzels	3	5	10	Trace	Trace	2	1	Trace	0	.01	.01	0
Rice, white, enriched:													
Instant, ready-to-serve, hot	1 cup	165	73	180	4	Trace	40	5	1.3	0	.21	—	0
Long grain, cooked, served hot	1 cup	205	73	225	4	Trace	50	21	1.8	0	.23	.02	0
Rolls, enriched:													
Commercial:													
Brown-and serve	1 roll	26	27	85	2	2	14	20	.5	Trace	.10	.06	Trace
Cloverleaf or pan, 2½-in diam., 2 in high	1 roll	28	31	85	2	2	15	21	.5	Trace	.11	.07	Trace
Frankfurter and hamburger	1 roll	40	31	120	3	2	21	30	.8	Trace	.16	.10	Trace
Hoagie or submarine	1 roll	135	31	390	12	4	75	58	3.0	Trace	.54	.32	Trace
Spaghetti, enriched, cooked:	1 cup	130	64	190	7	1	33	14	1.4	0	.23	.13	0
Spaghetti (enriched) in tomato sauce with cheese	1 cup	250	80	190	6	2	39	40	2.8	930	.35	.28	10
Spaghetti (enriched) with meat balls and tomato sauce	1 cup	250	78	260	12	10	29	53	3.3	1,000	.15	.18	5
Toaster pastries	1 pastry	50	12	200	3	6	36	54	1.9	500	.16	.17	—
Waffles	1 waffle	75	42	205	7	8	27	179	1.0	170	.14	.22	Trace
Legumes (Dry), Nuts, Seeds; Related Products													
Almonds, shelled:													
Chopped	1 cup	130	5	775	24	70	25	304	6.1	0	.31	1.20	Trace
Beans, dry:													
Cooked, drained:													
Great Northern	1 cup	180	69	210	14	1	38	90	4.9	0	.25	.13	0
Pea (navy)	1 cup	190	69	225	15	1	40	95	5.1	0	.27	.13	0
Canned, solids and liquid:													
White with													
Frankfurters (sliced)	1 cup	255	71	365	19	18	32	94	4.8	330	.18	.15	Trace
Pork and tomato sauce	1 cup	255	71	310	16	7	48	138	4.6	330	.20	.08	5
Pork and sweet sauce	1 cup	255	66	385	16	12	54	161	5.9	—	.15	.10	—
Red kidney	1 cup	255	76	230	15	1	42	74	4.6	10	.13	.10	—
Lima, cooked, drained	1 cup	190	64	260	16	1	49	55	5.9	—	.25	.11	—
Blackeye peas, dry, cooked	1 cup	250	80	190	13	1	35	43	3.3	30	.40	.10	—
Brazil nuts, shelled	1 oz	28	5	185	4	19	3	53	1.0	Trace	.27	.03	—
Cashew nuts, roasted in oil	1 cup	140	5	785	24	64	41	53	5.3	140	.60	.35	—
Coconut meat, fresh:													
Piece, about 2 by 2 by ½ in	1 piece	45	51	155	2	16	4	6	.8	0	.02	.01	1

Continued.

APPENDIX A NUTRITIVE VALUE OF THE EDIBLE PARTS OF FOODS—cont'd

Foods, Approximate Measures, Units, and Weight (Edible Part Unless Footnotes Indicate Otherwise)	(Grams)	Water (Percent)	Food Energy (Calories)	Protein (Grams)	Fat (Grams)	Carbohydrate (Grams)	Calcium (Milligrams)	Iron (Milligrams)	Vitamin A Value (International Units)	Thiamin (Milligrams)	Riboflavin (Milligrams)	Ascorbic Acid (Milligrams)
Legumes (Dry), Nuts, Seeds; Related Products—cont'd												
Coconut meat, fresh:—cont'd												
Shredded or grated, not pressed down	80	51	275	3	28	8	10	1.4	0	.04	.02	2
Lentils, whole, cooked	200	72	210	16	Trace	39	50	4.2	40	.14	.12	0
Peanuts, roasted in oil, salted	144	2	840	37	72	27	107	3.0	—	.46	.19	0
Peanut butter	16	2	95	4	8	3	9	.3	—	.02	.02	0
Peas, split, dry, cooked	200	70	230	16	1	42	22	3.4	80	.30	.18	—
Pecans, chopped or pieces	118	3	810	11	84	17	86	2.8	150	1.01	.15	2
Pumpkin and squash kernels	140	4	775	41	65	21	71	15.7	100	.34	.27	—
Sunflower seeds, dry, hulled	145	5	810	35	69	29	174	10.3	70	2.84	.33	—
Walnuts:												
Black, chopped or broken kernels	125	3	785	26	74	19	Trace	7.5	380	.28	.14	—
Persian or English, chopped	120	4	780	18	77	19	119	3.7	40	.40	.16	2
Sugars and Sweets												
Cake icings:												
Uncooked:												
Chocolate made with milk and butter	275	14	1,035	9	38	185	165	3.3	580	.06	.28	1
Creamy fudge from mix and water	245	15	830	7	16	183	96	2.7	Trace	.05	.20	Trace
White	319	11	1,200	2	21	260	48	Trace	860	Trace	.06	Trace
Candy:												
Caramels, plain or chocolate	28	8	115	1	3	22	42	.4	Trace	.01	.05	Trace
Chocolate:												
Milk, plain	28	1	145	2	9	16	65	.3	80	.02	.10	Trace
Semisweet, small pieces	170	1	860	7	61	97	51	4.4	30	.02	.14	0
Chocolate-coated peanuts	28	1	160	5	12	11	33	.4	Trace	.10	.05	Trace

Nutrients in Indicated Quantity

The approximate measures are: 1 cup, 1 cup, 1 tbsp, 1 cup, 1 cup, 1 cup, 1 cup, 1 cup, 1 cup, 1 cup, 1 cup, 1 cup, 1 oz, 1 oz, 1 cup or 6-oz, 1 oz.

Fondant, uncoated (mints, candy corn, other)	1 oz	28	8	105	Trace	1	25	4	.3	0	Trace	Trace	0
Fudge, chocolate, plain	1 oz	28	8	115	1	3	21	22	.3	Trace	.01	.03	Trace
Gum drops	1 oz	28	12	100	Trace	Trace	25	2	.1	0	0	Trace	0
Hard	1 oz	28	1	110	Trace	Trace	28	6	.5	0	0	0	0
Marshmallows	1 oz	28	17	90	1	Trace	23	5	.5	0	Trace	Trace	0
Chocolate-flavored beverage powders (about 4 heaping tsp per oz):													
With nonfat dry milk	1 oz	28	2	100	5	1	20	167	.5	10	.04	.21	1
Without milk	1 oz	28	1	100	1	1	25	9	.6	—	.01	.03	0
Honey, strained or extracted	1 tbsp	21	17	65	Trace	0	17	1	.1	0	Trace	.01	Trace
Jams and preserves	1 tbsp	20	29	55	Trace	Trace	14	4	.2	Trace	Trace	.01	Trace
Jellies	1 tbsp	18	29	50	Trace	Trace	13	4	.3	Trace	Trace	.01	1
Syrups:													
Chocolate-flavored syrup or topping:													
Thin type	1 fl oz or 2 tbsp	38	32	90	1	1	24	6	.6	Trace	.01	.03	0
Fudge type	1 fl oz or 2 tbsp	38	25	125	2	5	20	48	.5	60	.02	.08	Trace
Molasses, cane	1 tbsp	20	24	50	—	—	13	33	.9	—	.01	.01	—
Table blends, chiefly corn, light and dark	1 tbsp	21	24	60	0	0	15	9	.8	0	0	0	0
Sugars:													
Brown, pressed down	1 cup	220	2	820	0	0	212	187	7.5	0	0	.07	0
White:													
Granulated	1 cup	200	1	770	0	0	199	0	.2	0	0	0	0
	1 tbsp	12	1	45	0	0	12	0	Trace	0	0	0	0
	1 packet	6	1	23	0	0	6	0	Trace	0	0	0	0
Powdered, sifted	1 cup	100	1	385	0	0	100	0	.1	0	0	0	0
Vegetable and Vegetable Products													
Asparagus, green:													
Canned, spears ½-in diam. at base	4 spears	80	93	15	2	Trace	3	15	1.5	640	.05	.08	12
Beans:													
Lima													
Thick-seeded types (Fordhooks)	1 cup	170	74	170	10	Trace	32	34	2.9	390	.12	.09	29
Thin-seeded types (baby limas)	1 cup	180	69	210	13	Trace	40	63	4.7	400	.16	.09	22

Continued.

APPENDIX A   NUTRITIVE VALUE OF THE EDIBLE PARTS OF FOODS—cont'd

Foods, Approximate Measures, Units, and Weight (Edible Part Unless Footnotes Indicate Otherwise)	(Grams)	Water (Percent)	Food Energy (Calories)	Protein (Grams)	Fat (Grams)	Carbohydrate (Grams)	Calcium (Milligrams)	Iron (Milligrams)	Vitamin A Value (International Units)	Thiamin (Milligrams)	Riboflavin (Milligrams)	Ascorbic Acid (Milligrams)
Vegetable and Vegetable Products—cont'd												
Beans—cont'd												
Snap:												
Green:												
Cooked, drained:												
From raw (cuts and French style)	1 cup	92	30	2	Trace	7	63	.8	680	.09	.11	15
From frozen:												
Cuts	1 cup	92	35	2	Trace	8	54	.9	780	.09	.12	7
French style	1 cup	92	35	2	Trace	8	49	1.2	690	.08	.10	9
Canned, drained solids	1 cup	92	30	2	Trace	7	61	2.0	630	.04	.07	5
Bean sprouts (mung):												
Raw	1 cup	89	35	4	Trace	7	20	1.4	20	.14	.14	20
Cooked, drained	1 cup	91	35	4	Trace	7	21	1.1	30	.11	.13	8
Beets:												
Cooked, drained, peeled:												
Whole beets, 2-in diam.	2 beets	91	30	1	Trace	7	14	.5	20	.03	.04	6
Diced or sliced	1 cup	91	55	2	Trace	12	24	.9	30	.05	.07	10
Canned, drained solids:												
Whole beets, small	1 cup	89	60	2	Trace	14	30	1.1	30	.02	.05	5
Diced or slided	1 cup	89	65	2	Trace	15	32	1.2	30	.02	.05	5
Blackeye peas, immature seeds, cooked and drained:												
From raw	1 cup	72	180	13	1	30	40	3.5	580	.50	.18	28
From frozen	1 cup	66	220	15	1	40	43	4.8	290	.68	.19	15
Broccoli, cooked, drained:												
From raw:												
Stalk, medium size	1 stalk	91	45	6	1	8	158	1.4	4,500	.16	.36	162

APPENDIX

A-21

Food	Unit												
From frozen:													
Stalk, 4½ to 5 in long	1 stalk	30	91	10	1	Trace	1	12	.2	570	.02	.03	22
Chopped	1 cup	185	92	50	5	1	9	100	1.3	4,810	.11	.22	105
Brussels sprouts, cooked, drained:													
From raw, 7-8 sprouts	1 cup	155	88	55	7	1	10	50	1.7	810	.12	.22	135
From frozen	1 cup	155	89	50	5	Trace	10	33	1.2	880	.12	.16	126
Cabbage:													
Raw, finely shredded or chopped	1 cup	90	92	20	1	Trace	5	44	.4	120	.05	.05	42
Cooked, drained	1 cup	145	94	30	2	Trace	6	64	.4	190	.06	.06	14
Red, raw, coarsely shredded or sliced	1 cup	70	90	20	1	Trace	5	29	.6	30	.06	.04	43
Carrots:													
Raw, without crowns and tips, scraped:													
Whole	1 carrot or 18 strips	72	88	30	1	Trace	7	27	.5	7,930	.04	.04	6
Cooked (crosswise cuts)	1 cup	155	91	50	1	Trace	11	51	.9	16,280	.08	.08	9
Canned, sliced, drained solids	1 cup	155	91	45	1	Trace	10	47	1.1	23,250	.03	.05	3
Cauliflower:													
Raw, chopped	1 cup	115	91	31	3	Trace	6	29	1.3	70	.13	.12	90
Cooked, drained:													
From raw (flower buds)	1 cup	125	93	30	3	Trace	5	26	.9	80	.11	.10	69
From frozen (flowerets)	1 cup	180	94	30	3	Trace	6	31	.9	50	.07	.09	74
Celery, Pascal type, raw:													
Stalk, large outer, 8 by 1½ in. at root end	1 stalk	40	94	5	Trace	Trace	2	16	.1	110	.01	.01	4
Pieces, diced	1 cup	120	94	20	1	Trace	5	47	.4	320	.04	.04	11
Collards, cooked, drained:													
From raw	1 cup	190	90	65	7	1	10	357	1.5	14,820	.21	.38	144
From frozen (chopped)	1 cup	170	90	50	5	1	10	299	1.7	11,560	.10	.24	56
Corn, sweet:													
Cooked, drained:													
From raw, ear 5 by 1¾ in	1 ear	140	74	70	2	1	16	2	.5	310	.09	.08	7
From frozen:													
Ear, 5 in long	1 ear	229	73	120	4	1	27	4	1.0	440	.18	.10	9
Kernels	1 cup	165	77	130	5	1	31	5	1.3	580	.15	.10	8
Canned:													
Cream style	1 cup	256	76	210	5	2	51	8	1.5	840	.08	.13	13
Whole kernel:													
Vacuum pack	1 cup	210	76	175	5	1	43	6	1.1	740	.06	.13	11
Wet pack	1 cup	165	76	140	4	1	33	8	.8	580	.05	.08	7

Continued.

APPENDIX A   NUTRITIVE VALUE OF THE EDIBLE PARTS OF FOODS—cont'd

Foods, Approximate Measures, Units, and Weight (Edible Part Unless Footnotes Indicate Otherwise)		(Grams)	Water (Percent)	Food Energy (Calories)	Protein (Grams)	Fat (Grams)	Carbohydrate (Grams)	Calcium (Milligrams)	Iron (Milligrams)	Vitamin A Value (International Units)	Thiamin (Milligrams)	Riboflavin (Milligrams)	Ascorbic Acid (Milligrams)
Vegetable and Vegetable Products—cont'd													
Cucumber slices	6 large or 8 small slices	28	95	5	Trace	Trace	1	7	.3	70	.01	.01	3
Lettuce, raw:													
Butterhead, as Boston types:													
Head, 5-in diam.	1 head	220	95	25	2	Trace	4	57	3.3	1,580	.10	.10	13
Crisphead, as Iceberg:													
Head, 6-in diam.	1 head	567	96	70	5	1	16	108	2.7	1,780	.32	.32	32
Pieces, chopped or shredded	1 cup	55	96	5	Trace	Trace	2	11	.3	180	.03	.03	3
Looseleaf	1 cup	55	94	10	1	Trace	2	37	.8	1,050	.03	.04	10
Mushrooms, raw, sliced or chopped	1 cup	70	90	20	2	Trace	3	4	.6	Trace	.07	.32	2
Onions:													
Raw:													
Chopped	1 cup	170	89	65	3	Trace	15	46	.9	Trace	.05	.07	17
Sliced	1 cup	115	89	45	2	Trace	10	31	.6	Trace	.03	.05	12
Cooked (whole or sliced)	1 cup.	210	92	60	3	Trace	14	50	.8	Trace	.06	.06	15
Parsley, raw, chopped	1 tbsp	4	85	Trace	Trace	Trace	Trace	7	.2	300	Trace	.01	6
Parsnips, cooked	1 cup	155	82	100	2	1	23	70	.9	50	.11	.12	16
Peas, green:													
Canned	1 cup	170	77	150	8	1	29	44	3.2	1,170	.15	.10	14
Frozen, cooked, drained	1 cup	160	82	110	8	Trace	19	30	3.0	960	.43	.14	21
Peppers, hot, red	1 tsp	2	9	5	Trace	Trace	1	5	.3	1,300	Trace	.02	Trace
Peppers, sweet													
Raw	1 pod	74	93	15	1	Trace	4	7	.5	310	.06	.06	94
Cooked, boiled, drained	1 pod	73	95	15	1	Trace	3	7	.4	310	.05	.05	70
Potatoes, cooked:													
Baked, peeled after baking	1 potato	156	75	145	4	Trace	33	14	1.1	Trace	.15	.07	31
Boiled:													
Peeled after boiling	1 potato	137	80	105	3	Trace	23	10	.8	Trace	.12	.05	22
Peeled before boiling	1 potato	135	83	90	3	Trace	20	8	.7	Trace	.12	.05	22

Nutrients in Indicated Quantity

Food	Measure	Weight (g)	Water (%)	Food energy	Protein	Fat	Carbohydrate	Calcium	Iron	Vitamin A	Thiamin	Riboflavin	Ascorbic acid
French-fried, strip, 2 to 3½ in long:													
Prepared from raw	10 strips	50	45	135	2	7	18	8	.7	Trace	.07	.04	11
Frozen, oven heated	10 strips	50	53	110	2	4	17	5	.9	Trace	.07	.01	11
Hashed brown, prepared from frozen	1 cup	155	56	345	3	18	45	28	1.9	Trace	.11	.03	12
Mashed, prepared from Raw:													
Milk added	1 cup	210	83	135	4	2	27	50	.8	40	.17	.11	21
Milk and butter added	1 cup	210	80	195	4	9	26	50	0.8	360	0.17	0.11	19
Potato chips, 1¾ by 2½ in oval cross section	10 chips	20	2	115	1	8	10	8	.4	Trace	.04	.01	3
Potato salad, made with cooked salad dressing	1 cup	250	76	250	7	7	41	80	1.5	350	.20	.18	28
Pumpkin, canned	1 cup	245	90	80	2	1	19	61	1.0	15,680	.07	.12	12
Radishes, raw	4 radishes	18	95	5	Trace	Trace	1	5	.2	Trace	.01	.01	5
Sauerkraut, canned, solids and liquid	1 cup	235	93	40	2	Trace	9	85	1.2	120	.07	.09	33
Spinach:													
Raw, chopped	1 cup	55	91	15	2	Trace	2	51	1.7	4,460	.06	.11	28
Cooked, drained:													
From raw	1 cup	180	92	40	5	1	6	167	4.0	14,580	.13	.25	50
From frozen:													
Chopped	1 cup	205	92	45	6	1	8	232	4.3	16,200	.14	.31	39
Leaf	1 cup	190	92	45	6	1	7	200	4.8	15,390	.15	.27	53
Canned, drained solids	1 cup	205	91	50	6	1	7	242	5.3	16,400	.04	.25	29
Squash, cooked:													
Summer	1 cup	210	96	30	2	Trace	7	53	.8	820	.11	.17	21
Winter	1 cup	205	81	130	4	1	32	57	1.6	8,610	.10	.27	27
Sweet potatoes:													
Baked in skin, peeled	1 potato	114	64	160	2	1	37	46	1.0	9,230	.10	.08	25
Boiled in skin, peeled	1 potato	151	71	170	3	1	40	48	1.1	11,940	.14	.09	26
Candied, 2½ by 2-in piece	1 piece	105	60	175	1	3	36	39	.9	6,620	.06	.04	11
Canned, solid pack (mashed)	1 cup	255	72	275	5	1	63	64	2.0	19,890	.13	.10	36
Tomatoes:													
Raw	1 tomato	135	94	25	1	Trace	6	16	.6	1,110	.07	.05	28
canned, solids and liquid	1 cup	241	94	50	2	Trace	10	14	1.2	2,170	.12	.07	41
Tomato catsup	1 tbsp	15	69	15	Trace	Trace	4	3	.1	210	.01	.01	2
Tomato juice, canned	1 glass (6 fl oz)	182	94	35	2	Trace	8	13	1.6	1,460	.09	.05	29
Vegetables, mixed, frozen, cooked	1 cup	182	83	115	6	1	24	46	2.4	9,010	.22	.13	15

Continued.

APPENDIX A   NUTRITIVE VALUE OF THE EDIBLE PARTS OF FOODS—cont'd

Foods, Approximate Measures, Units, and Weight (Edible Part Unless Footnotes Indicate Otherwise)		(Grams)	Water (Percent)	Food Energy (Calories)	Protein (Grams)	Fat (Grams)	Carbohydrate (Grams)	Calcium (Milligrams)	Iron (Milligrams)	Vitamin A Value (International Units)	Thiamin (Milligrams)	Riboflavin (Milligrams)	Ascorbic Acid (Milligrams)
Miscellaneous Items													
Barbecue sauce	1 cup	250	81	230	4	17	20	53	2.0	900	.03	.03	13
Beverages, alcoholic:													
Beer	12 fl oz	360	92	150	1	0	14	18	Trace	—	.01	.11	—
Gin, rum, vodka, whisky (86-proof)	1½-fl oz jigger	42	64	105	—	—	Trace	—	—	—	—	—	—
Wines													
Dessert	3½-fl oz glass	103	77	140	Trace	0	8	8	.4	—	.01	.02	—
Table	3½-fl oz glass	102	86	85	Trace	0	4	9		—	Trace	.01	—
Beverages, carbonated, sweetened, nonalcoholic:													
Carbonated water	12 fl oz	366	92	155	0	0	29	—	—	0	0	0	0
Cola type	12 fl oz	369	90	145	0	0	37	—	—	0	0	0	0
Fruit-flavored sodas and Tom Collins mixer	12 fl oz	372	88	170	0	0	45	—	—	0	0	0	0
Ginger ale	12 fl oz	366	92	115	0	0	29	—	—	0	0	0	0
Root beer	12 fl oz	370	90	150	0	0	39	—	—	0	0	0	0
Chocolate, bitter or baking	1 oz	28	2	145	3	15	8	22	1.9	20	.01	.07	0
Gelatin, dry	1, 7-g envelope	7	13	25	6	Trace	0	—	—	—	—	—	—
Gelatin dessert prepared with gelatin dessert powder and water	1 cup	240	84	140	4	0	34	—	—	—	—	—	—
Mustard, prepared, yellow	1 tsp	5	80	5	Trace	Trace	Trace	4	.1	—	—	—	—
Olives, pickled, canned:													
Green	4 medium	16	78	15	Trace	2	Trace	8	.2	40	—	—	—
Ripe, Mission	3 small	10	73	15	Trace	2	Trace	9	.1	10	Trace	Trace	—
Pickles, cucumber:													
Dill, medium, whole, 3¾ in long, 1¼-in diam.	1 pickle	65	93	5	Trace	Trace	1	17	.7	70	Trace	.01	4

Nutrients in Indicated Quantity

Food	Measure	Grams	Water (%)	Food energy (cal)	Protein (g)	Fat (g)	Carbohydrate (g)	Calcium (mg)	Iron (mg)	Vitamin A (IU)	Thiamin (mg)	Riboflavin (mg)	Ascorbic acid (mg)
Fresh-pack, slices	2 slices	15	79	10	Trace	Trace	3	5	.3	20	Trace	Trace	1
Sweet, gherkin, small	1 pickle	15	61	20	Trace	Trace	5	2	.2	10	Trace	Trace	1
Relish, finely chopped, sweet	1 tbsp	15	63	20	Trace	Trace	5	3	.1	—	—	—	—
Popsicle, 3-fl oz size	1 popsicle	95	80	70	0	0	18	0	Trace	0	0	0	0
Soups:													
Canned, condensed:													
Prepared with equal volume of milk:													
Cream of chicken	1 cup	245	85	180	7	10	15	172	.5	610	0.05	0.27	2
Cream of mushroom	1 cup	245	83	215	7	14	16	191	.5	250	.05	.34	1
Tomato	1 cup	250	84	175	7	7	23	168	.8	1,200	.10	.25	15
Prepared with equal volume of water:													
Bean with pork	1 cup	250	84	170	8	6	22	63	2.3	650	.13	.08	3
Beef broth, bouillon	1 cup	240	96	30	5	0	3	Trace	.5	Trace	Trace	.02	—
Beef noodle	1 cup	240	93	65	4	3	7	7	1.0	50	.05	.07	Trace
Clam chowder, Manhattan type	1 cup	245	92	80	2	3	12	34	1.0	880	.02	.02	—
Cream of chicken	1 cup	240	92	95	3	6	8	24	.5	410	.02	.05	Trace
Cream of mushroom	1 cup	240	90	135	2	10	10	41	.5	70	.02	.12	Trace
Minestrone	1 cup	245	90	105	5	3	14	37	1.0	2,350	.07	.05	—
Split pea	1 cup	245	85	145	9	3	21	29	1.5	440	.25	.15	1
Tomato	1 cup	245	91	90	2	3	16	15	.7	1,000	.05	.05	12
Vegetable beef	1 cup	245	92	80	5	2	10	12	.7	2,700	.05	.05	—
Vegetarian	1 cup	245	92	80	2	2	13	20	1.0	2,940	.05	.05	—
Dehydrated:													
Bouillon cube, ½ in	1 cube	4	4	5	1	Trace	Trace	—	—	—	—	—	—
Mixes:													
Unprepared:													
Onion	1½-oz pkg	43	3	150	6	5	23	42	.6	30	.05	.03	6
Prepared with water:													
Chicken noodle	1 cup	240	95	55	2	1	8	7	.2	50	.07	.05	Trace
Onion	1 cup	240	96	35	1	1	6	10	.2	Trace	Trace	Trace	2
Tomato vegetable with noodles	1 cup	240	93	65	1	1	12	7	.2	480	.05	.02	5
White sauce, medium, with enriched flour	1 cup	250	73	405	10	31	22	288	.5	1,150	.12	.43	2

APPENDIX B NUTRITIVE VALUE OF FAST-FOOD ITEMS

	Kcal	Protein (g)	Fat (g)	Cho (g)	Calcium (mg)	Iron (mg)	Vit. A (IU)	Vit. C (mg)	Thiamin (mg)	Riboflavin (mg)	Sodium (mg)
Dairy Queen*											
Big Brazier Deluxe	470	28	24	36	111	5.2	—†	<2.5	0.34	0.37	—
Big Brazier Regular	184	27	23	37	113	5.2	—	<2.0	0.37	0.39	—
Big Brazier w/Cheese	553	32	30	38	268	5.2	495	<2.3	0.34	0.53	—
Brazier w/Cheese	318	18	14	30	163	3.5	—	<1.2	0.29	0.29	—
Brazier Cheese Dog	330	15	19	24	168	1.6	—	—	—	0.18	—
Brazier Chili Dog	330	13	20	25	86	2.0	—	11.0	0.15	0.23	—
Brazier Dog	273	11	15	23	75	1.5	—	11.0	0.12	0.15	—
Brazier French Fries, sm.	200	2	10	25	tr	0.4	tr	3.6	0.06	tr	—
Brazier French Fries, lg.	320	3	16	40	tr	0.4	tr	4.8	0.09	0.03	—
Brazier Onion Rings	300	6	17	33	20	0.4	tr	2.4	0.09	tr	—
Brazier Regular	260	13	9	28	70	3.5	—	<1.0	0.28	0.26	—
Fish Sandwich	400	20	17	41	60	1.1	tr	tr	0.15	0.26	—
Fish Sandwich w/Cheese	440	24	21	39	150	0.4	100	tr	0.15	0.26	—
Super Brazier	783	53	48	35	282	7.3	—	<3.2	0.39	0.69	—
Super Brazier Dog	518	20	30	41	158	4.3	tr	14.0	0.42	0.44	1552
Super Brazier Dog w/Cheese	593	26	36	43	297	4.4	—	14.0	0.43	0.48	1986
Super Brazier Chili Dog	555	23	33	42	158	4.0	—	18.0	0.42	0.48	1640
Banana Split	540	10	15	91	350	1.8	750	18.0	0.60	0.60	—
Buster Bar	390	10	22	37	200	0.7	300	tr	0.09	0.34	—
Choc. Dipped Cone, sm.	150	3	7	20	100	tr	100	tr	0.03	0.17	—
Choc. Dipped Cone, med.	300	7	13	40	200	0.4	300	tr	0.09	0.34	—
Choc. Dipped Cone, lg.	450	10	20	58	300	0.4	400	tr	0.12	0.51	—
Choc. Malt, sm.	340	10	11	51	300	1.8	400	2.4	0.06	0.34	—
Choc. Malt, med.	600	15	20	89	500	3.6	750	3.6	0.12	0.60	—
Choc. Malt, lg.	840	22	28	125	600	5.4	750	6.0	0.15	0.85	—
Choc. Sundae, sm.	170	4	4	30	100	0.7	100	tr	0.03	0.17	—
Choc. Sundae, med.	300	6	7	53	200	1.1	300	tr	0.06	0.26	—
Choc. Sundae, lg.	400	9	9	71	300	1.8	400	tr	0.09	0.43	—
Cone, sm.	110	3	3	18	100	tr	100	tr	0.03	0.14	—

Cone, med.	230	6	7	35	200	tr	300	tr	0.09	0.26	—
Cone, lg.	340	10	10	52	300	tr	400	tr	0.15	0.43	—
Parfait	460	10	11	81	300	1.8	400	tr	0.12	0.43	—
Dilly Bar	240	4	15	22	100	0.4	100	tr	0.06	0.17	—
Float	330	6	8	59	200	tr	100	tr	0.12	0.17	—
Freeze	520	11	13	89	300	tr	200	tr	0.15	0.34	—
Sandwich	140	3	4	24	60	0.4	100	tr	0.03	0.14	—
Fiesta Sundae	570	9	22	84	200	tr	200	tr	0.23	0.26	—
Hot Fudge Brownie Delight	570	11	22	83	300	1.1	500	tr	0.45	0.43	—
Mr. Misty Float	440	6	8	85	200	tr	120	tr	0.12	0.17	—
Mr. Misty Freeze	500	10	12	87	300	tr	200	tr	0.15	0.34	—
Hardee's‡											
Hamburger	305	16	13	29	23	3.6	57	<2.0	0.55	0.58	682
Cheeseburger	335	17	17	29	48	2.7	749	<2.0	0.51	0.32	789
Big Deluxe	546	29	26	48	98	6.7	398	42	0.50	0.73	1083
¼ lb. Cheeseburger	506	28	41	41	103	6.9	508	33	0.35	0.60	1950
Roast Beef Sandwich	377	20	17	36	56	6.3	542	3.2	0.93	0.19	1030
Big Roast Beef	418	28	19	34	74	8.0	648	7.6	1.03	0.22	1770
Hot Dog	346	11	22	26	43	2.5	tr	0	0.29	0.22	744
Hot Ham and Cheese	376	23	15	37	207	3.8	178	0.1	0.37	0.74	1067
Big Fish Sandwich	514	20	26	49	88	5.1	1152	4.9	—	1.51	314
Chicken Fillet	510	27	26	42	83	4.8	1098	13.2	0.63	0.63	360
Biscuit	275	5	13	35	149	2.4	44	0.03	0.34	0.24	650
Sausage Biscuit	413	10	26	34	138	2.8	45	0.1	0.36	0.22	864
Sausage Biscuit w/egg	521	16	35	34	169	4.0	755	0.1	0.41	0.37	1033
Steak Biscuit	419	14	23	41	121	4.6	62	0.1	0.34	0.43	803
Steak Biscuit w/egg	527	20	31	41	151	5.8	772	0.1	0.39	0.58	973
Ham Biscuit	349	12	17	37	181	3.2	127	0.1	0.60	0.42	1414

Continued.

From Anderson, J., & others. (1982). *Teens, foods, fitness and sports.* Raleigh, NC: Division of Child Nutrition.
*Source: International Dairy Queen, Inc., Minneapolis, Minn. 1978. Dairy Queen stores in the State of Texas do not conform to Dairy Queen approved products.
Any nutritional information shown does not necessarily pertain to their products.
†Dashes indicate information not provided by sources.
‡Source: Hardee's Food Systems, Inc., September 1, 1981.

APPENDIX B NUTRITIVE VALUE OF FAST-FOOD ITEMS—cont'd

	Kcal	Protein (g)	Fat (g)	Cho (g)	Calcium (mg)	Iron (mg)	Vit. A (IU)	Vit. C (mg)	Thiamin (mg)	Riboflavin (mg)	Sodium (mg)
Dairy Queen—cont'd											
Ham Biscuit w/egg	458	19	26	37	211	4.4	837	0.1	0.65	0.57	1584
Biscuit w/egg	383	11	22	35	179	3.6	754	0.03	0.39	0.39	819
French fries (sm)	239	3	13	28	13	0.8	tr	9.9	0.07	0.03	121
French fries (lg)	381	5	21	44	21	1.4	tr	15.8	0.11	0.05	192
Apple Turnover	282	3	14	37	19	0.9	tr	0	0.03	0.04	—
Milkshake	391	11	10	63	450	0.6	0	0	0.20	0.78	—
Kentucky Fried Chicken*											
Original Recipe Dinner†	830	52	46	56	150	4.5	750	27.0	0.38	0.56	—
Extra Crispy Dinner†	950	52	54	63	150	3.6	750	27.0	0.38	0.56	—
Individual Pieces (Original Recipe)											
Drumstick	136	14	8	2	20	0.9	30	0.6	0.04	0.12	—
Rib	241	19	15	8	55	1.0	58	<1.0	0.06	0.14	—
Thigh	276	20	19	12	39	1.4	74	<1.0	0.08	0.24	—
Wing	151	11	10	4	—	0.6	—	<1.0	0.03	0.07	—
9 pieces	1892	152	116	59	—	8.8	—	—	0.49	1.27	—
McDonald's‡											
Egg McMuffin	352	18	20	26	187	3.2	361	1.6	0.36	0.60	885
English Muffin, Buttered	186	6	6	28	87	1.6	106	<0.7	0.22	0.14	318
Hot Cakes, w/Butter & Syrup	472	8	9	89	54	2.4	255	<2.1	0.31	0.43	1070
Sausage (Pork)	184	9	17	tr	13	0.9	36	<0.5	0.22	0.13	615
Scrambled Eggs	162	12	12	2	49	2.2	514	<0.8	0.07	0.60	205
Big Mac	541	26	31	39	175	4.3	327	2.4	0.35	0.37	1010
Cheeseburger	306	16	13	31	158	2.9	372	1.6	0.24	0.30	767
Filet-O-Fish	402	15	23	34	105	1.8	152	4.2	0.28	0.28	781
French Fries	211	3	11	26	10	0.5	<52	11.0	0.15	0.03	109
Hamburger	257	13	9	30	63	3.0	231	1.8	0.23	0.23	520
Quarter Pounder	418	26	21	33	79	5.1	164	2.3	0.31	0.41	735
Quarter Pounder w/Cheese	518	31	29	34	251	4.6	683	2.9	0.35	0.59	1236
Cherry Pie	298	2	18	33	12	0.4	213	1.3	0.02	0.03	427

Chocolate Shake	364	11	9	60	338	1.0	318	<2.9	0.12	0.89	300
Strawberry Shake	345	10	9	57	339	0.2	322	<2.9	0.12	0.66	207
Vanilla Shake	323	10	8	52	346	0.2	346	<2.9	0.12	0.66	201
Hot Fudge Sundae	310	7	11	46	215	0.6	230	2.5	0.07	0.31	175
Caramel Sundae	328	7	10	53	200	0.2	279	3.6	0.07	0.31	195
Strawberry Sundae	289	7	9	46	174	0.4	230	2.8	0.07	0.30	96
Apple Pie	300	2	19	31	12	0.6	<69	2.7	0.02	0.03	398
Taco Bell‖											
Bean Burrito	343	11	12	48	98	2.8	1657	15.2	0.37	0.22	272
Beef Burrito	466	30	21	37	83	4.6	1675	15.2	0.30	0.39	327
Beefy Tostada	291	19	15	21	208	3.4	3450	12.7	0.16	0.27	138
Bellbeefer	221	15	7	23	40	2.6	2961	10.0	0.15	0.20	231
Bellbeefer w/cheese	278	19	12	23	147	2.7	3146	10.0	0.16	0.27	330
Burrito Supreme	457	21	22	43	121	3.8	3462	16.0	0.33	0.35	367
Combination Burrito	404	21	16	43	91	3.7	1666	15.2	0.34	0.31	300
Enchirito	454	25	21	42	259	3.8	1178	9.5	0.31	0.37	1175
Pintos 'N' Cheese	168	11	5	21	150	2.3	3123	9.3	0.26	0.16	102
Taco	186	15	8	14	120	2.5	120	0.2	0.09	0.16	79
Tostada	179	9	6	25	191	2.3	3152	9.7	0.18	0.15	101
Wendy's¶											
Single Hamburger	470	26	26	34	84	5.3	94	0.6	0.24	0.36	774
Double Hamburger	670	44	40	34	138	8.2	128	1.5	0.43	0.54	980
Triple Hamburger	850	65	51	33	104	10.7	220	2.0	0.47	0.68	1217
Single w/cheese	580	33	34	34	228	5.4	221	0.7	0.38	0.43	1085
Double w/cheese	800	50	48	41	177	10.2	439	2.3	0.49	0.75	1414
Triple w/cheese	1040	72	68	35	371	10.9	472	3.4	0.80	0.84	1848
Chili	230	19	8	21	83	4.4	1188	2.9	0.22	0.25	1065
French Fries	330	5	16	41	16	1.2	40	6.4	0.14	0.07	112
Frosty	390	9	16	54	270	0.9	355	0.7	0.20	0.60	247

*Source: Nutritional Content of Average Serving, Heublein Food Service and Franchising Group, June 1976.

†Dinner comprises mashed potatoes and gravy, cole slaw, roll, and three pieces of chicken.

‡Source: "Nutritional analysis of food served at McDonald's restaurants." WARF Institute, Inc., Madison, Wisc., June 1977.

‖Sources: Menu Item Portions, July 1976, Taco Bell Co., San Antonio, Tex. Adams CF: Nutritive Value of American Foods in Common Units, USDA Agricultural Research Service, Agricultural Handbook No. 456, November 1975. Church CF, Church HN: Food Values of Portions Commonly Used, ed 12. Philadelphia, J.P. Lippincott Co. 1975. Valley Baptist Medical Center, Food Service Department Descriptions of Mexican-American Foods, NASCO, Fort Atkinson, Wisc.

¶Source: Wendy's International, Inc., Dublin, Ohio. Nutritional analysis by Medallion Laboratories, Minneapolis, Minnesota.

APPENDIX C   COLLEGE PHYSICAL FITNESS RESOURCES

This discussion is intended to make you aware of college and university physical fitness and health programs that are available to most college students. Low levels of physical and health fitness may be due in part to the lack of students' knowledge or use of services that are provided by many colleges and universities to help create a physically fit student body.

College resources to enhance and protect the health and fitness of students commonly include a health center that provides immediate care to physically ailing students: health-related programs that provide seminars and training sessions relating to such things as cardiorespiratory function, medical self-help, and childbirth; a broad range of activities in the physical education program for both "normal" and "handicapped" students; intercollegiate and intramural athletics; and sports medicine and health education clinics.

PHYSICAL EDUCATION PROGRAMS

The Physical Education program in most colleges and universities provides a basic instructional class or service program, an adapted physical education program, and an intramural and extramural athletic program. In some cases the intercollegiate athletic program is also a part of the total physical education program.

Physical Education Instructional Service Program

The instructional service program in physical education is the program in which skills, strategies, understandings, and essential knowledge concerning the relation of physical activity to physical, mental, emotional, and social development take place. Participants are also provided with some of the ways to develop and maintain an optimal state of physical fitness. An important part of the instructional program is the teaching of sport-related skills. The instructional service program is available to all students, meets the needs of each person, stresses lifetime skills, is concerned with health-related physical fitness, and is conducted by qualified faculty members.

Some physical education programs are required and some are elective. Classes generally meet twice a week. The trend is toward an emphasis on recreation and fitness activities and on coeducational classes. Coeducation frequently exists at the college level in such activities as tennis, dancing, swimming, badminton, volleyball, golf, racquetball, aquatics, bowling, table tennis, skating, archery, horseback riding, mountaineering, orienteering, snow skiing, judo, hiking, tumbling, and camping. Several colleges have introduced "Foundations" courses that get at the why of the activity as well as the activity itself.

Physical achievement tests are often used in college physical education programs to assess student needs and to better assure progress. Special help and prescribed programs are provided for physically underdeveloped students.

Many 2-year colleges require students to take physical education both years. Most programs require 2 hours of activity each week and stress the importance of the successful completion of the service program as a requirement for graduation. Activities commonly required include aquatics, archery, badminton, bowling, fencing, folk and square dance, golf, ice skating, modern dance, sailing, social dance, tennis, tumbling gymnastics, trampoline, and volleyball.

Adapted Physical Education Programs

An adapted physical education program refers to that phase of physical education that meets the needs of a person who, because of some physical inadequacy, functional deficit capable of being improved through physical activity, or other deficiency, is temporarily or permanently unable to take part in the regular physical education program, or in which special provisions are made for handicapped students in regular physical education classes. It also provides service to students who do not fall into the "average" or "normal" classification for their age group. These students deviate from their peers in physical, mental, emotional, or social characteristics or in a combination of these traits.

All colleges have students who, because of heredity, environment, disease, or accident, have physical, mental, or emotional impairments. The responsibility of physical education programs is to help each person; even though a person may be handicapped, this is not cause for neglect. It should represent an even greater challenge to see that he or she enjoys the benefits of participating in physical education activities adapted to his or her needs. Provision for a sound adapted program has been a shortcoming of physical education throughout the nation because of the lack of properly trained teachers, the financial cost of remedial instruction, and physical educators who are unaware of their responsibility and the contribution they can make in this program. These obstacles, however, are gradually being overcome as the public and educators become aware of the need to physically educate all persons in all phases of an education program.

Intramural, Club, and Extracurricular Activities

A program of various leisure-time activities is frequently provided for all enrolled students in a college or university. The program is usually financed by the central administration or student government. In many cases the students direct the programs. A wide variety of activities are commonly provided to accomodate varied student interests. Activities are also conducted on a men's, women's, or coeducational basis. The most common intramural activities are flag football, volleyball, basketball, water polo, darts, billiards, softball, bowling, swimming, hockey, racquetball, tennis, floor hockey, ultimate frisbee, canoeing, surfing, windsurfing, and soccer.

Extracurricular activities other than intramural sports may include clubs, common interest groups, and extramural sports. The extramural programs may include activities such as bowling, fencing, karate, chess, sailing, rugby, snow skiing, scuba, water skiing, and soccer. Club activities usually have a faculty advisor and qualified personnel to train and teach the activity.

INTERCOLLEGIATE ATHLETICS

The function of an intercollegiate athletic program is to provide student-athletes with an environment in which they are able to pursue excellence in selected extracurricular, educationally-related athletic activities. The athletic department sponsors a number of activities for men such as baseball, basketball, cross-country running, football, golf, soccer, swimming and diving, tennis, wrestling, hockey, fencing and track and field. Activities for women include basketball, gymnastics, field hockey soccer, fencing, cross-country running, softball, tennis, swimming and diving, and volleyball. The objective of the intercollegiate athletic program is to pursue excellence of performance within the structure of the rules and within the budgetary framework imposed by the funding provided.

SPORTS MEDICINE CLINICS

The term *sports medicine* encompasses many different but closely related areas, all having to do with human performance in sport. The fields of exercise physiology, biomechanics, kinesiology, physical education, athletic training, and physical therapy all contribute to this broadly defined field of sports medicine. However, when you hear someone refer to a sports medicine clinic, you generally think more of the medically related aspects of human performance.

Sports medicine clinics are usually staffed with persons who deal exclusively with sport-related injuries. A typical sports medicine clinic has one or more physicians on staff. These physicians generally have their training and background in either internal medicine, orthopedics, or occasionally pediatrics. If the sports medicine clinic is located on a college or university campus, it is generally under the direction of the student health service. The physicians are usually team physicians who oversee the health care of the competitive athletes by supervising athletic trainers and physical therapists. Students who go to the student health service with any injury that is related to physical activity may be referred directly to the sports medicine clinic for evaluation by a team physician.

Sports medicine clinics also employ athletic trainers or physical therapists to handle the therapy and rehabilitation for the injured athlete. If these are private clinics located outside of the university setting, they will usually see all types of patients, whether young or old, competitive or recreational athletes.

The philosophy of injury management in sports medicine clinics is usually relatively aggressive. Physicians, trainers, and therapists do whatever is necessary to return the patient to activity as quickly as possible with minimal risk to patient health and safety.

HEALTH EDUCATION

Another clinic that may be of great value to students involved in physical activity programs is the health education clinic. Most health education clinics are staffed by professional health educators who hold advanced degrees in public health. These persons are prepared to deal with a variety of health-related problems by providing counseling and referral, if necessary, to additional medical personnel.

The function of the Health Education Clinic is to conduct health education programs specifically designed for special needs of the students, staff, and other members of the university community on matters such as:

Weight control and eating disorders
Nutritional counseling
Stress management
Smoking cessation
Management of alcohol and drug abuse
Handicapped needs
Use of contraceptives and birth control
Transmission of sexual diseases
Personal hygiene
Physical fitness and prevention of cardiovascular heart disease

The health education clinic prepares informative handouts and brochures that discuss health-related problems for distribution among the student population. They are also responsible for conducting seminars and various outreach efforts promoting positive health behaviors and wellness. The health educators are trained counselors who deal on a one-to-one basis with students who may be experiencing problems in one or more of the areas listed above. Persons seeking assistance in a health education clinic are assured of strict confidentiality and are referred to additional medical personnel only when consultation will benefit the student.

Health education clinics, like sports medicine clinics, can play an important role in the overall health care of the student who is involved in some type of regular physical activity.

STUDENT HEALTH CENTER

The college and university student health center provides medical care on an outpatient and limited inpatient basis for students and their dependents. Admission to the college or university is usually contingent on receipt of a personal health history and a physical examination, and this information becomes part of the student's health record.

Student health centers are usually open 24 hours a day and a medical professional is on duty at least during school hours. The staff may include physician(s), physician assistants, nurses, supporting professionals, and technical and administrative personnel such as x-ray technicians, pharmacists, social workers, gynecologists, dentists, or physical therapists. Facilities and clinics that are included in representative student health centers surveyed include:

Facility	Function
Outpatient clinic	Primarily emergency care
Inpatient	Minor surgery, sickness
Trauma	Students experiencing a disordered state resulting from mental or emotional stress or physical injury
General medical consultation	Students seeking medical advice concerning their health problems
Gynecology	Female students having problems involving sexual reproduction system
Dental	Prevention of dental problems and treatment in some cases
Pharmacy	Drugs provided on a limited basis
Emergency	Open for health problems that need immediate attention
X-ray	For such problems as bone fracture
Optometric clinic	Eye examinations for defects and prescriptions for corrective lenses
Sports medicine clinic	Prevention, treatment, and rehabilitation of sport-related injuries

SEEKING THE MOST QUALIFIED HELP

Colleges and universities tend to attract persons who are considered experts in their fields. Students are generally fortunate to have so many of these highly trained professionals at their disposal. If you feel that you have a problem, whether it is concerned with physical education, physical fitness, a sport-related injury, a health problem, or other malady, do not hesitate to seek out the health-care professionals who are more than willing to provide assistance. There is no reason to depend on the advice or assistance of someone who thinks they know, when so many professionals are available who really do know.

Life at a college provides more than classrooms, calculators, and textbooks. The campus offers a wide variety of cultural, social, athletic, and recreational activities. In addition, many services are available to assist with the academic, personal, financial, and health concerns of students. The health and fitness resources that a higher education institution provides its students represents an important investment for every college and university.

APPENDIX D   WORKSHEETS

Worksheet For Calculation of Training Heart Rate

Estimation of Maximal Heart Rate	Example
220	220
− Age	− 20
Predicted maximal heart rate	200
× % Intensity	× 0.7
Training heart rate	140 beats/min

Karvonen Equation	Example
Maximal heart rate	200
− Resting heart rate	− 70
	130
× % Intensity	× 0.6
	78
+ Resting heart rate	+ 70
Training heart rate	148 beats/min

Sample Worksheet For Harvard Step Test

	Example
1. Look up the "Duration of effort" _____	1. 3½
2. Find the "Total heart beats" for 60 to 90 seconds following cessation of exercise _____	2. 60-64
3. Intersect the "Duration of effort" row with the score column _____	3. 57
4. Determine the fitness level _____	4. Average

Scoring For The Harvard Step Test

Duration of Effort (Minutes)	Total Heart Beats 1 to 1½ Minutes in Recovery											
	40-44	45-49	50-54	55-59	60-64	65-69	70-74	75-79	80-84	85-89	90-94	95-99
0-½	6	6	5	5	4	4	4	4	3	3	3	3
½-1	19	17	16	14	13	12	11	11	10	9	9	8
1-1½	32	29	26	24	22	20	19	18	17	16	15	14
1½-2	45	41	38	34	31	29	27	25	23	22	21	20
2-2½	58	52	47	43	40	36	34	32	30	28	27	25
2½-3	71	64	58	53	48	45	42	39	37	34	33	31
3-3½	84	75	68	62	57	53	49	46	43	41	39	37
3½-4	97	87	79	72	66	61	57	53	50	47	45	42
4-4½	110	98	89	82	75	70	65	61	57	54	51	48
4½-5	123	110	100	91	84	77	72	68	63	60	57	54
5	129	116	105	96	88	82	76	71	67	63	60	56

From Conzolazio, C.F., Johnson, R.E., & Pecora, L.J. (1963). *Physiological measurements of metabolic function in man*. New York: McGraw-Hill. Used by permission of McGraw-Hill Book Company.

Sample Worksheet For Åstrand Rhyming Nomogram Test

	Example
1. Count heart rate at end	
Of minute 5 _____ HR	168
Of minute 6 + _____ HR	164
_____ Total	272
÷ 2	÷ 2
= Mean HR	166
2. Note workload setting on ergometer _____	1200 kp/min
3. Find points on nomogram under "Pulse rate" and "Workload" columns and connect them with a straight line	
4. Predicted $\dot{V}O_2$max _____	3.6 L/min

Sample Worksheet For Cooper's 12-Minute Walking/Running Test

	Example
1. Measure distance covered and round off to nearest ⅛ mile _____	1. 1.50
2. Locate this distance in appropriate "Age" column _____	2. Age 20
3. Determine fitness level _____	3. Good

12-Minute Walking/Running Test

Distance (Miles) Covered in 12 Minutes

Fitness Category		13-19	20-29	30-39	Age (Years) 40-49	50-59	60+
I. Very poor	(men)	<1.30*	<1.22	<1.18	<1.14	<1.03	<.87
	(women)	<1.0	<.96	<.94	<.88	<.84	<.78
II. Poor	(men)	1.30-1.37	1.22-1.31	1.18-1.30	1.14-1.24	1.03-1.16	.87-1.02
	(women)	1.00-1.18	.96-1.11	.95-1.05	.88-.98	.84-.93	.78-.86
III. Fair	(men)	1.38-1.56	1.32-1.49	1.31-1.45	1.25-1.39	1.17-1.30	1.03-1.20
	(women)	1.19-1.29	1.12-1.22	1.06-1.18	.99-1.11	.94-1.05	.87-.98
IV. Good	(men)	1.57-1.72	1.50-1.64	1.46-1.56	1.40-1.53	1.31-1.44	1.21-1.32
	(women)	1.30-1.43	1.23-1.34	1.19-1.29	1.12-1.24	1.06-1.18	.99-1.09
V. Excellent	(men)	1.73-1.86	1.65-1.76	1.57-1.69	1.54-1.65	1.45-1.58	1.33-1.55
	(women)	1.44-1.51	1.35-1.45	1.30-1.39	1.25-1.34	1.19-1.30	1.10-1.18
VI. Superior	(men)	>1.87	>1.77	>1.70	>1.66	>1.59	>1.56
	(women)	>1.52	>1.46	>1.40	>1.35	>1.31	>1.19

From the Aerobics Program for Total Well-Being by Dr. Kenneth H. Cooper. Copyright © 1982 by Kenneth H. Cooper. Reprinted by permission of the publisher, M. Evans & Co., Inc., New York, NY 10017.
*<Means "less than"; >means "more than."

Strength Training Worksheet I

Upper Body Exercises

Date and Weight

Exercise	Reps	Sets		Date and Weight
Bench press	6-8	3	Date	
			Weight	
Military press	6-8	3	Date	
			Weight	
Lateral pulls	6-8	3	Date	
			Weight	
Flys	6-8	3	Date	
			Weight	
Reverse flys	6-8	3	Date	
			Weight	
Medial rotation	6-8	3	Date	
			Weight	
Lateral rotation	6-8	3	Date	
			Weight	
Bicep curls	6-8	3	Date	
			Weight	
Tricep extensions	6-8	3	Date	
			Weight	
Wrist curls	6-8	3	Date	
			Weight	
Wrist extensions	6-8	3	Date	
			Weight	

Strength Training Worksheet II

Date and Weight

Lower Body Exercises

Exercise	Reps	Sets	
Hip adduction	6-8	3	Date / Weight
Hip abduction	6-8	3	Date / Weight
Hip flexion	6-8	3	Date / Weight
Hip extension	6-8	3	Date / Weight
Hip internal rotation	6-8	3	Date / Weight
Hip lateral rotation	6-8	3	Date / Weight
Quadricep extensions	6-8	3	Date / Weight
Hamstring flexions	6-8	3	Date / Weight
Toe raises	6-8	3	Date / Weight
Ankle inversion	6-8	3	Date / Weight
Ankle eversion	6-8	3	Date / Weight
Ankle dorsiflexion	6-8	3	Date / Weight

Checklist For Individualized Stretching Program

Exercise	Hold Time (sec)	Repetitions	Day 1 2 3 4 5 6 7 8 9 10 11 12 13 14
Arm hang	30	5	
Shoulder towel stretch	10	5	
Upper trunk stretch	30	3	
Lower trunk stretch	30	3	
Upper back and neck	30	3	
Lower back stretch	30*	3	
Lower back twister	30	3	
Pelvic thrust	30	3	
Quadriceps stretch	30	3	
Hamstring stretch	30	3	
Hurdler's stretch	30	3	
Groin stretch	30	3	
Achilles heel cord stretch	30	3*	
Toe pointer	30	3	

*In each position.

Worksheet For Calculating Percentage Body Fat
From Skinfold Measurements

1. Triceps skinfold thickness _____ mm
2. Subscapular skinfold thickness _____ mm

Calculation of Percent Body Fat

Men

__ % Body fat = $(0.43) \times$ _____ $+ (0.58) \times$ _____ $+ 1.47$
　　　　　　　　　　　　　Triceps skinfold　　　　　　　Subscapular
　　　　　　　　　　　　　　　　　　　　　　　　　　skinfold

Women

__ % Body fat = $(0.55) \times$ _____ $+ (0.31) \times$ _____ $+ 6.13$
　　　　　　　　　　　　　Triceps skinfold　　　　　　　Subscapular
　　　　　　　　　　　　　　　　　　　　　　　　　　skinfold

Worksheet For Calculating Desired Body Weight

Method 1

1. _____ = _____ − _____
   % Body fat to   Present %   Desired % body fat
   be lost   body fat

2. _____ = _____ × _____
   Pounds to be   % Body fat to   Present body
   lost   be lost   weight

3. _____ = _____ − _____
   Desired body   Present body   Pounds to be lost
   weight   weight

Method 2

1. _____ = _____ × _____ % Body fat
   Fat weight   Present body   100
                     weight

2. _____ = _____ − _____
   Fat-free   Present body   Fat weight
   weight   weight

3. _____ = _____ ÷ _____
   Desired body   Fat-free weight   % Body fat desired
   weight

Worksheet For Calculating Basal Metabolic Rate (BMR)

1. Estimated body surface area (see Fig. 6-3) = _____
2. BMR factor (see Table 6-1) = _____
3. _____ × _____ = _____
   Estimated body   BMR factor   BMR
   surface area
4. _____ = _____ × 24 hours
   Basal metabolic   BMR
   needs for 1 day

Worksheet For Calculating Daily Energy Expenditure

| | Daily Activities Log | | | Date: |
Clock Time	Activity (see Table 6-2)	Total Minutes Spent in Activity	kcal/min/lb	Total kcal Expended

Total calories expended during activities _____

Add calories expended in basal metabolism _____

Total calories expended

Worksheet For Estimating Caloric Balance

_____ − _____ = _____

Number of calories   Number of calories expended   Caloric balance
consumed   during activities

If the caloric balance is positive, body weight will tend to increase.
If the caloric balance is negative, body weight will tend to decrease.

Worksheet For Calculating Daily Calorie Intake

Date:

Daily Food Intake Log

Time	Food Eaten	Amount	No. of Calories	How Cooked	Meal or Snack	Hunger Level (0-3)	Activity and Location When Eating	Mood (1-3)

Total number of calories consumed =

Worksheet For Monitoring Weekly Weight Loss

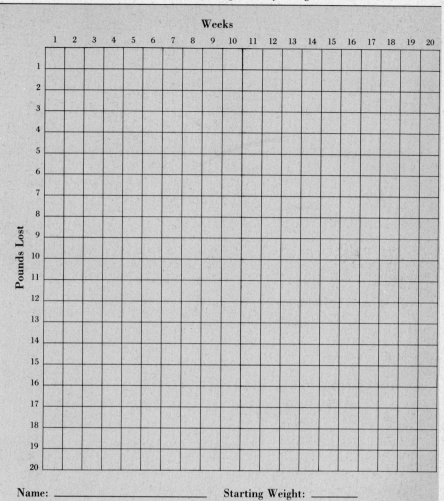

Name: _____   Starting Weight: _____

INDEX